UNDERSTANDING TEAMWORK IN HEALTH CARE

Gordon Mosser, MD, MLitt
Senior Fellow
Division of Health Policy & Management, School of Public Health
Adjunct Assistant Professor
Department of Medicine, Medical School
University of Minnesota

James W. Begun, PhD
James A. Hamilton Professor of Healthcare Management
Division of Health Policy & Management, School of Public Health
University of Minnesota

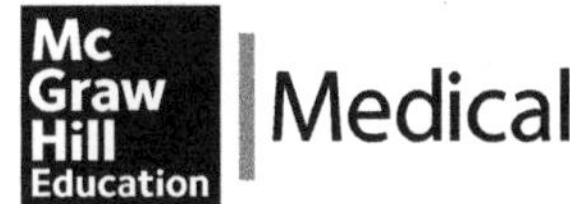

New York Chicago San Francisco Athens London Madrid Mexico City
Milan New Delhi Singapore Sydney Toronto

Understanding Teamwork in Health Care

1 2 3 4 5 6 7 8 9 0 DOC/DOC 18 17 16 15 14 13

ISBN 978-0-07-179195-3
MHID 0-07-179195-7

Notice

Medicine is an ever-changing science. As new research and clinical experience broaden our knowledge, changes in treatment and drug therapy are required. The authors and the publisher of this work have checked with sources believed to be reliable in their efforts to provide information that is complete and generally in accord with the standards accepted at the time of publication. However, in view of the possibility of human error or changes in medical sciences, neither the authors nor the publisher nor any other party who has been involved in the preparation or publication of this work warrants that the information contained herein is in every respect accurate or complete, and they disclaim all responsibility for any errors or omissions or for the results obtained from use of the information contained in this work. Readers are encouraged to confirm the information contained herein with other sources. For example, and in particular, readers are advised to check the product information sheet included in the package of each drug they plan to administer to be certain that the information contained in this work is accurate and that changes have not been made in the recommended dose or in the contraindications for administration. This recommendation is of particular importance in connection with new or infrequently used drugs.

This book was set in Minion by Cenveo® Publisher Services.
The editors were James F. Shanahan and Christina M. Thomas.
The production supervisor was Catherine Saggese.
Project management was provided by Sheena Uprety, Cenveo Publisher Services.
The cover designer was Thomas De Pierro.
RR Donnelley was printer and binder.

This book is printed on acid-free paper.

Library of Congress Cataloging-in-Publication Data

Mosser, Gordon.
Understanding teamwork in healthcare / Gordon Mosser, James W. Begun.
p. ; cm.
Includes bibliographical references and index.
ISBN 978-0-07-179195-3—ISBN 0-07-179195-7
I. Begun, James W. II. Title.
[DNLM: 1. Patient Care Team—organization & administration. 2. Clinical Competence. 3. Interdisciplinary Communication. 4. Interprofessional Relations. 5. Primary Health Care—organization & administration. WX 162.5]
RA971
362.1068—dc23

2013006957

Contents

Section IV. Advancing Teamwork In Health Care

Preface

We shall not cease from exploration
And the end of all our exploring
Will be to arrive where we started
And know the place for the first time.
—T.S. Eliot, *Little Gidding*, 1942

We all know teams. We work in teams. We use teams in community and leisure-time activities. We play or watch team sports. And yet there is a great deal of useful information about teamwork that is unknown to many people in health care. The aim of this book is to make that information more widely known and used. It is a book of exploration and explanation, which, hopefully, will enable the reader to be more effective as a team participant, team leader, and team manager.

Health care today requires teams. The rise of multiple healthcare professions, each with its own specialties, has brought a rich array of knowledge and skills to the tasks of preventing illness and caring for the sick, but it has also created risks. Health care has enormous power to heal, and yet it is complex and often uncoordinated, or simply fragmented. By using teams, we can decrease the risks of fragmentation and achieve effective delivery of care. But, of course, for team-based care to be successful, it must employ effective teamwork.

Understanding Teamwork in Health Care is a book about how to work proficiently in and with teams. Our emphasis is on interprofessional teams, but the concepts discussed apply also to teams composed of people from any single profession. The book aims to offset in some measure a deficiency in the education of almost all healthcare professionals in the United States, namely, the lack of training about working in teams composed of people from various professions. There are currently some indications that interprofessional education will in time become part of the education of nurses, physicians, and other healthcare professionals. Eventually, there may be no deficiency to address. However, at this point, nearly all professionals working in health care are obliged to puzzle out interprofessional teamwork on their own. This book is intended to help healthcare professionals in this effort.

We, the authors, each have over 30 years of experience in health care—one of us as a general internist and healthcare leader (GM) and one of us as a researcher and teacher (JWB). During this time, we have both had an enduring interest in teams and, more generally, in the interactions among patients, their families, people providing health care, and people leading and managing healthcare organizations. But we do not need to rely solely on our experience. Sociologists, organizational psychologists, management scientists, healthcare professionals, health services researchers, and other scholars have produced a great deal of knowledge about teams over the past 75 years, including knowledge of teams in health care. Unfortunately, most of this body of knowledge has not yet been put to use to improve the delivery of health care. In this book we strive to make some of this knowledge available for concrete use in improving health care through better teamwork.

THE AUDIENCE

This book is intended for people who are clinicians or managers of health care. In other words, we hope, first, that it will be useful to nurses, nurse practitioners, physicians, pharmacists, healthcare social workers, dentists, physician assistants, physical therapists, psychologists, and all others whom we call *clinicians* because they provide care directly to patients. We hope, second, that it will be useful to clerical staff, healthcare administrators, public health officials, and senior leaders in health care. We also hope that students in the health professions will find the book useful.

We have written about healthcare teams in the United States. However, the precepts and principles discussed are applicable in any country. Indeed, the literature cited originates not only from the United States but also from the United Kingdom, Canada, Finland, Australia, and elsewhere. We hope that the book will be helpful to healthcare professionals in these countries and others.

THE GOAL AND PLAN OF THE BOOK

The goal of *Understanding Teamwork in Health Care* is to advance the understanding and functioning of teams as they are used in health care, including both clinical teams and management teams.

Section I, Healthcare Teams and Team Members (Chapters 1-5), introduces the concept of a work team, explains different types of healthcare teams, describes the backgrounds of the professionals who comprise healthcare teams, and elucidates the distinctive roles of patients and administrators in teams. Section II, Working in Healthcare Teams (Chapters 6-12), explains how effective teams function and sets forth the competencies that individual team members and team leaders need to have to function effectively in teams. Decision making, creativity, and conflict management in teams are examined in detail. The final chapter in this section (Chapter12) explains the role and competencies of the team sponsor, the person to whom the team is accountable and through whom the team interacts with the larger organization in which it functions. Since sponsors are usually the designers of teams, principles of team design are explained in this chapter. Section III, Evaluating and Improving Healthcare Teams (Chapters 13-17), first explains how to assess team members and whole teams. It then explores 4 areas of action for improvement: training, team building, improving processes in teams, and troubleshooting of specific problems commonly encountered in teams. Section IV, Advancing Teamwork in Health Care (Chapters 18-19) addresses the role of senior leadership in advancing teamwork and looks to the future. Chapter 18 depicts the responsibilities of senior leaders in supporting teams and explains the senior leader competencies and the organizational culture needed to support teams. Finally, the conclusion (Chapter 19) speculates on the future of teams in health care and delineates near-term strategies for healthcare organizations and educational institutions to improve team-based care in the United States.

Our practical, larger purpose is to assist people working in health care to improve the performance of the teams they work in, lead, or manage so that the interests of patients are better served.

VIGNETTES

Writers about organizational behavior often use abstract concepts and terms. While abstract concepts and theory have their places in advancing knowledge of how people behave in organizations, they have limited utility for those who wish to use the knowledge in their day-to-day work providing and managing health care. To make the knowledge useful, a writer needs to render the concepts concrete and actionable. To this end, we make liberal use of vignettes throughout the book. Most of these vignettes are stories of clinical practitioners at work. Some of them are stories about managers or about clinicians and managers working together. We hope that these vignettes will make the material clearer and more immediately useful to clinicians and managers seeking to apply the book's ideas in their own settings.

The vignettes are based on our own experiences, the experiences of colleagues, or reports in the public media, healthcare literature, or management literature. Almost all of the vignettes are fictionalized to focus on the pertinent details and to assure privacy. In a few stories, the events are reported as they occurred, but the names and locales have been changed.

VOCABULARY

Much of the subject matter of this book is referred to as *interprofessional teamwork* or *interdisciplinary teamwork.* We see these 2 phrases as essentially synonymous and do not wish to mark any important distinction by using the phrases as labels for different ideas. We have chosen to use the phrase *interprofessional teamwork* for 2 reasons. First, for some readers, the phrase *interdisciplinary teamwork* suggests teamwork among people in different disciplines of medicine—pediatrics, internal medicine, surgery, and so on—or in different academic disciplines—physiology, anatomy, biochemistry, and so on. We are discussing teamwork across a broader range, that is, among individuals in wholly different professions—nursing, medicine, pharmacy, and others. Second, the phrase *interprofessional teamwork* appears to have become the favored phrase among people writing about this topic in recent years.

OUR VIEWPOINT

We come to the topic of healthcare teamwork with a viewpoint on the current state of affairs and what should be done to improve it. The reader will notice that our opinions have shaped various portions of the book. To eliminate any doubt about our position, we articulate our views here.

Teamwork Needs to Be Improved

A great deal of health care in now delivered by teams. In order to make care safer, more effective, less expensive, and more responsive to patients' values and choices, healthcare teams need to perform much better than they often do. Failures of communication, collaboration, and team management too often degrade patients' experience of care, their health outcomes, and the safety of their care while increasing costs. We can and must improve teamwork as part of our overall efforts to improve health care.

Healthcare Professionals Need to Understand Each Other's Professions

Some shortfalls in teamwork arise because healthcare professionals are not adequately familiar with their colleagues' professions. Too often the knowledge bases, skills, and values of people in other healthcare professions are not well known by physicians, nurses, social workers, and others. Sometimes they are barely known at all. In order for team members to make full use of each other's knowledge and skills, they must know what the other team members can contribute. Moreover, some team dysfunction results from differences in professional values, and these difficulties cannot be overcome unless team members understand the differences.

Patients Are in Charge If They Choose to Be

Patients have the right to make the decisions about their care if they choose to do so. In other words, if a patient wants to decide what his or her healthcare team does in providing care for him or her, then that patient should be permitted to make these decisions. Patients may also delegate decision making to their physicians or to other care providers—or to family members or to other people whom they trust to speak for them. Alternatively, they may be partners with their physicians and other care providers if they choose to be partners. But if they prefer to have the final word without partnering, they are entitled to have the final word. Of course, there are exceptions for patients who are incapacitated because of injury or illness, who have certain kinds of mental illness, or who are making decisions that will cause harm to them and are based on plainly false beliefs. However, these cases are unusual and do not undo the general rule that patients are in charge if they want to be.

Healthcare Administrators Should Become Team Members

When clinicians think about team-based health care, they ordinarily regard the members of the team to be the clinicians plus the patient and, sometimes, key clerical staff in the units where they work. They do not think of administrators as team members. Health care would be improved if administrators were brought into the team. Administrators have pertinent knowledge and skills that many clinicians do not have: skills in designing and improving workflow processes, project management skills, facility in managing people, and organizational political skills useful in mobilizing resources. To become members of the team, administrators will need to stop standing at a distance. They will need to understand the training, activities, and values of other healthcare professionals.

Teams Should Become Less Hierarchical

Large differences in authority and status between team members interfere with communication and inhibit participation by the junior members, leading to lost information, lost insights, and diminished contributions from the junior members. Flattening the hierarchy in commercial airline cockpits has made aviation safer. During the past 25 years, airlines have used intensive training to flatten hierarchies and make other improvements in teamwork.

As a result, they have achieved dramatic improvements in accident rates. In order to improve health care, we need to make hierarchies in healthcare teams less steep.

Roles of Physicians Are Changing and Should Change

For over a century, physicians have been presumed to be the leaders of most healthcare teams to which they have belonged. They have been presumed to be the final authorities on any questions that might arise. Having this authority makes sense when answering questions that require knowledge that only physicians have. However, it does not make sense to use the medical knowledge of physicians as a rationale for generalizing their authority to cover all healthcare and organizational questions. Health care already has teams that include physicians and are led by practitioners in other professions. In many teams, a professional who is not a physician will be better suited than any physician on the team to maintain the team's focus, develop the team's capacity over time, and coach team members. Considerations of suitability for leadership should determine whether a particular person is the team leader, not whether the person is a member of a particular profession.

Future Healthcare Organizations Will Be Able to Support Teams

Many of the activities discussed in this book can be pursued only by organizations large enough to have the economy of scale necessary to provide adequate funding and other resources. These activities include team training, coaching, and systematic improvement of performance. We believe that the current aggregation of medical practices and hospitals into larger units will continue to the point that solo practitioners, small clinical groups, and independent, small hospitals will be uncommon, in both urban and rural areas. Even those small practices and hospitals that persist will find it necessary to form associations to achieve economies of scale, permitting them to support teamwork better than they can now. Thus we believe that institutional support for teamwork will be increasingly available in the future.

ACKNOWLEDGEMENTS

We wish to thank Kendall Richardson and Isaiah Zirkle for background research on the health professions, Preethi Nakappan for research on team building and initial development of selected graphics, and Thaddeus Murray for contributions to editing of vignettes. Discussions with Susan Anderson, Paul Batalden, Mark Gildea, Nancy Jaeckels, Linda Lindeke, Shailey Prasad, Omer Sanan, Curt Wyman, Thomas Wyman, Ken White, and Andrew Zinkel on healthcare teamwork provided insight and inspiration. Ken White was a major contributor to the material in Chapter 5. The McGraw-Hill team of James Shanahan, Christina Thomas, and Laura Libretti was supportive and accommodating. Thomas Bodenheimer helped us greatly through his early enthusiasm and support for the project. Our spouses, Nina Mosser and Jean Wyman, sustained us with insights, patience, love, and grace throughout the long process of researching and writing this book.

Any errors or misinterpretations are, of course, our responsibility. We welcome comments and suggestions for improvement from readers.

CONCLUSION

This is a book about a facet of health care that has been neglected until recently, namely, teamwork among individuals in different healthcare professions. Better interprofessional teamwork promises to improve patient care, outcomes of care, and costs. Better teamwork also promises to make working in health care more collegial and gratifying for healthcare professionals and for those who support them. It is time to take up the challenge of improving our teams.

Gordon Mosser
James W. Begun
Minneapolis, Minnesota
April 2013

Work Teams and Teamwork Competencies

Section I of this book (Chapters 1-5) describes the concept of a work team, differentiates different types of teams in health care, introduces the professionals who comprise healthcare teams, and explains the roles of patients and administrators. This section introduces the team and the members of the team. It sets the stage for what follows. Sections II-IV then build on this foundation by examining how effective teams and team members work and how we can advance the effectiveness of teams throughout health care.

WHY HEALTHCARE TEAMWORK MATTERS NOW

Healthcare delivery is a specialized enterprise, and it promises to become more and more specialized as knowledge advances. Decades ago, most physicians in the United States were general practitioners. In 1940, 76% of physicians were general practitioners. By 1955, the proportion had declined to 56%; by 1969, it was 31% (Starr, 1982, pp. 358-359). In 2007, only 13.5% of physicians were family physicians or general practitioners, and 34.3% were practicing in all of the primary care fields combined—family medicine, general practice, internal medicine, and pediatrics (American Association of Medical Colleges, 2008). By then the American Medical Association was tracking counts of physicians in 33 specialties in addition to the primary care fields. Medicine has become highly specialized. Similar developments have occurred in nursing. Nursing now has registered nurses, licensed practical nurses, clinical nurse specialists in various fields, nurse practitioners, and doctors of nursing practice. Pharmacy has established specialties in nuclear pharmacy, pharmacotherapy, oncology pharmacy, and other fields. Social workers and physical therapists are also specialized. The care of most patients is provided by several people practicing different professions. This fragmentation calls for teamwork to assure that they work together effectively.

Calls for improved interprofessional teamwork date back to at least the mid-1950s (Garrett, 1955). However, progress has been slow for several reasons. First, in their training, physicians and nurses and many other clinicians are imbued with the notion that they are individually responsible for what happens to their patients and that performance must be flawless (Leape, 1994). Although a more complex and realistic viewpoint is now gaining sway, for more than a century, clinical professionals finished their training believing that good outcomes were the results of individual effort and that mishaps were caused by individual mistakes. Teamwork had nothing to do with it, or so it was believed. Second, the members of each healthcare profession are educated in isolation. Pharmacists are educated in Colleges of Pharmacy; nurses, in Schools of Nursing; physicians, in Medical Schools; and so on. They rarely meet. One result is that they embrace the values, vocabulary, and conceptual frameworks of their own professions without any exposure to this same socialization process as experienced by students in other healthcare professions (Hall and Weaver, 2001). These values, vocabulary, and concepts are different in different professions as explained in Chapter 3, and these differences hinder teamwork, especially when they are not understood. Separation during training also means that students do not learn how to work in interprofessional teams and are left to figure out teamwork (or not) once they are in practice. Change is stirring here too, but regular interprofessional education in the core curricula of healthcare professional schools is still distinctly uncommon. Third, rivalries between professions, especially medicine and nursing, have at times cooled enthusiasm for teams (Fagin, 1992). Controversy between physicians and nurse practitioners over leadership of medical homes (a team-based, patient-centered approach to primary health care in the United States) is a recent example of such rivalries (Lowes, 2012).

Nevertheless, the desirability of team-based care has not been seriously disputed in all these years. The problem has been that action was taken only in limited arenas—for example, mental health and developmental pediatrics—until the early 2000s. Interest in teamwork was reignited then by the widespread recognition that high quality health care is achieved not solely by the competent practice of individual healthcare professionals but also by the presence of systems—contexts, settings, processes—that enable and encourage good practice and protect against mishaps. A key event in building this recognition was the publication of *To Err Is Human: Building a Safer Health System* (Institute of Medicine, 2000). The foundation for that publication had been prepared by Donald Berwick, Paul Batalden, Lucian Leape, and others who had been writing and speaking for over 10 years about the importance of systems in determining the quality of health care (Batalden and Mohr, 1997; Berwick et al, 1990; Leape et al, 1995). *To Err Is Human* was widely discussed in newspapers, television, and radio—as well as in healthcare publications. Its impact was solidified by several other books issued by the Institute of Medicine over the next few years. Soon healthcare professionals across the country were discussing how systems might be changed to improve the safety and quality of care. And, of course, healthcare teams are important components of healthcare systems, as was emphasized in *To Err Is Human*. When *To Err Is Human* was published, interest in the quality and effectiveness of team-based health care increased, and it has continued to increase since that time.

This chapter begins our exploration of teamwork in health care by dealing with several foundational issues. How is the word *team* to be understood in the context of health care? What benefits do teams bring to health care, and what are the risks of working in teams? What evidence do we have that teams are more effective in making decisions and providing care than individuals working alone? What values must various people in clinical practices and hospitals have in order for healthcare teams to function well? What knowledge must these individuals have? What must team members be able to do? We begin by considering what a team is.

WORK GROUPS AND WORK TEAMS

To begin at the beginning, it is important to understand the word *team*. In ordinary conversation, the word is used to describe a wide variety of groups of people jointly engaged in one activity or another. There are sports teams, management teams, surgical teams, and so on. In some organizations, every employee is regarded as a team member so that the team consists of thousands of people, many of whom have never seen each other. For example, if you pick up a customer service telephone at a Target store and ask for help, you are told that a team member will be with you shortly. All of these uses of the word *team* make sense in their contexts, but in order to understand teamwork in health care, it is useful to define a term that refers to teams as they are encountered in the workplace, that is, teams of the kind that can provide team-based health care and can make decisions in healthcare organizations. We will call these teams *work teams*; and in this book, the term *team* means *work team*. It is somewhat arbitrary to use the phrase *work team* instead of *work group* for these entities. For the sake of clarity, we choose to think of *work group* as the name of a class or genus of groups of people and to think of *work team* as the name of a sub-class or species within that class (Figure 1–1).

It is Monday morning. The Chief Executive Officer (CEO) of Memorial Hospital has called a meeting to make an important announcement. The hospital is going to merge with another hospital across town. Attending the meeting are the Chief Nursing Officer (CNO), the Vice President of Medical Affairs, the Medical Staff President, the Chief Financial Officer (CFO), and about 25 others, including the head of the housekeeping service, the nurse manager of the emergency room, a prominent orthopedist who performs surgery at Memorial, and the hospital's in-house legal counsel. Everyone has known for months that merger talks are in progress, and many in the room have participated in them. However, only a small group knew before this meeting that the talks had reached a successful conclusion over the weekend.

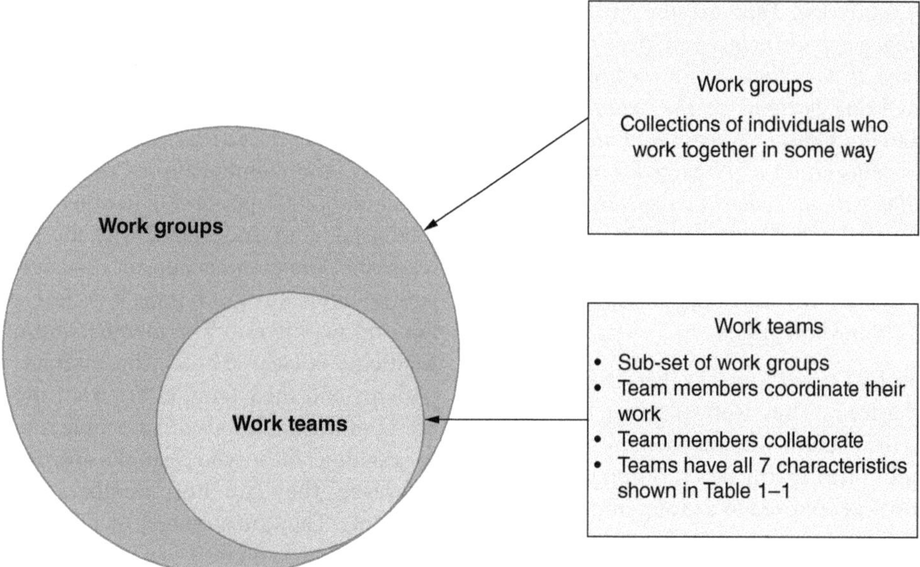

▲ Figure 1–1. Work groups and work teams.

The response to the announcement of the merger is jubilation. The merger will be very good for Memorial. The CFO and in-house counsel smile broadly and shake hands. The CNO and the Medical Staff President exchange looks of satisfaction—mingled with relief. All around there are signs of collegiality, pride, and anticipation of good things to come.

All of the people attending the meeting in the vignette work at Memorial Hospital. In some sense they are all on the same team. They may even call each other team members, meaning that they are all colleagues. There is no doubt that they all work together and that they all depend on each other to do their best so that Memorial can provide excellent health care to the people it serves.

But are they really a team? Describing the group of people at Memorial as a team stretches the concept. For example, many of the people do not interact. The CFO may recognize the head of housekeeping, but she never meets with him or communicates with him in any way. The group seems to be too large to be called a team. Within the broad scope of activity in the hospital, the people present in the room have specific objectives that they work toward each day without needing to know what many of the others are doing. Only some of them work interdependently on a daily or weekly basis.

Still, the Memorial Hospital employees and medical staff share a common general purpose, which is to provide health care, either directly or by supporting those who provide it directly. Each of them plays his or her part to serve that purpose. They collaborate in various sub-groupings. They identify with Memorial in its successes and difficulties. The group receiving the good news this Monday is certainly a work group.

But they are not a team except in some watered-down sense of the word. Why are they not a team? How does a work team differ from other work groups?

WHAT IS A WORK TEAM?

John Kimpell, MD, is a family physician. He works in a large medical group. His immediate colleagues are 3 other family physicians, Anna Gomez, MD, Allen Lewis, DO, and Jane Pearson, MD, and 1 nurse practitioner, Sarah Harris, RN, CNP. Penny Mills, RN, is a nurse who works closely with the physicians and the nurse practitioner. She receives patients' telephone calls and e-mail notes and assesses their needs for care, often meeting their needs herself without the need for a face-to-face visit. There are also 2 receptionists, who make appointments and greet patients as they arrive in the clinic, and 3 medical assistants, who bring patients to the examination rooms, take vital signs, and help the clinicians in other ways. This group of 11 cares for approximately 9000 patients who are registered with them. In the clinic, Dr. Kimpell and his colleagues are referred to as Red Family Medicine. *There are 3 other similar family medicine groups functioning within the medical group.*

Dr. Kimpell, Dr. Gomez, and the others in Red Family Medicine are a team. They work together to provide health care to the patients who see them in their clinic. What is it about them that makes it fitting to describe them as a team—as opposed to a group of people who simply work near one another in the same organization? A work team is commonly defined as a work group with several characteristics that mark it more specifically as a team (Hackman, 2002, pp. 41-59; Katzenbach and Smith, 2006, p. 45; Reeves et al, 2010, pp. 37-42; Scholtes et al, 2003, pp. 1-2; Sundstrom et al, 1990, p. 120; West, 2012, pp. 27-28, 65). There are 7 defining characteristics of a work team, listed in Table 1–1.

First, the members of the team have a shared goal or a set of goals. They are not pursuing their own individual aims while working nearby one another. Instead they are jointly seeking to achieve the same aim or perhaps a set of aims. In the case of Dr. Kimpell and his colleagues, the aim is to provide primary health care to the patients seen in the clinic. All of their work is oriented toward the task of achieving this aim.

Second, the team members share responsibility for achieving the goal. If the goal is reached, then all of the members share the credit for the achievement. And if the goal is not reached, all members of the team bear the burden of not succeeding. If Red Family Medicine provides health care with good outcomes, good patient experience, and efficient use of resources, then all of the individuals will share the credit, despite the fact that the roles of the various team members are different. All also will share the satisfaction.

Table 1–1. Defining characteristics of a work team

Shared team goal
Shared responsibility for achieving the goal
Defined membership
Authority for taking action to achieve the goal
Interdependency of members
Absence of independent sub-groups
Accountability to the larger organization

Third, the membership of the team is "bounded" (Hackman, 2002, pp. 44-50). In other words, it is clearly established and understood who the members of the team are. The membership may change over time, of course; but at any given time, it is clear who is a member and who is not. The membership of Red Family Medicine is clear. Those who interact directly with patients and their families are team members. There are 11 of them. Various other people support the team, for example, those who clean the offices in the evening. However, they are not members of Red Family Medicine. They are members of a different team.

Some writers on teams go further to say that a group larger than a certain size cannot be a team (Katzenbach and Smith, 2006, pp. 45-47; Reeves et al, 2010, p. 61; West, 2012, pp. 28). Sometimes this upper bound is said to be 25; some writers say that a team can be no larger than 10 or even smaller. We have more to say about the important consideration of team size in Chapter 12 where we consider the design of teams.

Fourth, the team has authority to carry out its task without needing to obtain approval for its decisions from someone outside of the team. In other words, it has autonomy in execution (West, 2012, pp. 27-28, 65). The team has sufficient capability in the pursuit of its goals to be able to take action without routinely seeking help and permission from people outside of the team. It has responsibility for achieving its goals, and it also has accountability as discussed below.

Fifth, the members of the team are interdependent. In order for the team to achieve its goal, the individuals depend on each other to carry out various portions of the work. Moreover, their dependency on one another is interactive. Dr. Gomez can do her work only if the medical assistants in Red Family Medicine do their work well, and her actions are often performed in response to what a medical assistant has done. For example, if a medical assistant brings a patient to an examination room but does not take the patient's blood pressure because the patient is agitated at that moment, then the assistant will tell Dr. Gomez, who will take the blood pressure later. The medical assistant has served the patient's psychological needs and has intentionally not gathered important physiological information with the usual timing, so Dr. Gomez fills the gap later. In health care, there is almost always some degree of skill specialization across the team members so that the members are not interchangeable, and the specialization makes the interdependency quite obvious. In other arenas other than health care, there are teams that consist of members who all have essentially the same skill set and do different pieces of the work depending on what is needed. For example, a carpentry crew erecting the structure for a new house could consist wholly of people who could substitute for each other if someone happens to be absent. In health care, teams with this ability to substitute team members are distinctly unusual, and so the dependence of one team member on another exercising his or her skills is usually very clear.

Sixth, the team functions as an undivided unit in working toward its goal. In other words, a work team does not have sub-groups operating separately, nor does it have an internal structure. This does not mean that sub-groups never meet or make decisions by themselves. Obviously, the 5 physicians and nurse practitioner in Red Family Medicine must decide how many of them can be on vacation and how many must be in the clinic to see patients each day. However, in making this decision they do not operate autonomously in that they are accountable to the team as a whole for their decision. For example, it is reasonable, even expected, that Ms. Mills, the registered nurse in the team, or one of the medical assistants would raise a question about staffing being too low for a given week because the clinicians have overlooked the fact that spring school vacation will mean that more children than usual will be brought in for care.

If what seems to be a team does have operational sub-groups, then each of these sub-groups is a team and the whole is a pair or a cluster of teams. If there is an internal structure through which some individuals are accountable to others but not to the team as a whole, then some individuals are not actually team members or there is more than one team at work. The members of Red Family Medicine all interact frequently. Although there is differentiation of function, no sub-group operates separately from the rest of the team.

Seventh, regardless of its authority and responsibility for carrying out its purpose, a work team is accountable to the larger organization of which it is a part. Dr. Kimpell's team is accountable for the team's performance, including its quality of care and its financial performance, to the head of primary care in the medical group and ultimately to the president of the medical group. The only exception to this rule is a team that is the whole organization, for example, a small primary care practice that is freestanding. But even then the team is accountable to the practice's governing board or partnership committee.

A work group is a work team only if it has all 7 of the characteristics listed in Table 1–1. This is not to say that a team with all 7 attributes is necessarily an effective team or a good team in any other sense. This is a separate question, one that is addressed in Chapter 6. For the moment, we are simply getting clear on what counts as a team, good or bad.

WORK TEAMS AND LOOK-ALIKES

Defining a work team as a work group with these 7 characteristics has several implications. Some of them may not be immediately obvious.

A group of individuals, each producing a product or service that contributes to a final goal, is not a team unless the individuals work interdependently, that is, unless the individuals adjust their outputs depending on the actions of other group members. In the vignette about Red Family Medicine, this adjustment is illustrated by the interactions of Dr. Gomez and the medical assistant with whom she works. In contrast, the individuals who wash and sterilize the laundry in a hospital, those who sterilize surgical instruments, and those who clean the operating rooms all contribute to effective, safe surgery, but they are not a single team because the members of each group work separately from all of the people in the other groups. Individuals performing the cleaning and sterilization of laundry, surgical instruments, and operating room cleaners constitute 3 separate teams.

Similarly, a group that appears to be an organizational leadership team may actually be a group of individual contributors and not a genuine team. The difference can be quite subtle. Leadership team members can meet together regularly and appear to be a team while they are actually performing their own functions without attending to the actions of the other team members and without any adjustment to assure that their respective portions of the organization work together effectively (Lencioni, 2002). A hospital leadership team consisting of a Vice President for Patient Care, a Chief Medical Officer, a Director of Human

Resources, and others may function in this way. If they do, they are not a team; they are some other kind of work group.

Because a team has the authority to carry out its task, a work group is not a team if it is closely supervised from outside the group. Thus, a group of nurses is not a team if they are given repeated, detailed direction by a supervisor who is not a member of the unit. This group does not have the latitude to work together collaboratively because individual members of the group are not permitted to interact with one another to make joint decisions and act on them.

Some large groups that are sometimes labeled *teams* are not work teams. For example, a football team is not a work team. Its large size and separation of players into different sub-units are inconsistent with the requirement that a team does not have components that operate independently. Within a football team, normally there are 3 sub-groups: an offensive group, a defensive group, and a special-teams group. A football team is a cluster of 3 teams, perhaps more. For similar reasons, the medical staff of a hospital is not a work team and a hospital's nursing staff is not a work team. And the employees of a Target store are not members of one work team; at any Target store there are multiple work teams.

These considerations are important because understanding the performance of a hospital or healthcare practice—or a football team or a Target store—requires attention to the real work teams in the organization and to those small groups that aspire to be work teams but have not yet succeeded. Attending to a cluster of work teams as if it were a single work team will obscure the function of the component work teams and frustrate attempts to improve the performance of both the component teams and the whole.

TRUE TEAMS

The reader may have noticed that stability of team membership is not among the characteristics listed in Table 1–1. Why not? Surely, a group of strangers who come together, carry out a task for an hour or less, and part company forever cannot be regarded as a team. Surprisingly, though, health care has many teams that function in exactly this way: code blue teams, emergency cesarean delivery teams, and even some routine operating room teams. To rule out these groups as teams would mean neglecting a good deal of health care. It is because of such teams that membership stability is not a defining feature of healthcare work teams.

Nonetheless, stability is a desirable team characteristic, something to encourage and maintain when circumstances permit. Teams that persist over time but must contend with ever-changing membership usually do not achieve levels of commitment and interdependency that are characteristic of the most highly performing teams. Moreover, only teams that are stable over long periods of time are likely to be able to attain mutual accountability; that is, only the members of stable teams are likely to actively hold each other accountable for their performance. And only stable teams are likely to develop in their members a sense of identity with the team and its goal. The advantages of stability in a team are discussed more fully in Chapters 2 and 6.

Red Family Medicine—with its long-serving members—does seem to be more fully a team, more like a genuine team than one that forms and carries out a task over an hour or even a month, then disbanding. Because Red Family Medicine has the 7 defining characteristics of a work team and, in addition, has stable membership, it is an example of an important archetype among healthcare teams. Our label for this type of team is *true team*. In Chapter 2, this archetype is contrasted with other team archetypes.

BENEFITS OF TEAMS

Why are teams used to provide health care? For many episodes of health care, given the specialization discussed earlier, there is no other way to provide the needed care. To meet the needs of many patients, the expertise of several people is required so that all of their expertise can be brought to bear on the problem, expertise that no one person has or could have. But beyond this consideration, what value do teams bring—generally and to health care in particular? What are the justifications for using teams in situations in which the work could be done by individuals working alone? There are actually many reasons for using teams (Katzenbach and Smith, 2006, pp. 15-19; West, 2012, pp. 17-20). Let us consider 4 important ones.

Bay Medical Group provides primary care to people of all ages in a coastal community 100 miles north of San Francisco. Its staff includes general internists, pediatricians, nurse practitioners, and many others. It is unusual in having a psychologist and a social worker therapist in the group. These 2 clinical professionals were added 2 years ago to improve the care provided for adults with mental health problems. Prior to that time, a patient with depression, for example, would be treated with medication by one of the physicians or would be referred to a mental health group nearby. There was nearly always a delay in getting an appointment for the patient with the mental health group. Often the information transferred would be incomplete, requiring another delay as the mental health provider obtained the information needed. Similarly, the information transferred back to Bay Medical Group was often incomplete or delayed.

Now that the primary care providers work as a team with their own mental health care providers, the sequence of events is much faster and easier. A patient presenting to a nurse practitioner with serious depression can usually be seen by the psychologist for brief initial assessment the same day. The primary care providers can seek guidance informally by walking down the hallway for a brief conversation with the psychologist or social worker. Often they learn then and there that a visit with a mental health provider is not needed because the problem can be handled by the primary care provider. Sometimes they learn that the situation is more urgent than they realized and that mental health care is needed immediately.

Teams are faster in performing many tasks. This advantage is graphically illustrated by the team arrangement at Bay Medical Group. When the care was provided by the various professionals providing their items of care serially, everything took much longer. The rapid interaction of people working in a team often saves both time and money.

Teams also enable individuals and organizations to learn. By working together closely, the primary care providers and mental health care providers at Bay Medical Group have learned a great deal from each other about providing high quality mental health care. They also have learned many routines for working together smoothly and effectively.

Moreover, these routines for referral, information transfer, and the like have become codified in the operation of the clinic. When the providers turn over as various people move away or retire, the lessons learned will be retained by the team even though the team members have changed. The team serves as a repository of useful knowledge.

Teams are also sources of innovation. When the psychologist and social worker first joined Bay Medical Group, they were disappointed that they were not consulted more frequently on an informal basis. In meetings with the primary care providers, the psychologist and social worker voiced their disappointment. This led to exploration of the issue and eventually to a discussion about the causes and solutions for a problem of lost opportunity. It was revealed that when the primary care providers began seeking informal consultation they had become frustrated because the mental health care providers seemed never to be available. The principal solution chosen was to schedule the mental health providers less tightly so that they had slack time available to be interrupted as their days progressed. This solution would have been unlikely to be discovered if the primary care and mental health care providers had been working separately.

Despite these and other advantages for teams, it is, however, important to note that not all tasks are suitable for teamwork. Some examples of tasks suitable for one person are obvious from the nature of task. A portrait painted by 2 people is likely to suffer from the division of labor rather than being enhanced—unless the styles of the 2 painters are identical (for example, because one painter trained the other). A prosthetic aortic valve can be sewn into place by only 1 surgeon. But even some tasks commonly performed by teams are often better done by individuals. Task force reports written by teams sometimes are stigmatized as "camels," that is, horses designed by committees. The decision as to whether a given task should be carried out by a team is an important consideration in designing teams. In other words, the first decision to make when designing a team is whether a team should be created for the task at hand. This issue is discussed more fully in Chapter 12.

RISKS OF TEAMS

Working in teams also carries some risks. The most frequently noted risk often is called *social loafing* (Thompson, 2011, pp. 28-31). Primarily because teams commonly have more than one person who can perform a given task, it becomes tempting for team members to stand by while someone else does the work.

For this reason, teams can have a demotivating effect on individual members. This problem is also called *freeloading* or *free riding*. The risk of social loafing is higher with larger teams since responsibility is diffused more widely when there are more people who might do the work.

In addition, decision making and action by individuals may be degraded when individuals work in a team rather than alone. A common cause of this problem is domination by hierarchy or personality so that team members set aside what they think is best and instead do what they think is expected of them by those they perceive to have more power in the team (Jelphs and Dickinson, 2008, p. 68; Reeves et al, 2010, pp. 60-61). Thus, in the operating room, where the surgeon and the anesthesiologist are the acknowledged leaders, often other members of the surgical team are reluctant to disagree with them. It is likely that some cases of wrong-site surgery could be prevented if team members did not feel inhibited about voicing their doubts about the course of action being taken (Clarke et al, 2008). So too, a physician with a forceful personality may intimidate the nurses and others with whom she works so that the other clinicians set aside their own insights into what would best serve the patient's interest—even if the physician would be most dismayed if she understood the effects of her manner on team performance.

Despite being sources of innovation, teams can actually be less creative than individuals working alone (West, 2012, pp. 23-25). Again, there are several causes for this diminished creativity. One of the most obvious causes is that offering novel ideas in a group carries the risk that one will be ridiculed (or criticized in gentler ways) because the idea offered is unfamiliar and, at least at first blush, implausible. A particularly interesting second cause goes by the name of *production blocking*. Despite the enthusiasm often expressed for the practice of multitasking, it is in fact not possible to switch back and forth between different trains of complex thought and maintain the quality of both (Thompson, 2011, pp. 212-215). In group discussions, the production of truly new ideas gets blocked when those who are formulating a novel thought get diverted by the need to attend to what other members of the group are saying. Production blocking is discussed further in Chapter 9. Still, innovation is fueled by the pooling of facts and insights that no one person possesses before the discussion begins. Fortunately, there are methods for overcoming fear of criticism, production blocking, and the other threats to team creative thinking and problem solving. We explore those methods in Chapter 10, which deals with creativity.

Table 1–2 summarizes the benefits and risks of teams.

Table 1–2. Benefits and risks of teams

Benefits	Risks
Perform tasks faster than individuals working alone	Social loafing (= freeloading, = free riding)
Enable individuals and organizations to learn	Degrading of decision making, for example, by hierarchy or personality
Enable organizations to retain lessons learned despite turnover of individuals	Diminished creativity if the team is not managed well
Enable innovation	

EVIDENCE FOR THE EFFECTIVENESS OF TEAMS

Teams have been shown to be more effective than individuals working alone in manufacturing, oil and gas, the apparel industry, and many other settings (West, 2012, pp. 17-20). The basic question of whether teams are effective is in fact no longer a focus of research by scholars in the field of organizational behavior. Instead, for 30 years or more, researchers have focused on various factors that influence the degree of a team's effectiveness. In financial services, team self-management has been found to increase effectiveness (Cohen and Bailey, 1997, p. 250). Performance feedback is associated with increased productivity in railway crews (Guzzo and Dickson, 1996, p. 315). In teams that conduct time-limited projects, for example, development of a new electronic device, group cohesion improves performance (Sundstrom et al, 2000, p. 59). Teams are widely used in manufacturing, commercial fishing, banking, software development, making movies, and many other sectors of the economy. Their usefulness was established and documented through research long ago.

Teams are not new to health care either. But they have become more common recently, and even more recently strong interest has developed in interprofessional teams.

Nonetheless, there already is ample evidence of team effectiveness in health care (Bosch et al, 2009; Lemieux-Charles and McGuire, 2006). As already noted, for many aspects of care, delivery by individuals working alone is simply not possible. In these cases, care is team-based by necessity. But in many other situations care could be provided by teams even though it is often provided by professionals working separately. In many of these situations, team-based care yields superior results. For example, several studies have shown improved outcomes when pharmacists join physicians, physician assistants, or nurse practitioners in a team-based approach instead of working separately (Bogden et al, 1998; Gattis et al, 1999). Interprofessional psychogeriatric teams were found to be more effective than general practitioners working alone in providing care for frail elderly people with depression (Banerjee et al, 1996). Teams of geriatricians, nurses, social workers, occupational therapists, physical therapists, and dieticians were able to decrease mortality, at least in the short term, in hospitalized elderly patients when team-based care was compared with care provided by physicians working alone (Hogan and Fox, 1990). For surgical patients, interprofessional medical emergency teams were found to decrease postoperative adverse events and deaths when introduced in a hospital that had previously used only a traditional cardiac arrest response system (Bellomo et al, 2004). Higher levels of nurse-physician collaboration, as reported by nurses, were associated with better outcomes among patients who were discharged from intensive care units (ICUs) and then followed to learn their rates of death and return to the ICU (Baggs et al, 1999). In a Scottish study, breast cancer patients receiving multidisciplinary care experienced lower mortality than breast cancer patients treated conventionally. In this study, multidisciplinary care was provided by an organized interprofessional team that followed written clinical guidelines, made collective decisions about treatment, and audited their results; conventional care was provided by surgeons and other clinicians practicing without any formal team organization (Kesson et al, 2012). Palliative care has been shown to be more effective when delivered by an interdisciplinary team compared with primary care physicians (PCPs) practicing alone (Rabow et al, 2004). One study showed superior performance of an interprofessional team versus attending physicians working alone in prescribing antibiotics in the hospital. Both length of stay and cost of care were improved without any ill effect on outcomes of care (Gums et al, 1999). As illustrated in Figure 1–2, collaborative care for people with depression has been shown

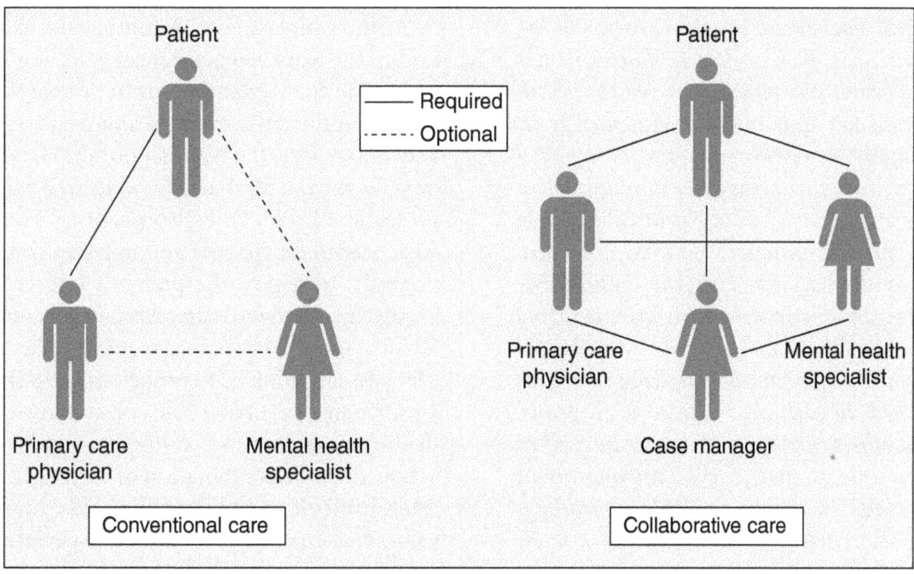

▲ **Figure 1–2.** Collaborative care for depression.

to be more effective than conventional care. Collaborative care is provided by a team that consists of a PCP, a case manager, and a mental health specialist; conventional care does not make use of case managers, and the physician may or may not refer the patient to a mental health specialist (Gilbody et al, 2006).

Of course, not all teams are effective in everyday health care or even when they function in research settings with special resources provided. And sometimes teams are used for purposes better served by individual practitioners who work alone and simply refer patients to another practitioner when it is warranted. As noted earlier, not all tasks are suitable for teams. Nonetheless there is solid evidence that teams can be effective in general and are effective for many specific clinical purposes in many different healthcare settings.

COMPETENCIES FOR TEAMWORK

Mary Jackson, RN, MHA, is Director of Surgery at North Valley Hospital. She worked as a scrub nurse for 8 years. During that time she completed a Master of Healthcare Administration degree online during evenings and weekends and in person during summer sessions at the University that offered the program. Since becoming the Director 4 years ago, Ms. Jackson has been a full-time administrator although she occasionally fills in for other nurses who are on vacation or absent for other reasons. There are 6 operating rooms in the surgical suite. Ms. Jackson has 15 nurses in her department as well as 8 technicians and 10 clerical staff. She and her staff interact with staff from Central Supply, Housekeeping, the Emergency Department, and other areas of the hospital. There are 23 surgeons who operate at North Valley. They are all in private practice, that is, none are employed by the hospital. Five anesthesiologists and 6 nurse anesthetists work in the operating room suite. All of them are employed by the hospital. In a typical day, about 35 surgical procedures are performed. In each case, a team of surgeons, nurses, and others carries out the procedure. After surgery, patients go first to the Post-anesthesia Care Unit (PACU), which is staffed and led by a group separate from Ms. Jackson's unit. Ms. Jackson reports to the Director of Nursing (DON) at North Valley, who in turn reports to the CEO.

In order for safe and effective surgery to be carried out at North Valley, a good deal of effective teamwork needs to take place. For that to happen, a large number of people need to have certain knowledge and skills that are relevant to working effectively in teams. They also need to have certain values. This knowledge, set of skills, and set of values go beyond what they need to practice in their own professions. In order to understand team-based care, it is necessary to understand the specific knowledge, skills, and values of teamwork.

These necessities are often called *competencies*. In recent decades, educators have developed the notion of competencies in their efforts to improve education in medicine, psychology, architecture, and many other fields (Calhoun et al, 2002). Defining competencies serves to establish objectives for training programs and to provide the basis for evaluating whether both students and practitioners have what it is needed to practice their professions effectively. In medicine, the Accreditation Council for Graduate Medical Education has defined competencies for residency training programs (Leach, 2008). In nursing, the American Association of Colleges of Nursing has taken the lead in defining competencies for nursing education (American Association of Colleges of Nursing, 2008). These lists of competencies specify what a healthcare professional needs to have learned to practice a given profession—regardless of whether the professional practices alone or in a team.

At the simplest level, a competency is an ability or skill, as the word *competency* suggests. For example, Ms. Jackson in the vignette needs to be able to assess nursing job applicants, make hiring decisions, and bring new nurses into the team smoothly. However, abilities or skills are not all that one needs to perform well in a professional role. One also needs to have the knowledge needed for the role and to have certain values, for example, to regard the patient's interest as centrally important. The word *competencies* is a convenient label for all of these performance requisites taken as a package. Thus we can think of a competency as a skill needed to perform in a particular role, or as knowledge in a particular domain, or as a value that can be expressed in action, or some combination of these 3. In practice, it is often difficult to separate the skills, knowledge, and values that enable a professional to perform well in carrying out a component of professional practice. For example, a nurse discussing with a patient what lies ahead in the patient's treatment and care for a newly diagnosed cancer exhibits skills, knowledge, and values all at once—skills in listening and talking with patients under emotional stress, knowledge about the cancer and its treatment, and values such as respect for the patient's feelings and preferences.

The concept of competency can be extended to teamwork. Teamwork competencies are abilities, knowledge, and values that professionals need in order to work effectively in teams—regardless of whether they are pharmacists, social workers, nurses, physicians, or other professionals. In the last few years, professional groups in the United States and Canada have devised competency models for interprofessional or collaborative healthcare practice. These competencies pertain to nurses, physicians, administrators, and others working as members of a healthcare team. Recently the American Association of Colleges of Nursing, the Association of American Medical Colleges, and 4 other associations of healthcare educators issued a joint statement of core competencies for interprofessional collaborative practice (Interprofessional Education Collaborative Expert Panel, 2011). Their report separates these competencies into 4 domains: values/ethics, roles/responsibilities, communication, and teamwork. In Chapter 7, we discuss this competency model and deal in more detail with competencies needed by team members.

But for teamwork to be effective, it is not enough for the members of the team to have the competencies that pertain specifically to team membership. Individuals in other roles also need competencies for the work they do. For example, Ms. Jackson in the North Valley Hospital vignette needs competencies not only as a team member but also as a team leader. As the leader, she must keep the team focused on its goal of providing safe and effective surgical procedures for patients. She must also build and maintain the team and assure that it has the resources it needs to do its work. We deal with the competencies of team leaders in Chapter 8.

Ms. Jackson reports to the DON. In this book, we refer to the person to whom the team leader is accountable as the *team sponsor*. The team sponsor must also have competencies specific to her role. For example, she must set the task for the team. In this case, the team sponsor has determined that the Director of Surgery's team provides surgical procedures but not PACU care, which is provided by a different team. She must also designate the composition of the team. Ms. Jackson may have her own views about how many people in various job categories should work in the operating room suite, but she needs to have the DON's approval for changes in the team's composition. We address the competencies of team sponsors in Chapter 12.

Finally, the senior leaders of the hospital have their roles to play and must have the competencies corresponding to their roles. Chief among these is the ability to mold the culture of the organization so that it supports teamwork. There are also other competencies pertinent to this level of the organization, for example, the ability to provide various supports for teamwork, including training and effective communication tools such as an electronic health record. In Chapter 18, we discuss the competencies needed by senior leaders with respect to teamwork.

In sum, competencies are needed at 4 levels: team member, team leader, team sponsor, and senior leader. Figure 1–3 lists the types of competencies needed at each level, and later chapters elaborate on them. In order for teamwork to proceed smoothly, individuals at all 4 levels need to know not only what is expected of them but also what they should expect from others.

CONCLUSION

Red Family Medicine provided an example of team-based health care and thus a way to see concretely the characteristics of a *work group* that make it a *work team*. Briefly, a work team is a defined group of interdependent individuals who share responsibility for achieving a common goal and have sufficient authority to take action to achieve the goal. Teams have advantages over individuals working alone, but there are also risks. The evidence for the effectiveness of healthcare teams in various situations is strong. Finally, for teamwork to be effective, thus enabling team-based care, team members, team leaders, team sponsors, and senior leaders all need to have competencies pertinent to their roles.

We have established what a healthcare team is, why teams are used, and, in general terms, what competencies among healthcare professionals are needed for effective teamwork to occur. Next, we explore the different types of teams encountered in health care as a prelude to understanding the differences in how these various teams function and the differences in what they require to perform well.

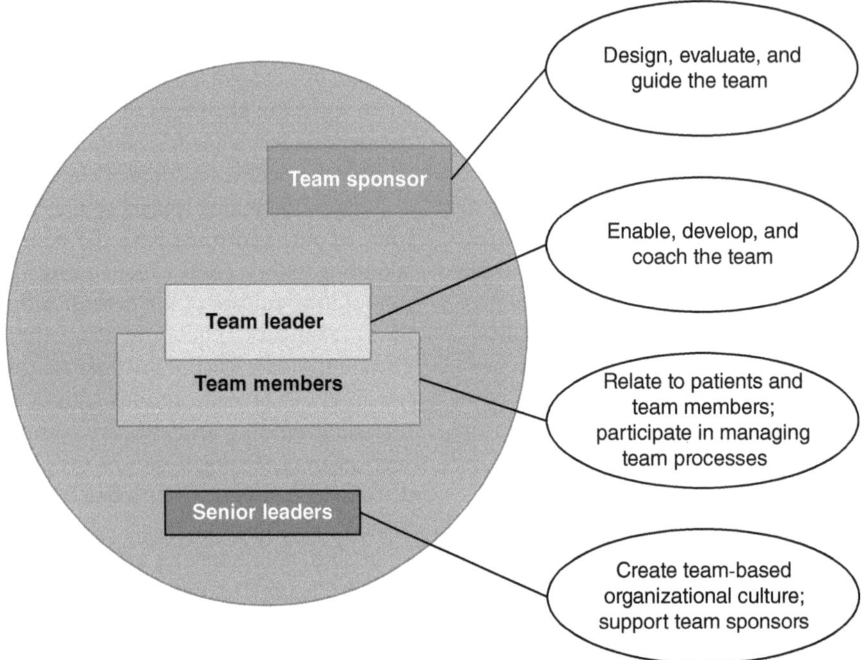

▲ **Figure 1–3.** Teamwork competencies needed at 4 levels.

REFERENCES

American Association of Colleges of Nursing. *The Essentials of Baccalaureate Education for Professional Nursing Practice.* Washington, DC: American Association of Colleges of Nursing; 2008. https://www.aacn.nche.edu/education-resources/BaccEssentials08.pdf. Accessed January 31, 2012.

American Association of Medical Colleges. *2008 Physician Specialty Data.* Washington, DC: American Association of Medical Colleges; 2008. https://www.aamc.org/download/47352/data/specialtydata.pdf. Accessed February 18, 2012.

Baggs JG, Schmitt MH, Mushlin AI, et al. Association between nurse-physician collaboration and patient outcomes in three intensive care units. *Crit Care Med.* 1999;27:1991-1998.

Banerjee S, Shamash K, Macdonald AJD, et al. Randomised controlled trial of effect of intervention by psychogeriatric team on depression in frail elderly people at home. *BMJ.* 1996;313:1058-1061.

Batalden PB, Mohr JJ. Building knowledge of health care as a system. *Qual Manag Health Care.* 1997;5:1-12.

Bellomo R, Goldsmith D, Uchino S, et al. Prospective controlled trial of effect of medical emergency team on postoperative morbidity and mortality rates. *Crit Care Med.* 2004;32:916-921.

Berwick DM, Godfrey AB, Roessner J. *Curing Health Care.* San Francisco, CA: Jossey-Bass; 1990.

Bogden PE, Abbott RD, Williamson P, et al. Comparing standard care with a physician and pharmacist team approach for uncontrolled hypertension. *J Gen Intern Med.* 1998;13:740-745.

Bosch M, Faber MJ, Cruijsberg J, et al. Effectiveness of patient care teams and the role of clinical expertise and coordination: a literature review. *Med Care Res Rev.* 2009;66(6 supplement):5S-35S.

Calhoun JG, Davidson PL, Sinioris ME, et al. Toward an understanding of competency identification and assessment in health care management. *Qual Manag Health Care.* 2002;11:14-38.

Clarke JR, Johnston J, Blanco M, et al. Wrong-site surgery: can we prevent it? *Adv Surg.* 2008;42:13-31.

Cohen SG, Bailey DE. What makes teams work: group effectiveness research from the shop floor to the executive suite. *J Manage.* 1997;23:239-290.

Fagin CM. Collaboration between nurses and physicians: no longer a choice. *Acad Med.* 1992;67:295-303.

Garrett JF. Social psychology of teamwork. In: Harrower M, ed. *Medical and Psychological Teamwork in the Care of the Chronically Ill.* Springfield, IL: Charles C Thomas, Publisher; 1955:67-70.

Gattis WA, Hasselblad V, Whellan DJ, et al. Reduction in heart failure events by the addition of a clinical pharmacist to the heart failure management team. *Arch Intern Med.* 1999;159:1939-1945.

Gilbody S, Bower P, Fletcher J, et al. Collaborative care for depression: a cumulative meta-analysis and review of longer-term outcomes. *Arch Intern Med.* 2006;166:2314-2321.

Gums JG, Yancy RW, Hamilton CA, et al. A randomized, prospective study measuring outcomes after antibiotic therapy intervention by a multidisciplinary consult team. *Pharmacotherapy.* 1999;19:1369-1377.

Guzzo RA, Dickson MW. Teams in organizations: recent research on performance and effectiveness. *Annu Rev Psychol.* 1996;47:307-338.

Hackman JR. *Leading Teams: Setting the Stage for Great Performances.* Boston, MA: Harvard Business School Press; 2002.

Hall P, Weaver L. Interdisciplinary education and teamwork: a long and winding road. *Med Educ.* 2001;35:867-875.

Hogan DB, Fox RA. A prospective controlled trial of a geriatric consultation team in an acute-care hospital. *Age Ageing.* 1990;19:107-113.

Institute of Medicine. *To Err Is Human: Building a Safer Health System.* Washington, DC: National Academy Press; 2000.

Interprofessional Education Collaborative Expert Panel. *Core Competencies for Interprofessional Collaborative Practice: Report of an Expert Panel.* Washington, DC: Interprofessional Education Collaborative; 2011. http://www.aacn.nche.edu/education-resources/IPECReport.pdf. Accessed January 29, 2012.

Jelphs K, Dickinson H. *Working in Teams.* Bristol, UK: The Policy Press; 2008.

Katzenbach JR, Smith DK. *The Wisdom of Teams: Creating the High-Performance Organization.* Collins Business Essentials, ed. New York, NY: HarperCollins Publishers; 2006.

Kesson EM, Allardice GM, Burns HJG, et al. Effects of a multidisciplinary team working on breast cancer survival: retrospective, comparative, interventional cohort study of 13,722 women. *BMJ.* 2012;344:e2718.

Leach DC. Changing education to improve patient care. *Postgrad Med J.* 2008; 84:437-441.

Leape LL. Error in medicine. *JAMA.* 1994;272:1851-1857.

Leape LL, Bates DW, Cullen DJ, et al. Systems analysis of adverse drug events: ADE Prevention Study Group. *JAMA.* 1995;274:35-43.

Lemieux-Charles L, McGuire WL. What do we know about health care team effectiveness? A review of the literature. *Med Care Res Rev.* 2006;63:263-300.

Lencioni P. *The Five Dysfunctions of Teams.* San Francisco, CA: Jossey-Bass; 2002.

Lowes R. NPs should not lead medical homes, AAFP says. *Medscape Medical News.* September 19, 2012. http://www.medscape.com/viewarticle/771179. Accessed October 22, 2012.

Rabow MW, Dibble SL, Pantilat SZ, et al. The comprehensive care team: a controlled trial of outpatient palliative medicine consultation. *Arch Intern Med.* 2004;164:83-91.

Reeves S, Lewin S, Espin S, et al. *Interprofessional Teamwork for Health and Social Care.* Chichester, UK: John Wiley & Sons, Ltd.; 2010.

Scholtes PR, Joiner BL, Streibel BJ. *The Team Handbook.* 3rd ed. Madison, WI: Oriel Incorporated; 2003.

Starr P. *The Social Transformation of American Medicine.* New York, NY: Basic Books; 1982.

Sundstrom E, De Meuse KP, Futrell D. Work teams: applications and effectiveness. *Am Psychol.* 1990;45:120-133.

Sundstrom E, McIntyre M, Halfhill T, et al. Work groups: from the Hawthorne studies to work teams of the 1990s and beyond. *Group Dyn.* 2000;4:44-67.

Thompson LL. *Making the Team: A Guide for Managers.* 4th ed. Upper Saddle River, NJ: Prentice Hall; 2011.

West MA. *Effective Teamwork: Practical Lessons From Organizational Research.* 3rd ed. Chichester, UK: John Wiley & Sons, Ltd.; 2012.

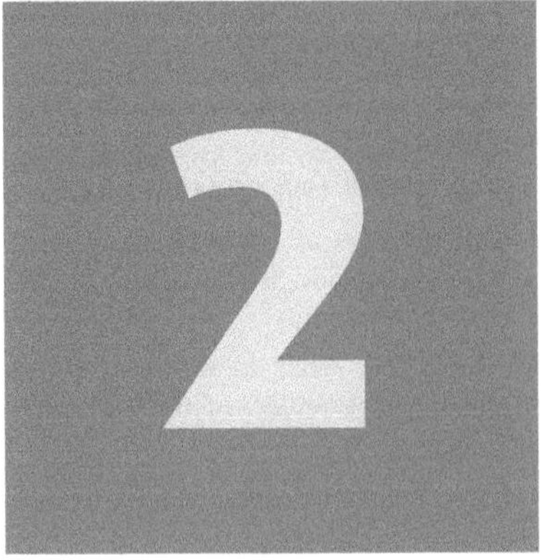

Types of Healthcare Teams

In this chapter, we explore the different types of work teams that are encountered in health care. This is not an exercise in classification for its own sake. Different types of teams have different capabilities, different limitations, and different needs for planning, participation, training, and management. Knowing the type of team at hand helps team members, leaders, and sponsors to ensure that the team is performing as effectively as it can. As they seek to perform well in their own roles, team members, leaders, and sponsors as well as senior leaders all benefit from understanding the characteristics of different types of teams.

THE VALUE OF CLASSIFYING TEAMS

Many different taxonomies have been offered by writers on teams. An early and influential classification was offered by Sundstrom and colleagues (1990), who proposed 4 categories: (a) advice and involvement teams, (b) production and service teams, (c) project and development teams, and (d) action and negotiation teams. An example of an advice and involvement team in health care is a quality improvement team, which serves to recommend process changes in a healthcare practice or hospital and to engage people in making the changes successfully. Sundstrom's category of production and service teams includes all clinical teams. Project or development teams are exemplified by teams charged with implementing electronic health records in hospitals. And a team of health system executives and attorneys seeking a merger with another system is an action or negotiation team. Sundstrom's interest was in identifying very general factors that influence team effectiveness and, in particular, in showing that factors beyond internal team processes affect team performance. His 4 categories—and examples under each heading—served to make his analysis concrete and plausible. With respect to teams in health care, however, this classification will not provide much help in understanding the functions and needs of different teams. For example, all clinical teams, from primary care teams to international air ambulance teams, are lumped into the single category of production and service teams. The needs of primary care teams and air ambulance teams are quite different. It is helpful to tease out the characteristics that make them different and place these teams in different categories in order to clarify the differences in their needs.

Taxonomies are devised for a variety of purposes. Sometimes the purpose is simple description. For example, real estate listings commonly classify houses for sale as single-family homes, duplexes, townhouses, and so on. These categories enable potential buyers to decide quickly whether they wish to consider a particular house. Researchers usually use team taxonomies to formulate hypotheses and eventually to generate new knowledge about team functioning and about factors that affect team performance. If a researcher studies a sample of teams with widely differing characteristics, he or she is not likely to obtain results that are reproducible, much less results that are useful in improving the performance of any particular kind of team. The researcher needs to focus on a single kind of team or to take the differences among teams into account by using multiple categories or more sophisticated quantitative methods (Hollenbeck et al, 2012). For example, research findings about the performance of healthcare software installation teams will probably offer little guidance in understanding the performance of surgical teams.

No classification of teams is compelling in itself, that is, independently of its utility in serving a given purpose. The purpose of this book is to convey knowledge useful to people delivering and managing health care as they plan, participate in, lead, and support healthcare teams, especially interprofessional teams. We present a classification that serves the purpose of helping teams to improve their functioning, that is, to improve their capacities to achieve their goals. The classification needs to have categories that are familiar and credible to clinicians and managers. It also needs to distinguish among teams that differ with respect to their needs for planning, participation, training, and management. At the same time, the classification needs to be kept as simple as possible, avoiding a proliferation of categories that might be conceptually interesting but carry no implications for action to improve team performance.

In sum, the value of classifying teams is to make clear the characteristic strengths, vulnerabilities, and needs of teams in each category. This clarification enables team members to participate in a way that optimizes team performance. Also, team leaders are provided with more explicit guidance for leading teams of different kinds. Team sponsors gain more well-defined methods for designing and guiding teams. And, finally, senior leaders have a more clearly delineated set of considerations to use in supporting teams and providing for their organizational needs.

We begin with a general division of healthcare teams into clinical teams and management teams.

CLINICAL TEAMS

Clinical teams are, of course, teams that provide clinical care. To be more precise, they are teams that provide care directly in the sense that they interact directly with patients and families. A clinical team may include people who are not clinicians, for example, the Health Unit Coordinators or HUCs who are central to the function of all hospital wards. Conversely, the presence of a clinician in a healthcare team does not make it a clinical team. The executive leadership team of a large health system typically includes at least 1 nurse and 1 physician, but these teams do not provide health care directly, and so they are not clinical teams.

True Teams

The U.S. Preventive Services Task Force recommends screening for colorectal cancer beginning at age 50, using either colonoscopy or one of a few alternative methods. Sam Murphy turned 50 about a year ago. After some delay (not at all unusual), he decided to undergo colonoscopy after discussing the options with his general internist. His internist referred him to a gastroenterology group to have the procedure performed. After spending a largely sleepless night while prescribed laxatives cleansed his colon, Mr. Murphy arrived at the outpatient endoscopy facility early the next morning. There he met Kevin Leon, MD, the gastroenterologist to whom he had been referred. Dr. Leon performed the colonoscopy, working along with Susan Wallace, RN, and a technician expert in the function and maintenance of the equipment. Mr. Murphy later remembered nothing of the procedure itself since he was sedated with midazolam, administered intravenously by Ms. Wallace. After the procedure, Mr. Murphy recovered while attended by Ms. Wallace. He learned from her that she, Dr. Leon, and the technician had been working together for 5 years performing colonoscopies and other endoscopic procedures. Occasionally one of them is absent for various reasons, but whenever possible the same 3 work together. They prefer this approach even though it complicates scheduling because it has enabled them to know each other's work preferences, communication styles, and skill levels for different procedures.

This colonoscopy team, like Red Family Medicine in Chapter 1, is a true team. *True team* is a technical term. Other writers have used the terms *long-term teams* (Joshi and Roh, 2009, pp. 610-611) or *intact teams* (Salas et al, 2008, pp. 909-910) for similar teams. The distinctive and defining feature of these teams is that, in addition to having all of the 7 attributes of work teams (Table 1–1 in Chapter 1), they possess stability of membership over time. They also have clear leaders. The characteristics of true teams are shown in Table 2–1 along with the characteristics of other types of clinical teams, which are discussed below.

True teams have many strengths, which, taken together, constitute an advantage for true teams

Table 2–1. Characteristics of clinical teams

Team Type	Purpose	Characteristics: All 7 Characteristics of Work Teams (Table 1-1 in Chapter 1)?	Stable Membership?	Clear Leader?	Shared Responsibility?
True team	To provide clinical care over extended periods of time or for repeated, time-limited episodes	Yes	Yes	Yes	Yes
Template team	To provide clinical care for time-limited episodes	Yes	No	Yes	Yes
Knotwork[a]	To provide clinical care for a particular patient's specific need	Often no	No	No	Yes
Network[b]	To provide information & support to network clinicians in providing care to patients	No	No	No	No

[a]Knotworks commonly do not fit the definition of a work team, but they have some of the same characteristics.
[b]Networks are not work teams, but they are similar in some respects.

compared with other teams. These strengths are listed in Table 2–2.

When people work together frequently over extended periods, they normally develop deep commitment to their shared purpose. This level of commitment usually comes only with time. Of course, some teams are dysfunctional and do not develop in this way, but a team of short duration never even has the opportunity, whether it functions smoothly or not. Members of stable teams also typically come to know one another in their work roles and to trust one another to a degree not possible at the outset.

Table 2–2. Strengths of true teams

Potential for strong commitment to shared purpose
Members' mutual knowledge of each other as team members
Potential for high levels of trust
Higher likelihood of mutual accountability than teams of other types
Potential for strong identification by members with the team
Potential for a high level of interdependency
Opportunity to fit roles to individuals' interests and skills
Potential for lower error rates than teams of other types

The members of true teams usually come to know one another well. They learn about each other's strengths, knowledge bases, values, and skills. They also learn each other's vulnerabilities and limits of toleration for difficult situations. This knowledge permits true teams to develop advantages that can contribute to good performance.

Over time, the members of true teams also commonly develop high levels of trust in one another. This trust also provides the basis for tangible functional advantages.

Because they are work teams, true teams by definition share responsibility for achieving their goals, but the commitment, mutual knowledge, and trust that develop with time often enable the team members to go beyond simply sharing responsibility. They can come to hold one another accountable for performing their roles well. In other words, true teams often achieve mutual accountability. In the vignette, it is easy to imagine that Dr. Leon and Ms. Wallace could point out to each other without awkwardness or offense that he or she is about to take action without having gone through all the steps required for full safety. For example, Ms. Wallace might forget to state aloud (or "call out," to use a common teamwork term) the dose of midazolam before administering it. If Ms. Wallace were to choose the wrong dose, "calling out" the dose would enable the other 2 team members to recognize the dose as atypical. One can imagine that Dr. Leon might tactfully remind her to call out the dose and that she would regard his prompt with gratitude, not annoyance. Mutual accountability is one of the marks of a particularly high-performing team. Some writers on teams regard mutual accountability as a defining feature of a work team (Katzenbach and Smith, 2006, pp. 60-61). Using this definition, a work group does not count as a team unless the members actually take action, when appropriate, to hold each other accountable for performance. This high standard commonly is not achieved in health care. True teams are more likely to rise to this standard than are teams with changing membership or short duration. The issue of mutual accountability is discussed more fully in Chapter 6.

Members of a team who stay together for a long period of time also often develop a strong sense of identification with the team and its goals, especially if the team's activities comprise substantial parts of their work lives. Identifying with the team means that members see the team as a reflection of themselves. Under these circumstances, the value or esteem of the team becomes merged with the members' self-esteem, and their motivation to perform well is heightened.

As trust develops over time among team members, they become more deeply interdependent. In other words, as their confidence in each other's skills and reliability grow, there is less need for the team members to second-guess and check each other's work. This leads to faster action, less duplication, and more parallel action when possible. Because Dr. Leon has full confidence in the technician on his team, he does not need to watch the technician assemble the equipment or take it down; he can instead use this time to talk with the patient or to perform other tasks.

Members of true teams can also clarify their roles and communication routines over time, taking full advantage of the idiosyncrasies of the members' personalities, knowledge bases, and skill sets. In a stable endoscopic team, it is not necessary for roles and routines to be fully defined in advance of each procedure. Early in the life of a true team, the speed with which members accomplish a procedure will be slower because they need to take time to clarify who does what. But eventually the assignment of tasks will fit the individual team members better than it would if the assignments were made in advance. For example, if the team in the vignette learns that Ms. Wallace is more effective in reassuring anxious elderly patients while Dr. Leon is more effective in reassuring middle-aged males, they can perform these more specialized roles routinely instead of one of them chatting with all patients before the procedure begins. They might even develop a means for signaling each other that an attempt to reassure a patient is not succeeding and that the other team member should take over the task because he or she is more likely to succeed. A team that is composed of different individuals each time it performs its task does not enjoy this opportunity to fit roles to individuals.

Health care has numerous teams that are composed of different individuals each time the teams go into action, for example, labor and delivery teams and many others as mentioned in Chapter 1. For many of these teams, there is no practical alternative to frequent changes in personnel. For staffing operating room (OR) suites, for example, frequently there are too many team members with duties in geographically dispersed places to be able to keep teams intact from one surgical procedure to another. Some observers have even suggested that these teams with variable composition are superior to stable teams because stable teams are vulnerable to complacency and other faults, leading to poor decision making and errors (Wachter, 2012, pp. 153-154). If we can extrapolate from the evidence in aviation, this suggestion is highly doubtful. Newly formed airplane cockpit crews experience more major accidents than do crews who have flown together before—in fact, many more (National Transportation Safety Board, 1994). Similarly, hospital-specific mortality rates for cardiac surgery are lower for surgeons who have performed more procedures recently at a given hospital, regardless of how many procedures they have performed recently at other hospitals. Operating consistently at one hospital improves a surgeon's performance at that hospital but not at other hospitals, suggesting that stability of the OR team (and perhaps stability of the work setting) has a beneficial effect (Huckman and Pisano, 2006).

Writers on teams sometimes regard membership stability as a defining feature of teams (Thompson, 2011, p. 4). J. Richard Hackman, a prominent researcher on teams, regarded membership stability as so important that only stable teams were worthy of his label *real teams* (Hackman, 2002, pp. 54-59). (This was not

Table 2–3. Vulnerabilities of true teams

Poor leadership
Decision making that does not engender the support of members for decisions made
Inadequate resolution of relationship conflicts

Hackman's only requirement for a team to be a real team.) As explained in Chapter 1, a definition drawn this tightly does not work well in health care because we have many groups plausibly called *teams* despite their routine turnover of membership. In health care, we have no choice about using many teams with fluctuating membership, and we can make them safe and effective—as will be discussed in the next section. Nonetheless, stable teams do have several advantages, and they should be used in preference to teams with variable membership when it is practical.

Even so, true teams are vulnerable in many ways, including some ways that do not pertain to variable teams. Outside of health care, true teams are the norm, and this had led to a great deal of research about their pitfalls. We consider these vulnerabilities in several later chapters. However, 3 points of vulnerability are so commonly encountered that they merit mention here (Table 2–3). First, all teams require effective leadership, and they may not have it. We deal with this topic in Chapters 8-11. Second, in a true team, it is important for decisions to be made in a way that secures team members' support for the decisions. A team member who does not agree with an important decision will experience diminished identification with the team. If this happens occasionally, it will be unimportant. But, if there are frequent disagreements, over time the team member will cease to identify with the team and may become alienated. She may continue to perform in her customary role, but full engagement will be lost and performance quality is likely to suffer even if the loss of engagement is not overt. In fact, a disengaged team member often has reason to hide the change, for example, to avoid conflicts or to maintain employment. Third, true teams need to be able to resolve interpersonal or relationship conflicts. Relationship conflicts in short-lived teams often can be ignored—by the people who have the conflict and by others in the team. If there is an end in sight, team members can usually suppress their interpersonal disagreements. But in a true team, the members work together over long periods of time. Under these circumstances, the relationship conflicts are very likely, eventually, to cause dysfunction in the team.

Because of these 3 vulnerabilities, true teams have 3 corresponding critical needs. Table 2–4 depicts the critical needs of true teams as well as the critical needs of the other types of clinical teams. The critical needs for each type of team arise from corresponding points of vulnerability that have special importance for that type.

We turn next to the second type of clinical team. These teams differ from true teams in that substantial changes in their membership are expected to occur often.

Table 2–4. Critical needs for clinical teams

	Critical Need						
Team Type	Effective Leadership	Decision Making That Secures Team Support	Effective Management of Relationship Conflicts	Definition of Roles & Procedures Prior to Team Beginning to Function	Training	Agreement on Approach to Leadership & Other Roles	Agreement on Expectations for Communication
True team	✔	✔	✔				
Template team	✔			✔	✔		
Knotwork[a]	✔					✔	✔
Network[b]							

[a]Knotworks commonly do not fit the definition of a work team, but they have some of the same characteristics.
[b]Networks are not work teams, but they are similar in some respects.

Template Teams

It was Friday night in the Emergency Department (ED). County General Hospital is located in a large, urban area. It is one of 4 Level I trauma centers serving a population of 3.5 million people. On this particular Friday evening, traffic on the area's freeways was heavy and brisk. It was raining, and numerous traffic accidents had occurred in the vicinity of County General.

At 6:30 p.m., a middle-aged woman was brought in by ambulance. She had sustained trauma to her chest in a front-to-side collision. She was taken from the ambulance into the ED on a stretcher, attended by Patricia Sterns, RN, CNS. Almost immediately Ms. Sterns was joined by Roy Collins, MD, a trauma surgeon, and within minutes another nurse and 2 technicians joined them. Ms. Sterns listened to the patient's chest with her stethoscope and found that no breath sounds were audible on the left, suggesting that the lung on that side was collapsed. A chest x-ray confirmed that fluid (not air) filled most of the left chest cavity. With the help of Ms. Sterns and one of the technicians, Dr. Collins inserted a chest tube between 2 of the patient's ribs. Bloody, yellow fluid began to fill a drainage bag.

At 9:15 p.m., a 22-year-old man was brought in unconscious. The car he was driving had hit another car from behind. He was not using a seat belt and was thrown through the windshield of his car, sustaining injuries to his head, left shoulder area, and chest. Again, Ms. Sterns met the patient and the Emergency Medical Technicians (EMTs) at the door. This time she was joined by James Anderson, MD, a trauma surgeon. One more nurse and 2 technicians joined them shortly. One of the technicians had participated in the care of the woman brought in earlier; the other technician had not. Ms. Sterns checked the position of the head immobilizer put in place by the EMTs while Dr. Anderson did a quick physical examination and ordered a computed tomography (CT) scan of the patient's head.

This ED, like all other EDs, uses template teams. Like true teams, template teams have all 7 attributes of a work team (Table 1–1 in Chapter 1). They also have clear leaders. What is distinctive about this type of team? In contrast to true teams, template teams do not have stable membership. In Table 2–1, the characteristics of template teams are compared and contrasted with the characteristics of other clinical teams. Template teams typically provide time-limited episodes of health care such as the episodes of emergency care described in the vignette. The defining characteristic of template teams is their changing membership. If a team repeatedly provides time-limited episodes of care without any change in the individuals who comprise the team, then it is a true team, for example, an emergency rescue team of EMTs that remains intact from one rescue to the next.

Although the individuals in a template team change and may change every time the team provides clinical care, the roles and procedural routines in template teams *are* stable. Each time a template team is called into action, it performs in essentially the same way even though the particular individuals comprising the team change. In this story of County General's ED, 2 instances of a template team are described. The task of both teams was to provide health care to the patients who had traumatic injuries from car accidents. The composition of the team was the same in both cases, that is, as specified by the inclusion of 2 nurses, 2 technicians, and 1 trauma surgeon. However, the particular people on the team changed. Dr. Collins was the trauma surgeon on the first team, and Dr. Anderson had this role on the second team. One of the 2 technicians was on both teams, but the other slot was filled by one person on the first team and a different person on the second team.

The term *template team*, like *true team*, is technical. Other writers use different terms for this team type or similar types: *short-term team* (Joshi and Roh, 2009, p. 610), *crew* (Morey et al, 2002), *fluid team* (Wachter, 2012, p. 153), *stable role-variable personnel* team (Andreatta, 2010. p. 349), and *ad hoc team* (Salas et al, 2008, p. 910). The advantage of the term *template team* is that it suggests an analogy with a document template. In a document template such as a form letter, the format and most of the text are fixed, but crucial words or phrases used at particular points in the template are expected to change each time the template is used to produce a new document. Similarly, a template team remains much the same each time it is reconstituted, but the individual team members can change. The team is not entirely variable—far from it—but it is variable with respect to team composition. As one

Table 2–5. Strengths of template teams

Potential for reliable processes and outcomes
Capacity for swift trust
Rapid responsiveness to the needs of the patients whom they serve
Resistance to deterioration of performance due to changes in personnel

author aptly wrote, "teamwork is sustained by a shared set of teamwork skills rather than permanent assignments that carry over from day to day" (Morey et al, 2002, p. 1555). One might expand this comment to say that clear role definitions, standardized communication routines, common behavioral expectations, and shared values also contribute to sustaining teamwork in template teams despite turnover in the team's membership.

Template teams have several strengths, which are listed in Table 2–5. Because of their standardized roles and processes, they can have highly reliable processes and outcomes. As described by Meyerson and colleagues (1996), they also have the capacity for *swift trust.* In other words, when members of a template team assemble, assuming that they are familiar with the purpose of the team and the roles of the various team members, they can quickly establish trust that is adequate for the team to perform well. In general, template teams need little lead time to respond to the needs of the patients whom they serve. And template teams are resistant to deterioration in their performance when they undergo changes in personnel.

Template teams also have characteristic vulnerabilities, which are listed in Table 2–6. First, like true teams, template teams need effective leadership, and may not have it. But the role of the leader in a template team is different from that of a leader in a true team. Briefly, in a template team, the leader usually deals directly with short-term, operational issues. A template team leader is ordinarily an operational manager rather than a true leader. This difference is discussed in Chapter 8. Also, despite the urgent circumstances under which template teams commonly operate, the leadership is often shared. For example, the surgeon and anesthesiologist often share the leadership in an OR team.

Table 2–6. Vulnerabilities of template teams

Poor leadership
Unclear role definitions
Inadequate training

Second, unlike true teams, template teams do not enjoy the luxury of being able to refine the members' roles over time. When a motor vehicle accident victim is brought into the ED, there is no time to work out who will put in the intravenous line, who will measure the patient's blood pressure, and so on. All of these tasks need to be assigned in advance. Even in situations in which time pressure is not so great, for example, at the beginning of an elective surgical procedure such as a mastectomy, it would be quite inefficient to work out the assignment of tasks anew each time the operation is done. Surgeons, scrub nurses, circulating nurses, and nurse anesthetists all know their roles in considerable detail before they enter the OR, and they have no need to negotiate their roles with the other team members. This standardization permits different OR teams to be composed of different people. At the same time, standardization of roles carries with it a degree of rigidity that is unnecessary in true teams and would often hinder achievement of optimal performance. Recall that over time Dr. Leon and Ms. Wallace in the earlier vignette about colonoscopy had the latitude to define their different roles in reassuring different groups of patients undergoing colonoscopy. They could even switch roles on short notice. In contrast, template teams have a higher need for clear and reliable role definitions from task to task.

Third, template teams are especially vulnerable to inadequate training. New template team members must be brought into the pool of team members with close attention to their orientation and initial training. All team members need periodic updates or refreshers of their training. In ED teams, surgical teams, and most other template teams, important parts of the necessary role definitions arise from professional education. Physicians perform certain tasks; nurses perform other tasks; pharmacists perform their tasks; and so on. However, educational differences do not fully assure that role differences in a template team will be clear because there are significant overlaps in what people in the various professions do. For example, both physicians and nurses do physical examinations of patients. It is only through training that team members acquire a clear and common understanding of their roles in a template team—as well as the role of the leader.

Standardization of communication processes is one important objective of template team training. Through training, various techniques become legitimized and expected. For example, *check-backs* become established as expected behavior. A check-back is a repetition by one team member of the answer just received from another team member. In other words, the person who asked for an important piece of information, say, how many units (bags) of blood are needed for a transfusion, repeats back to the person answering the question what that person said. The purpose of this routine is to confirm that the answer was received and that it was received correctly. With training, check-backs become an expected mode of behavior. Without the training, repeating someone's answer might seem puzzling, awkward, or even sarcastic. The use of several other communication routines can also help in assuring that communication is standardized and reliable.

Communication routines are concrete and easily explained and taught. More abstract lessons can also be conveyed through team training, namely, behavioral expectations and the values underlying them. For example, in teams with steep hierarchy gradients, the junior members often will be reluctant to challenge the senior members because such challenges might be taken to imply disrespect. To cite an example from education, a freshman student in a chemistry laboratory session will be reluctant to tell the chemistry professor that she is about to add the wrong solution to a beaker, even if the risk at hand is a fire. Similarly, in an OR, a young and inexperienced circulating nurse may be reluctant to raise the question of whether the surgeon is about to operate on the wrong knee. Through training, everyone—including surgeons, nurses, and technicians—can come to understand that the good of the patient requires people to voice their concerns when they see an error in the making and that suggesting that an error might occur does not imply disrespect for anyone.

We deal with more aspects of communication, behavior change, and other aspects of team training in Chapter 14. Training is central to achieving the "set of teamwork skills" mentioned earlier as necessary for sustaining teamwork in template teams.

The existence of these 3 vulnerabilities of template teams—poor leadership, unclear role definition, and inadequate training—implies corresponding critical needs. In Table 2–4, the critical needs of template teams are compared and contrasted with the critical needs of teams of other types.

Beyond their differences with respect to needs for upfront role definition and training, the differences between true teams and template teams are less pronounced. As mentioned, both true teams and template teams require effective leadership. True teams can eventually develop deep commitment to their goals among their members, and many template teams can also enjoy deep commitment—even immediately, simply because of the nature of the task. It is difficult to imagine that the commitment of trauma teams would increase with time. The urgent needs of the patients engender strong commitment straightaway.

In true teams, team members achieve familiarity and mutual knowledge over time. Template teams can also achieve familiarity and mutual knowledge, especially if the pool from which the team members are drawn is relatively small and stable. For example, an ED might employ 30 nurses, 35 technicians, and 15 physicians. These professionals constitute the pool from which various individuals are drawn to make up the specific template teams providing care to the stream of patients arriving at the ED. Over time, all of the members of the pool will work with all of the other members; if necessary, this interaction can be deliberately planned. By working together, the members of the pool will become familiar with each other even if this happens more slowly than it would in a stable team of 5 or 6 who always work together. As the size of the pool increases, achieving this familiarity becomes more difficult.

Template teams are capable of swift trust, but deeper levels of trust are largely determined by mutual knowledge. This mutual knowledge—assuming that competence and reliability are present in the various team members—engenders confidence in each member that every other member can be relied upon even if he or she is departing from his or her customary role in the team. Since the potential for mutual knowledge is present in template teams, they can also achieve trust in addition to the high levels of commitment noted earlier. If the hierarchy gradient can be made less steep, through training or otherwise, template teams can also achieve mutual accountability. Mutual accountability is harder to achieve in template teams than in true teams because of the residual unfamiliarity of team members in most template teams, but it can be achieved. If it is not achieved throughout the whole team, it can sometimes be achieved between various pairs of team members who have worked together more frequently and for a longer duration.

Strong identification with the team and its goals can also be achieved by template teams, especially if the pool of team members is relatively small and stable. Those who work in an ED, for example, do develop a sense of identification with their ED. They are identifying not with specific template teams in which they participate but instead with the whole pool of people from which the specific teams are drawn. If the size of the whole group is large or if the group experiences high turnover, this identification will be more difficult to achieve.

Finally, the factors that determine whether mutual accountability is achieved also affect the level of interdependency in a template team. If commitment, mutual knowledge, and trust are high, then the level of interdependency will be high. As in true teams, this results in faster action, decreased second-guessing, and decreased duplication of effort.

Knotworks

Most clinical teams are either true teams or template teams. However, these 2 categories do not account for all clinical teams. There are 2 other categories of clinical teams, although these other teams are not fully team-like as they do not have all of the 7 attributes of work teams (Table 1–1 in Chapter 1). The teams in one of these 2 additional categories are called *knotworks* (Engeström et al, 1999).

Hakim Ghazzi was a 45-year-old Iraqi refugee who presented to George Walker, DO, his family physician, with weight loss and vague abdominal pain that sometimes went through to his back. Physical examination and a CT scan of his abdomen quickly established that Mr. Ghazzi probably had a cancer of his pancreas. The diagnosis was confirmed by taking a biopsy, that is, sampling tissue from his pancreas. Several additional tests were performed. None of them showed any spread of the tumor outside of his pancreas.

Mr. Ghazzi felt that he had lost much of his life to the turmoil in Iraq and that he had only recently been able to start again after a long hiatus. He was determined to undergo any treatment that might extend his life, regardless of how unlikely the treatment was to be successful.

Dr. Walker set about arranging for Mr. Ghazzi to see a surgeon and a medical oncologist, who would talk with him about treatment options. Although Mr. Ghazzi spoke English reasonably well, he requested to see specialists who spoke Arabic because he anticipated that the discussions would be complex and because he wanted his wife to join in the conversations. His wife spoke almost no English. Fortunately, Mr. Ghazzi lived in a large urban area, and Dr. Walker was able to identify suitable Arabic-speaking specialists. Appointments were made with both the surgeon and the medical oncologist. Dr. Walker agreed to continue as the coordinator for Mr. Ghazzi's care.

Within 3 weeks, Mr. Ghazzi underwent surgery. The surgeon then referred him to a radiation oncologist for radiation therapy. (The radiation oncologist did not speak Arabic.) After the radiation therapy was completed, he received chemotherapy from the medical oncologist for several months. During this time, Dr. Walker continued to receive reports from the other physicians, and Mr. Ghazzi saw him every few weeks so that Dr. Walker could monitor him to detect signs and symptoms of depression or other complications.

Mr. Ghazzi's physicians and the nurses who worked with them were working as a team—more or less. However, this was not a template team and certainly not a true team. The 4 physicians came together specifically to pursue the goal of eliminating Mr. Ghazzi's pancreatic cancer. The surgeon and radiation oncologist had shared patients many times in the past, but the group as a whole had never worked together before and most likely would never work together again. They constituted a *knotwork*, tied together temporarily as the word *knot* suggests.

By definition, a knotwork has shared responsibility for the care of a patient but does not have a clear leader or stable membership. These characteristics are depicted in Table 2–1 along with the characteristics of true teams and template teams.

Knotworks are very common in health care. The example described here is largely within one profession, but there are many interprofessional knotworks as well. For example, a knotwork could be composed of a general internist, psychiatrist, clinical nurse specialist, and psychologist who do not work together normally but who have come together to provide care for a patient with bipolar disorder. Another interprofessional knotwork might be comprised of a pediatrician, pediatric neurologist, psychologist, and social worker, all caring for an autistic child and the child's family—again, assuming that they have joined together to serve this particular child and family and do not ordinarily work together. A teacher at the child's school might also be a member of the knotwork. A knotwork serving a teenager with disruptive behavior disorder might include police officers as participants.

Knotworks differ from true teams and template teams in several ways. As mentioned, they lack clear leaders and stable memberships. In addition, while some knotworks have all of the characteristics of a work team, most of them lack one or more of these characteristics. A knotwork does have a shared goal, shared responsibility for achieving the goal, authority for taking action, and interdependency of members. However, a knotwork's membership is often not clearly defined. In Mr. Ghazzi's story, the original team did not include a radiation oncologist, who was invited in by the surgeon without foreknowledge or approval by the family physician or medical oncologist although, of course, they would not have objected and did not object later. Similarly, as Mr. Ghazzi's illness progresses, a psychologist, a visiting nurse, or various other professionals might be added to the knotwork, all in response to Mr. Ghazzi's needs as perceived by him and by one or another member of the existing knotwork. In knotworks, there is also often independence of sub-groups, that is, sub-groups who are not accountable to the whole team. For example, the medical oncologist and the visiting nurse might make various decisions together without seeking the agreement of the family physician even though the family physician might want to participate. For some decisions, the oncologist and the nurse might not even notify the surgeon, and the surgeon might not expect to be notified since he might regard his work for Mr. Ghazzi as finished. And knotworks often are not accountable to anyone outside of the knotwork because commonly the group crosses organizational boundaries and there is no supervisor or governing board to which all of the members are accountable.

The group caring for Mr. Ghazzi is in fact not a team as defined in Chapter 1. Instead it is an appropriately fluid group, evolving over time. Whether or not they are regarded as work teams, it is desirable for knotworks to achieve teamwork if the patients' interests are to be well served. For this reason, knotworks warrant discussion along with genuine work teams. In fact, knotworks frequently are thought to be teams but are not distinguished from template teams, leading to neglect of how knotworks' special characteristics affect their performance.

Table 2–7. Strengths of knotworks

Flexibility of membership
Rapid responsiveness to patient and family needs

Knotworks have certain strengths, which are listed in Table 2–7. First, they are highly flexible. New knotwork members can be added easily, normally at the request of one of the existing professional members and sometimes at the request of the patient or family. Second, because of their flexibility, knotworks are quickly responsive to the needs of patients and families. No team decision-making process needs to be followed to revise the membership of the knotwork or its plan of care. In fact, often there is no unified plan of care. Instead, individual knotwork members or pairs of members commonly have separate plans.

Knotworks also have important vulnerabilities, listed in Table 2–8. First, like true teams and template teams, knotworks need good leadership, and may not have it. Leadership in a knotwork is almost always shared, and shared leadership always poses risks. Thus the leadership of a network is often deficient because it is shared.

Second, there is often no common agreement across the members of a knotwork about the definitions of their roles beyond the components of their roles that are defined by their professions. This lack of common understanding usually pertains to the leadership as well as other roles. A knotwork usually does not have a recognized leader, at least not one who is acknowledged as the leader of all the knotwork members. Sometimes the absence of a clear leader results in a pair of team members becoming rivals for the leadership, and this rivalry usually serves the patient very poorly. At the other end of the spectrum, sometimes no one in the

Table 2–8. Vulnerabilities of knotworks

Poor leadership, often compromised because it is shared
Lack of agreement on leadership and other roles
Absence of common expectations for communication among knotwork members

knotwork takes the initiative for a while because each person thinks that someone else is acting to assure that progress is being made. The resulting pauses in care sometimes cause distress or even harm to the patient. Other role definitions can also be problematic and are often difficult to address. For example, when a patient is receiving psychotherapy, the role of the primary care provider often becomes unclear. Also, when a patient is admitted to a hospital for a joint replacement procedure, it is often unclear who should do the admission history taking and physical examination. Should it be the primary care physician or the orthopedist—or perhaps a hospitalist called in for this particular task?

Third, knotworks have no established communication routines or defined communication roles beyond those that are characteristic of their professions. Communications are commonly arranged ad hoc and can misfire because one member expects and prefers one form of communication while another member prefers something different. For example, a surgeon or other consultant may prefer to receive a letter to explain the patient's situation while the referring knotwork member may prefer to speak by telephone or to use a secure e-mail system. Sometimes a clinician diagnosing and treating a patient on referral, for example, a rheumatologist or other internal medicine specialist, will not plan to send information to the referring primary care physician until a diagnosis has been established and treatment has been started. The referring physician, however, may want information about the specialist's diagnostic impression immediately after the patient's first visit to the specialist. Similarly, a physical therapist may communicate with the referring physician when the treatment plan is established but not communicate again until the treatment is completed, not knowing that the physician would prefer to receive progress reports while the treatment is in progress.

These 3 special points of vulnerability—poor leadership, lack of agreement on roles, and lack of common expectations for communication—are reflected in 3 critical needs for knotworks, which are depicted in Table 2–4 along with the critical needs for other types of clinical teams.

Good teamwork means effective interaction of team members in pursuit of the common goal, respectful interaction among the members, clear and timely communication, reasonable harmony, and effective problem solving—among other features of effective teams, discussed in Chapter 6. It is more difficult to achieve good teamwork in a knotwork than it is in a true team or a template team. Knotworks usually do achieve good teamwork, but they are more vulnerable. Unfortunately the pitfalls cannot be avoided by training because it would be inefficient (and simply impractical) to train a group that works together perhaps only once a year or even less often. In any case, unless all members of the knotwork are parts of the same healthcare system, there is no institutional common ground for organizing the training.

Knotworks are usually constructed and revised in response to particular patient and family needs. They are usually not planned in advance. In the case of Mr. Ghazzi in the vignette, advance planning would have been impossible. His need for Arabic-speaking physicians could not have been anticipated by Dr. Walker, and this requirement meant that the members of the knotwork were very likely not to have worked together before. Dr. Walker's reactive and piecemeal approach to initiating the knotwork is the norm.

However, there are exceptions. Sometimes knotworks are repeatedly formed by members of one healthcare organization reaching out to work with members of one or two other organizations. For example, a primary care group could choose to work with one general surgery group in caring for patients who need abdominal, breast, or skin surgery. Or a general surgery group could choose to work with one medical oncology group when caring for patients with malignancies. In these situations, the pairs of medical groups benefit from devising written agreements on roles and communication routines. These agreements are called *care agreements* (Engeström et al, 1999, pp. 356-362), *referral agreements* (Murray, 2002), or *service agreements.* They can be used not only for standardizing the interactions between medical groups but also for standardizing the interactions of medical groups with hospitals or surgical centers. Such agreements can be used even for knotworks that exist wholly within a single, very large healthcare system such as Mayo Clinic or Kaiser Permanente. The referral agreements serve the purpose of institutionalizing the knotworks that can be confidently predicted to form in the future. The agreements help to promote good teamwork by dealing in advance with some of the ambiguities in role definition and communication procedures. In other words, the referral agreements have the effect of making knotworks function more like template teams. (Chapter 12 deals more fully with the desirability of converting knotworks to template teams and template teams to true teams.) When referral agreements are in place, training makes sense for the purpose of making sure that all physicians, nurse practitioners (NPs), and others in each of the practices know the provisions of the agreements and the procedures that have been established.

Additional supports for effective teamwork in knotworks are available in situations in which the members of the knotwork are all within the same large healthcare organization. Delivery organizations need not be as large as the Cleveland Clinic or other very large systems of care for knotworks to be formed within them. For example, in an integrated system with a 250-bed hospital and a 400-physician medical group, a family physician, orthopedist, physical therapist, and a visiting nurse might join together to care for a 70-year-old man undergoing spine surgery and subsequent rehabilitation. Even if they have not worked together before as a group of 4 and will not work together again, their ability to function as a knotwork can be enhanced by the organizational context that they share, for example, a team-oriented culture, a unified electronic health record, additional communication methods used by all of the clinicians in the organization, and standardized training that they all have received to aid them in participating in teams in their usual settings within the organization.

Aside from using referral agreements and taking advantage of a shared organizational setting when possible, the best that one can do to avoid the pitfalls of knotworks is to be mindful that the team is a knotwork and therefore certain difficulties are likely to be encountered. If it is possible to negotiate role definitions, it should be done. In particular, it will be useful to agree on an approach to leadership. When the issue is explicitly addressed, the approach most commonly chosen is shared leadership, but agreement that one member of the knotwork is the leader is also common. For example, in a knotwork comprised of a cardiologist, a clinical nurse specialist, a cardiac surgeon, and a family physician, all collaborating to care for a patient with an artificial heart valve, the natural leader in the medium term will usually be the cardiologist; but in the long term, if all goes well for the patient, the family physician could become the leader. The knotwork members should make their expectations or wishes known as events progress. Often handling the role issues, especially the question of who is assuring coordination, requires considerable tact.

Communication expectations can be handled more easily. For example, a primary care physician, NP, or physician assistant making a referral to a specialist can state whether the first referral visit is for the purpose of identifying options for treatment or for initiating treatment. He or she can also indicate whether the patient intends to stay with the specialist indefinitely for all needed care or to return to the referring clinician after a certain interval. Similarly, different knotwork members can indicate to each other the information they expect to receive plus the preferred communication vehicle (in person, letter, phone, or e-mail) and the preferred frequency of updates.

Knotworks are extremely common and often present challenges to participants. Because they are barely teams, teamwork can be difficult to achieve. In particular, knotworks require attention to the potential ill effects of undefined roles and ad hoc communication. They must also cope without a clearly acknowledged single leader in many cases. They represent one end of the spectrum of teams considered as integrated functional units.

We now take one more step away from tightly integrated clinical teams to deal with groups that are not teams at all, although they do have some characteristics in common with teams and are sometimes thought to be at least team-like.

Networks

Andrew McWhirter, MD, is a hematologist and an expert in bone marrow transplantation. He practices medicine in the Bone Marrow Transplant Program at a southeastern U.S. academic medical center. The program includes hospital and outpatient nurses, hematologists, medical oncologists, radiation oncologists, transplant technicians, and others. The work is generally carried out in template teams. Dr. McWhirter participates in these teams and also interacts with many of the program's staff in other ways. He also has many contacts throughout the world, that is, other clinicians who also do bone marrow transplantation. He and they have connected over the years by attending conferences, by doing research together, and by informal communications engendered by common interests.

Patients undergoing bone marrow transplantation have temporarily compromised immune systems. They are vulnerable to unusual viral, bacterial, fungal, and parasitic infections that are rare in people with normal immunity. On one particular Tuesday morning, Dr. McWhirter and his colleagues were seeking a way to treat a 38-year-old transplant recipient who had developed a bloodstream fungal infection and was not responding to standard treatment. The patient had a lymphoma (lymph node cancer), for which he had received high-dose chemotherapy and a bone marrow transplant 3 weeks earlier. His situation was complicated by the presence of diabetes and impaired kidney function. After discussing the few available options with his colleagues and not reaching a very promising conclusion, Dr. McWhirter telephoned Dr. Mariana Martinez, a colleague in at another academic medical center in Philadelphia. Dr. Martinez is also a bone marrow transplantation expert. She has a particular interest in fungal infections in transplant patients. Dr. McWhirter telephoned her to test out his thinking and to solicit any suggestions that she might have for the treatment of his patient.

Dr. McWhirter and Dr. Martinez are members of a *network*. Knotworks are tightly formed for the sake of a given patient. As the contrast between the words *knot* and *net* suggests, networks are looser. Networks have none of the characteristics of work teams They lack shared responsibility, clear leaders, and stable membership, as depicted in Table 2–1.

Networks are "complexes of links between individuals and organizations, driven largely by the interests of the parties and their recognition of the value of working together" (Southon et al, 2005, p. 318). Networks are not authorized by anyone or any organization beyond the participants themselves. They are not accountable to any larger organization. However, they do exhibit cooperation, and the participants share interests and similar purposes despite the fact that the members of the network do not share responsibility for achieving a specific goal. Dr. McWhirter and Dr. Martinez share the general aims of using bone marrow transplantation to cure disease and doing research to improve the effectiveness of bone marrow transplantation, but they treat different patients and have different research programs.

Clinical networks differ from true teams and template teams in many ways. One of the most striking differences is that, unlike both true teams and template teams, a network does not have a defined membership. The members of a network come and go, and usually no one keeps track of these changes. Unlike a template team, a network has no standardized roles to be filled. A network is similar to a knotwork in that both have fluid membership and typically have no single leader. A network differs from a knotwork in that members of a knotwork share responsibility for achieving a goal—improvement of a particular patient's health—whereas the members of a network have no such shared responsibility.

Dr. McWhirter and Dr. Martinez, if asked, might say that they are on the same team, meaning that both are dedicated to the use and improvement of bone marrow transplantation and are engaged in some joint activities that serve these ends. But the network in which they participate is not a work team as defined in Chapter 1—despite the fact that the network might appear to be a loose team and might sometimes be described in this way. The members of the network to which Drs. McWhirter and Martinez belong share common interests and have similar expertise. They find it useful to interact with one another in order to be more effective in achieving their individual goals. The network would not be useful to the members if it did not exhibit responsiveness, cooperation, openness, and trust. But these features alone do not make the network a team. Nevertheless, clinical networks can provide great value to their participants. They often serve to aid clinicians and clinical teams in serving patients. Compared with true teams, template teams, and knotworks, little is expected of them. They do not have collective tasks to carry out. They also do not have special vulnerabilities or critical needs, as reflected in the empty cells in the bottom line of Table 2–4.

We turn next to healthcare teams that do not deliver care but are instead concerned with managing care. Clinicians generally spend most of their time working in clinical teams, but they also often participate in various kinds of management teams and need to understand their natures and functions—as do healthcare administrators.

MANAGEMENT TEAMS

Health care uses management teams as well as clinical teams. Management teams manage healthcare delivery or activities that support delivery, but they do not provide care directly. As noted earlier, management teams often have members who are clinicians, but their presence does not make the team a clinical team. In fact, a management team can consist wholly of clinicians. Usually, however, management teams include managers—or supervisors, administrators, or leaders—who are not clinicians, who have administrative experience, and who often have postgraduate degrees in management or administration.

As discussed earlier, the rationale for a taxonomy is its utility in serving a chosen purpose. The purpose of this book is to elucidate team-based health care for those who work in healthcare teams, plan them, or guide them so that they can improve team effectiveness. In classifying management teams, this purpose leads to a taxonomy that is quite different from the one discussed earlier for clinical teams.

In understanding clinical teams, the most important considerations are whether the team has stable membership, a clear leader, and shared responsibility. Using these team characteristics, we can draw distinctions among true teams, template teams, knotworks, and networks. True teams have all 3 characteristics; template teams do not have stability of membership but do have clear leaders and shared responsibility; knotworks do not have stability of membership or clear leaders but do have shared responsibility; networks lack all 3 characteristics and are not actually teams at all. True teams, template teams, and knotworks have different needs for conduct of the team's activities, for planning, for training, and for management. The value of the distinctions among these 3 types of clinical teams lies in making clear the needs of the different teams, thus encouraging action leading to improved performance for teams of each type.

When devising a classification for management teams, membership stability, clarity of leadership, and shared responsibility are not particularly useful considerations. Management teams are nearly always stable; they have clear leaders; and they have shared responsibility. In other words, management teams are almost always true teams. On first reflection, it may seem that there are many exceptions to this rule. Some management teams are not stable because they have high turnover. But high turnover does not make them template teams or knotworks; they are simply true teams with problems. Some management teams are not stable because they have poorly defined membership, but again this does not mean that we are dealing with 2 different types of management teams, one with well-defined membership and one without well-defined membership. Poorly defined membership is a problem, and management teams can eliminate it—unlike clinical knotworks, which must cope with poorly defined and shifting membership because the members are not organized to be able to do otherwise. And some management teams are self-managed, suggesting that there is no leader. In fact, self-managed teams do have leaders as is explained in Chapter 8.

There are only a few exceptions to the rule that management teams are true teams, not template teams or knotworks. The most visible exceptions are template teams used in times of crisis. For example, hospital emergency management teams are used for managing responses to major emergencies such as airplane crashes or bridge collapses, and disaster recovery teams are used for managing the restoration of a system-wide information system when the computer hardware has been damaged by a fire, an earthquake, or some other disaster. Knotworks are also occasionally used in management. For example, a hospital purchasing manager might connect with a specialized manufacturer and a trucking firm with special expertise in order to obtain an unusual airflow handler for an OR, expecting that he or she will never again have occasion to work with this manufacturer and trucking firm again. Aside from these few exceptions, management teams are true teams.

If we used considerations of stability, the presence of a leader, and shared responsibility to construct a taxonomy of management teams, nearly all of the teams would be classified in one category, that is, they would be classified as true teams. We would fail to make clear the distinctions among management teams that are useful for understanding the needs of different types of teams. A different basis is needed for classifying management teams.

The core of a useful alternative approach is consideration of the purpose of the team. Clinical teams all have the same purpose, namely, providing care to particular patients. In contrast, management teams have a variety of purposes. It is also useful to distinguish between management teams that are ongoing and those that have a predetermined end. These 2 considerations provide the basis for devising a taxonomy that is useful in improving the performance of management teams.

Teams in business, manufacturing, and services industries have been studied far more than teams in health care. Numerous classifications of teams in these various sectors have been suggested, and these classifications always include management teams (Hollenbeck et al, 2012). Most of the classifications use the purpose of the team as the primary defining characteristic although various other characteristics are also used by some writers, for example, whether the team members have been assembled from different parts of an organization. Sundstrom's classification, discussed earlier, is one example of a classification that includes management teams. There are at least 20 other classifications. We present categories with features taken from several of these classifications while seeking to define the categories so that they are familiar, credible, and useful to people working in health care.

Operational Teams

Nancy Klein, RN, CNS, is the nurse manager of the Medical Intensive Care Unit (MICU) in a 350-bed urban hospital. Greg Weingarten, MD, is the medical director. Diane Westover, PharmD, is the lead pharmacist. Twenty-four registered nurses work in the MICU along with 8 critical care physicians, 3 critical care clinical pharmacists, 20 respiratory therapists, and many others. While Dr. Weingarten is the official head of the unit, he and Ms. Klein function in effect as partners. Dr. Westover has more recently joined them in directing the unit and has a less prominent role, but none of them regard this as a problem. The 3 of them meet every Tuesday morning for 30-45 minutes. Most of their meetings are devoted to troubleshooting the day-to-day function of the unit. For example, on this Tuesday morning they are discussing options for increasing pharmacist participation in the interprofessional rounds that are held each morning. Later they will share their perceptions about whether there is a performance problem with one of the nurses, who has come to work an hour late 3 times in the past month.

Dr. Weingarten, Ms. Klein, and Dr. Westover are an operational team. They are responsible for managing a unit that provides a service or product directly to patients. In other words, they are in charge of the day-to-day and week-to-week operations of the MICU. Their team is ongoing, that is, their task will continue until some distant time when the unit is merged or closed. The defining characteristics of operational teams are depicted in Table 2–9 along with the defining characteristics of the other 3 types of management teams.

The effectiveness of all management teams depends on the suitability of the team's composition for its purpose, the quality of its leadership, and the relationship of the team to other parts of the organization. In this team, the question of composition is a matter of balancing the need for adequate multiprofessional input against the need for simplicity in decision making. Simplicity in decision making enables the team to respond quickly to problems that arise. Ms. Klein and Dr. Weingarten had discussed the composition of the team many times before they invited Dr. Westover to join them on a regular basis. Previously, they had consulted her only when pharmacy issues arose. The 3 team members now sometimes discuss whether a respiratory therapist also should be added to the team. The leadership of the

Table 2–9. Characteristics of management teams

	Characteristics	
Team Type	Purpose	Duration
Operational team	To manage an organizational unit that either provides a service or product directly to patients, or supports patient care	Perpetual
Project team	To accomplish a specific goal within a specified time frame	Time-limited
Consultative team	To provide advice to managers and leaders on a specified topic	Often time-limited but not always
Leadership team	To set goals and guide a whole organization or part of it but not to manage directly any unit that provides a service or product to patients or supports patient care	Perpetual

team rests with Dr. Weingarten and Ms. Klein as co-leaders. Both of them need to exhibit the leadership characteristics that are explored in Chapters 8-11. The relationships crucial to this team's success are, first, the relationship between the team and those who work in the ICU and, second, the relationship of the team to the leadership of the whole hospital, through which the ICU obtains the resources it needs to do its work well.

Beyond sound composition, good leadership, and functional intra-organizational relationships, there are 3 more particularly important needs for operational teams. They need to be able to make decisions in a way that secures team members' support. They need to have autonomy to implement decisions made by the team. And they need to be able to manage interpersonal or relationship conflicts within the team. Securing team members' support for decisions is important because the operational team members are the ones who act on the decisions, working with other people who work in the MICU. For some other types of management teams, securing team members' support for decisions is less important as is discussed in the next sections of this chapter. Having autonomy in execution is a point of vulnerability for operational teams because they are susceptible to interference by people higher in the organizational hierarchy. When individuals higher in the hierarchy interfere, the members of an operational team begin to back away from taking responsibility; and, if the interference is extreme, the team will stop making decisions and simply seek direction from the interfering party. Some other management teams are also vulnerable in this way, but not all. Settling relationship conflicts is crucial to operational teams because these conflicts degrade the give-and-take that leads to good decision making. Persistent conflicts also undercut support for decisions made. Settling relationship conflicts is desirable in all teams, but it is less important in some team types than it is in operational teams.

In sum, an operational team—like all other management teams—has a critical need for a suitable composition, effective leadership, and sound relationships with other parts of the organization in which the team functions. In addition, an operational team has a trio of critical needs that is unique to this team type. It needs to be able to secure support for decisions, to be truly autonomous in execution, and to be able to resolve relationship disputes effectively. Table 2–10 displays these 6 critical needs of operational teams as well as the critical needs of the other types of management teams.

We move next to consider management teams that have a well-defined, concrete goal and a limited lifespan.

Project Teams

Eric Shelstad, MHA, is the Director of Emergency Department Services at a suburban hospital. For the past few months, he has been leading a project to plan an expansion of the ED. Due to a steady increase in volume over several years, the hospital has outgrown its ED space. In addition, Mr. Shelstad and others have concerns about patient privacy in the existing space, where many patients

Table 2–10. Critical needs for management teams

	Critical Need							
Team Type	Suitable Composition	Effective Leadership	Sound Intra-organizational Relationships	Clarity of Task	Decision Making That Secures Team Support	Autonomy in Execution	Effective Management of Interpersonal Conflict	Training
Operational team	✔	✔	✔		✔	✔	✔	
Project team	✔	✔	✔	✔		✔		✔
Consultative team	✔	✔	✔	✔				✔
Leadership team	✔	✔	✔		✔		✔	

are separated only by curtains. The space is also impersonal and does not permit optimal experience by patients. For example, there is very little room for chairs for family members who accompany patients.

Mr. Shelstad leads a planning team. Other team members are the nurse manager of the ED, 2 staff nurses, 3 physician assistants, 1 pharmacist, 1 ED scribe, 1 radiology technician, 1 laboratory technician, 1 ED health unit coordinator, the materials manager for the hospital, 1 housekeeping supervisor, a financial analyst from the Chief Financial Officer's office, and an architect from the firm engaged for the project.

The team has met every 2 weeks for 5 months. It has worked with the architectural firm, solicited input from the hospital's patient advisory council, made progress reports to the hospital's executive committee, projected the cost of the construction, and so on. The team is working under some time pressure in that the onset of construction is now 8 weeks away.

Mr. Shelstad's team is a project team. The characteristics of project teams are shown in Table 2–9. Mr. Shelstad's team is charged with accomplishing a specific goal, and once that goal is achieved, the team will be disbanded.

As with the MICU operations team in the previous vignette, the composition, leadership, and intra-organizational relationships of the team are critical to its success. With respect to the composition of a project team, especially a planning team, the main risk is that the team will become too large—as has happened with the planning team in this vignette. Commonly many different parties will be affected by a planning project, and often a large fraction of these parties want representation on the team. If the team is too large, discussions at the meetings become drawn out and lose focus. Coming to conclusions becomes difficult. A good rule of thumb is to keep the team size to 12 or fewer people. The brief rationale for this rule is that groups larger than about 12 people generally experience deterioration in the quality of careful, analytical discussion—the kind of discussion needed to make good decisions. In Chapter 12 we deal with the topic of team size at greater length. The characteristics of good leadership in a project team are similar to those needed in an operational team and are discussed in Chapters 8-11. With respect to intra-organizational relationships, the 2 that are critical to success for a project team are the relationship with the people who will use the project's product—in this case, those who work in the ED—and the relationship with senior management, who have a grasp of the project in the context of the whole organization and who have hold of the purse strings.

Points of special need for project teams are task clarity, autonomy to pursue the project, and training. Mr. Shelstad's planning team needs to know very clearly what it is expected to produce. Is planning for the telephone system in the ER part of its charge? What about planning for the enlargement of the ED staff and recruiting new staff members? The team needs clear direction from management. If there is a mismatch between the team's understanding of its task and what other people expect, the project may be near its deadline before it is discovered that important pieces of the project (or pieces that need to be coordinated with the project) have not been attended to. In contrast, the task for an operational team is ordinarily quite clear without the need for any carefully crafted statement. For example, the Medical ICU operational team is in charge of providing care to patients in the ICU, and the team managing the billing department is responsible for sending out bills. Both project teams and operational teams are vulnerable to meddling by more senior people in the organization. This causes disengagement of team members, who may devote their best efforts elsewhere or stop participating altogether. Project teams very often require special training, if they are to perform well. For example, the ED planning team in the vignette needed to be instructed in the requirements of the municipal building code for hospitals. They also needed to learn about changes in other hospitals that have made EDs more family friendly and less stark and intimidating than EDs have been in past decades.

Project teams have less need than operational teams for strong support of decisions across the whole team. Project team members do not have ongoing management responsibility as part of their role because the team disbands when the task is accomplished. It is far more important that those whose work is affected by the project find the end-product satisfactory. If the end-users—those who work in the ED or, for other projects, those who will use the new electronic health record or those who will interact with a supplier through the terms of a new contract—find that the project team's product meets their needs, it will not be important whether some members of the project team disagree.

Project teams also have less need for harmony. In an operational team, relationship conflicts will eventually interfere with the team's function. Since project teams are limited in time, members can often suppress their antagonisms and carry on with the task, knowing that the conflicts will last only as long as the team lasts. There are exceptions. If relationship conflicts are severe, project team function may be affected adversely even in the short run. And if the life-span of a project team is expected to be long, say, 2-3 years or more, then the conflicts will need to be settled; otherwise they are likely to affect the team's ability to function before the team reaches its goal.

The 6 critical needs of project teams are depicted in Table 2–10, which compares and contrasts the critical needs of all 4 types of management teams.

Consultative Teams

It is the third Thursday of the month, and Ben Pender is chairing a meeting of the Patient and Family Advisory Council at East Shore Community Hospital. Margery Blatt, MHA, the hospital's Chief Executive Officer (CEO), asked him to take this position 2 years ago. He had become devoted to the hospital when his daughter was treated there for a severe asthma attack many years ago. For 10 years, he has been an active member of East Shore Volunteers, the organization of people who volunteer to direct hospital visitors, deliver flowers, and help in many other ways. There are 10 other members of the Council, some recommended by hospital staff and some recruited by people already on the Council.

The Council meets monthly. Members rarely miss a meeting. Ms. Blatt sometimes attends, but usually the hospital's senior leadership is represented by Polly Jackson, MSN, RN, Director of Patient Care Services, including nursing, social work, physical therapy, and a few other services. Two secretaries also assist the Council by preparing agenda packets, keeping meeting minutes, and assuring follow-up on recommendations made by the Council.

At this month's meeting, the Council is discussing a proposal by Ms. Jackson and other hospital leaders to change the volunteer program at East Shore. The proposal includes writing job descriptions for volunteers, instituting formal training, and—most controversial—establishing qualifications for becoming a volunteer. The discussion is delicate because several members of the Council volunteer in the hospital and became volunteers when there were no required qualifications for the role.

Mr. Pender's committee is a consultative team. Its purpose is to advise managers and leaders on a specified topic. The characteristics of this type of team are shown in Table 2–9. In this vignette, the team exists to aid in making the hospital more responsive to the needs of patients and families. As the word *advisory* in its name clearly implies, the team provides advice to the management of the hospital and has no executive authority of its own. In this case, the team is not limited in time since the Council continues indefinitely, taking up a series of different topics over time.

Other consultative teams are time-limited. An example of a time-limited team is a quality improvement team aimed at improving the ordering of x-rays and rapid reporting of results needing urgent action. A quality improvement team typically immerses itself in its topic, devises recommendations, and disbands—possibly coming together at some later time to assess progress in the implementation of its recommendations. Action on the recommendations made by a quality improvement team remains the responsibility of the managers and clinicians who have the authority to change procedures or establish new ones. Other common consultative teams are task forces that consider which ambulatory electronic health record to purchase and make recommendations to senior leaders in medical groups. Sometimes a health system CEO will create a consultative task force to review the health system's competitive situation and recommend changes in business strategy for the system.

As with other management teams, a consultative team's composition, leadership, and intra-organizational relationships are key determinants of its success. In the case of the Council in the vignette, the membership needs to be representative of the patient population served by East Shore Hospital. The Council also needs to be sufficiently confident and independent of the hospital's management to be able to assert patients' interests when the implications are unwelcome to the management. The leader needs to be seen by the other

Council members as speaking his own mind and not serving as an agent for hospital management, and in general the leader needs to exercise the competencies of an effective leader that are discussed in Chapters 8-11. The important relationships for this consultative team are the relationship with the patient population served by the hospital and the relationship with the hospital's management, who retain authority to accept or reject recommendations made by the Council.

As with project teams, consultative teams require clarity in the definition of their tasks. The Council has been asked to advise on improving the experience of patients and families at the hospital. Would it be suitable for the Council to offer advice on the hospital's business strategy? Presumably not. Hospital management and Mr. Pender need to be clear with the Council about the intended scope of topics to be considered. Still, there are bound to be gray areas. Would it be suitable for the Council to raise questions about whether too many antibiotic-resistant infections are occurring in the hospital? This would be uncertain territory. The Council, speaking for the hospital's patients, has a legitimate interest in this question, but the members are not likely to have the knowledge to reach any well-supported conclusions on their own. Ms. Jackson and others would need to respond carefully and without evasion to an inquiry about hospital infections—lest the relationship with the Council be damaged, impairing the ability of the Council and hospital management to work together effectively. Besides being vulnerable to misunderstandings about scope, consultative teams, like project teams, will usually need special training pertaining the topic on which they are asked to advise. For example, the Council would need to be briefed on the privacy requirements of the federal Health Insurance Portability and Accountability Act (HIPAA).

Consultative teams are, however, less vulnerable than other management teams with respect to needs for broad team support for decisions, autonomy in execution, and management of relationship conflicts. Consultative teams are by definition advisory, so it is not crucial, for example, for the Council to resolve all disagreements about a recommendation. It is the hospital leaders and mangers, not the Council members, who need to be committed to action if they take up a Council recommendation. Autonomy in execution is also unimportant since a consultative team does not take action. And relationship conflicts, unless extreme, can be and usually are suppressed by the team members themselves because they usually wish to move ahead with the team's tasks and do not regard the team's activities as central to their self-esteem or work lives. If a consultative team is time-limited, avoidance of interpersonal conflict is especially easy to achieve.

As for the other types of management teams, the critical needs of consultative teams are shown in Table 2–10.

Leadership Teams

James Caldwell, MBA, meets with his direct reports every other week. He is the CEO of St. Andrew's Health System, which includes 9 hospitals and a medical group of 650 physicians. Reporting directly to him are the Chief Operating Officer, Chief Financial Officer, Chief Medical Officer, the CEOs of the 2 largest hospitals in the system, and the President of St. Andrew's Medical Group. Together this team is responsible for the vision, strategy, and management of the whole system, which served 650,000 patients last year and had operating revenues of $2.7 billion.

Mr. Caldwell's executive team considers a wide variety of strategic and operational questions. At their last meeting, they discussed whether to grow the internal medical group to serve a new geographical area or instead to partner with an existing multispecialty group practice in that area. Earlier in the year they considered whether to continue with the current electronic health record or to switch to the electronic record used by many other hospitals and systems in the region. Although this was an operational decision, it was made at the most senior level of the organization because of the large costs involved.

This team is a leadership team. Its purpose is to set goals and guide the whole organization but not to manage directly any unit that provides patient care or supports patient care. The characteristics of leadership teams are shown in Table 2–9. Even though Mr. Caldwell's team does not manage directly the provision or support of patient care, it is actually quite similar to the MICU operational team described in an earlier vignettte. The main difference is that this team resides at the apex of an organizational hierarchy rather than at a lower operational level. There are also many leadership teams that fall in between, for example, the executive teams at each of the 9 hospitals in the St. Andrew's system.

Again, the composition, leadership, and intra-organizational relationships of this team must be sound if the team is to succeed. The chief objective in composing a leadership team is to encompass the whole organization—or, for a team at a lower level than the organization's apex, to encompass the whole of that part of the organization that is led by the team. At the same time, the team must not be too large because excessive size interferes with the quality and speed of decision making—just as it does in operational teams and project teams.

The leadership provided by a senior leadership team is leadership of the whole organization. Leadership teams at lower levels in an organization provide leadership for their respective segments of the organization. Leadership of whole organizations or large segments of organizations is outside the scope of this book. There exists a large literature on the general topic of organizational leadership, especially senior leadership (Katzenbach and Smith, 2006, pp. 212-258; Kouzes and Posner, 2012; Wageman et al, 2008). However, the leadership of teams, including leadership teams, is a central topic of this book. The contributions of team leaders are discussed in Chapters 8-11. Chapters 18 discusses the contributions of senior leaders to the effectiveness of all teams in their organizations.

The intra-organizational relationships that are most crucial for a senior leadership team are those with the organization's governing board and those with the people who work in the organization, quite generally. At lower levels, the crucial relationships for a leadership team are those with the next highest level in the organization and with the people who work in the organizational segment led by the team.

The other important needs for leadership teams are almost the same as those for operational teams. They need to make decisions in such a way that all team members are committed to implementing them. And they must deal effectively with relationship conflicts so that these conflicts do not hamper the team's function. There is one obvious difference between leadership teams and operational teams. The issue of autonomy in execution is less pressing for leadership teams because they are generally less vulnerable to outside meddling. To be more precise, the risk of interference decreases as the location of the team gets closer to the apex of the organization. But even a senior leadership team can lose some of its proper autonomy—for example, when a governing board fails to confine itself to policy issues and begins directing the operations of the organization.

For most leadership teams, the risk of task ambiguity and the need for team training are not points of special vulnerability. The task of a leadership team is to set goals and guide the organization or some portion of it. Teams that are leading parts of organizations may occasionally be unclear about how their authority meshes with that of teams leading other parts, and these questions will need to be settled if they arise. A leadership team's task is a general task, not a technical one, and so the team as a whole will rarely require special training although particular members of the team are almost always expected to have technical expertise, for example, in nursing, finance, supply chain management, or other aspects of health care.

The critical needs of leadership teams as well as comparisons with the needs of other management teams are shown in Table 2–10.

Knotworks, Networks, and Virtual Teams

Management can be carried out using management analogues of clinical knotworks and networks in addition to the 4 types of management teams discussed here. An example of a knotwork used for purchasing equipment was cited earlier. Management knotworks and networks function in much the same ways as their clinical counterparts. No fundamentally new issues arise. Knotworks are less common in management work than they are in clinical care. Networks, on the other hand, are used extensively, more frequently than they are used in clinical care. Maintenance of network connections is commonly seen as very important for managers and leaders of healthcare organizations.

The reader may have noticed that the phrase *virtual teams* has not appeared as the name of a team type. This is because *virtual* refers to a method for handling communication in a team, namely, using electronic means to communicate at a distance. There are virtual teams included in every category of clinical and management teams discussed earlier, even among true teams and template teams providing clinical care directly. For example, the advent of telemedicine has made it possible for critical care physicians to work closely with critical care nurses in the care of particular patients even though the physicians and nurses are separated by hundreds of miles. Virtual teams do not stand apart as a category of their own. They do need special handling, as we discuss in Chapter 6. However, being virtual is a less important team characteristic than being stable, having a clear leader (or not), having operational responsibility, and the other characteristics that distinguish the various types of clinical and management teams discussed in this chapter.

CONCLUSION

Healthcare teams can be classified in many ways. This chapter offers a taxonomy that aims to aid in identifying the important needs of different teams. Clinical teams are classified as true teams, template teams, knotworks, and—reaching somewhat beyond the notion of a team—networks. Management teams are classified as operational teams, project teams, consultative teams, and leadership teams—plus management knotworks and networks. Knowing that a given team falls into a particular category helps in understanding how it will function, what it needs, and what pitfalls one must keep in mind.

"All models are wrong but some are useful," wrote the statistician George E. P. Box (1979). The taxonomy offered here has limitations. For example, group cohesion is important for many teams (Thompson, 2011, pp. 106-109), but it does not feature in the taxonomy as a critical need. Despite this and other limitations, if the taxonomy helps team members, team leaders, and team sponsors to understand how to make their teams function more effectively, it will have served its purpose.

We are now ready to take a close look at the different professions represented in healthcare teams, that is, to see how the education, values, and roles of different professionals affect the way teams function. We will also consider how the roles of some healthcare professionals are changing and how these changes are affecting the nature of teamwork in health care.

REFERENCES

Andreatta PB. A typology for health care teams. *Health Care Manage Rev.* 2010;35:345-354.

Box GEP. Robustness in the strategy of scientific model building. In: Launer RL, Wilkinson GN, eds. *Robustness in Statistics.* New York, NY: Academic Press; 1979:202.

Engeström Y, Engeström R, Vähäaho T. When the center does not hold: the importance of knotworking. In: Chalkin S, Hedegaard, Jensen UJ, eds. *Activity Theory and Social Practice: Cultural-Historical Approaches.* Aarhus, Denmark: Aarhus University Press; 1999:345-374.

Hackman JR. *Leading Teams: Setting the Stage for Great Performances.* Boston, MA: Harvard Business School Press; 2002.

Hollenbeck JR, Beersma B, Schouten ME. Beyond team types and taxonomies: a dimensional scaling conceptualization of team description. *Acad Manage Rev.* 2012;37:82-106

Huckman RS, Pisano GP. The firm specificity of individual performance: evidence from cardiac surgery. *Manage Sci.* 2006;52:473-488.

Joshi A, Roh H. The role of context in work team diversity research: a meta-analytic review. *Acad Manage Rev.* 2009;52:599-627.

Katzenbach JR, Smith DK. *The Wisdom of Teams: Creating the High-Performance Organization.* Collins Business Essentials ed. New York, NY: HarperCollins Publishers; 2006.

Kouzes JM, Posner BZ. *The Leadership Challenge.* 5th ed. San Francisco, CA: John Wiley & Sons; 2012.

Meyerson D, Weick, KE, Kramer RM. Swift trust and temporary groups. In: Kramer RM, Tyler TR, eds. *Trust in Organizations: Frontiers of Theory and Research.* Thousand Oaks, CA: Sage Publications, Inc.; 1996:166-195.

Morey JC, Simon R, Jay GD, et al. Error education and performance improvement in the emergency department through formal teamwork training: evaluation results of the MedTeams Project. *Health Serv Res.* 2002;37: 1553-1581.

Murray M. Reducing waits and delays in the referral process. *Fam Pract Manag.* 2002;9(3):39-42.

National Transportation Safety Board. *A Review of Flightcrew-involved Major Accidents of U.S. Air Carriers, 1978 through 1990.* Report No. NTSB/SS-94/01. Washington, DC: National Transportation Safety Board; 1994.

Salas E, DiazGranados D, Klein C, et al. Does team training improve team performance? A meta-analysis. *Hum Factors.* 2008;50:903-933.

Southon G, Perkins R, Galler D. Networks: a key to the future of health services. *Aust Health Rev.* 2005;29:317-326.

Sundstrom E, De Meuse KP, Futrell D. Work teams: applications and effectiveness. *Am Psychol.* 1990;45:120-133.

Thompson LL. *Making the Team: A Guide for Managers.* 4th ed. Upper Saddle River, NJ: Prentice Hall; 2011.

Wachter RM. *Understanding Patient Safety.* 2nd ed. New York, NY: McGraw-Hill; 2012.

Wageman R, Nunes DA, Burruss JA, et al. *Senior Leadership Teams: What It Takes to Make Them Great.* Boston, MA: Harvard Business School Press; 2008

Roles, Education, and Values of Healthcare Professionals

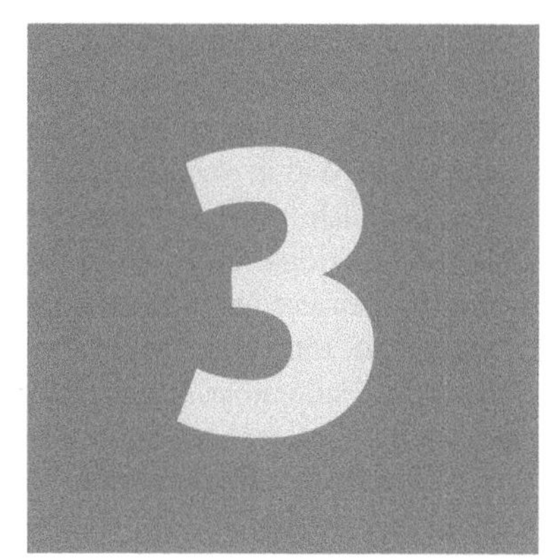

Healthcare delivery involves a diverse and amazing tapestry of highly specialized professions. This makes teamwork in healthcare delivery more challenging than in virtually any other sphere of human work activity. It requires that professionals go to extra lengths to learn about the other members of their teams so that each team member can call on all the others to contribute everything they are able to offer in the service of patients or in the support of patient care. In this chapter we describe and compare the roles, education, and values of the professionals who are the most common members of healthcare teams.

WHY UNDERSTAND OTHER PROFESSIONS?

Newly graduated with the Doctor of Pharmacy (PharmD) degree and employed by Community Medical Center for 1 month, pharmacist Jerry Young turned to his colleague, Nancy Burns, BSPharm, for advice. Ms. Burns had worked at Community Medical Center for all of her 30-year career. Dr. Young asked, "How often do the physicians and nurses in the hospital call you for advice? I've been here a month now, and I've only talked to you and other pharmacists and patients. I think I could contribute more by giving more input into decisions about prescriptions and side effects. It would prevent some issues that I think some patients will have down the road." Ms. Burns thought awhile and carefully commented, "I get several inquiries a week from physicians, and a few from nurses. I imagine you will get some calls, once people get to know you. We don't have a lot of opportunities to share our knowledge with the clinical staff, though, so it may take a few years. Nurses and physicians are becoming more receptive to suggestions by pharmacists, but change is slow. Many physicians and some nurses still think that we spend our days counting pills, sad to say."

Dr. Young's dilemma is a common one in healthcare delivery. Changes in knowledge occur more and more rapidly, and workplace roles in several healthcare professions are undergoing transformation as newly trained graduates become qualified to dispense new knowledge and provide new services. As a recent PharmD graduate, Dr. Young may have different expectations for his role than his colleague Ms. Burns has. Indeed, Dr. Young holds a doctoral-level degree, now the entry-level degree for pharmacists, compared to Ms. Burns' baccalaureate degree (therefore the appellation *Dr.* for Jerry Young). Ms. Burns was educated, trained, and worked in an earlier era of healthcare delivery. New practitioners enter a workforce in which old patterns of interaction are difficult to change. Practitioners are focused on mastering their own specialized work domains. Their images of other professionals and the training received by them are often formed early in their experience base, and the images may be difficult to change. Dr. Young will have to work hard to communicate and demonstrate the value of his pharmacy knowledge to some practitioners and patients. The benefits of specialized knowledge will be lost if practitioners are unable to convey that knowledge to other professionals and patients. In teams, the benefits of specialization can be lost if team members are not aware of the specialized knowledge bases of their colleagues.

The challenges to teamwork caused by the specialization of team members can be understood in a broader sense with an analogy to work processes in the whole organization. Within organizations, *differentiation* is the degree to which individual employees are divided into different functional units of similar employees. Large healthcare delivery organizations have functional units of workers dealing with financial management, nutrition services, laboratory services, human resource management, nursing services, and information technology (IT), for example. When employees are grouped together because they do similar work, they are less connected to employees doing different work. Differentiation is a powerful driver of economy and productivity within the functional units, though, as employees within each unit can improve quality and efficiency by interacting and sharing ideas with other employees who "speak the same language." For example, the IT unit workers share a common vocabulary and view of the "outside" or "non-IT" workplace, in the same way that nurses in a patient care unit share a common vocabulary and view of the "non-nursing" workplace.

Differentiation in organizations comes at a high cost to the whole organization, however, if activities of one unit need to be integrated or coordinated with those of other units. As a result, organizational researchers have long observed a positive correlation between the level of differentiation and the level of *integration* in effective organizations (Lawrence and Lorsch, 1967). Integration is the degree to which harmony of effort exists among different units. Integration of work processes is intensified when individual members of each unit know what the other units are doing. This requires interaction, sharing of information, and joint decision making about strategies and goals among the relevant units. For example, delivery of nutritious meals to hospital inpatients requires integration among nutrition services, nursing services, and admission and discharge services, at the least. In organizations, frequent communication and meetings, liaisons, cross-functional committees, cross-training, and co-leadership are examples of ways that different units use to share information and make joint decisions.

Differentiation among organizational units serves as a model for understanding differentiation within teams based on the professional identities of the team members. The various healthcare professionals are influenced by the roles, education, and values ingrained in the process of education, training, and socialization into their own profession—they are highly differentiated. If the team's services require more than one profession, integration among the members of the different professions is needed to produce effective and efficient services.

One important tool for integration that can be applied to teams is *cross-understanding*. Cross-understanding as applied to groups of people is defined formally as "the extent to which group members have an accurate understanding of one another's mental models" (Huber and Lewis, 2010, p. 7). Mental models affect the way that individuals make decisions and define and solve problems. Improved understanding of others' mental models has 3 main effects. First, it improves the quality of communication. Cross-understanding allows group members to use terminology that is both known and respectful to other group members. Otherwise, messages can be perceived to be politically charged, technically incorrect, or confusing. Second, cross-understanding deepens and enriches one's interpretation of another group member's contribution. With cross-understanding, members are comfortable revealing their unique knowledge and beliefs, increasing the likelihood that the group "will discover or more fully understand relevant facts and cause-effect relationships" (Huber and Lewis, 2010, p. 11). Indeed, members in groups with high cross-understanding are more likely to consider information that is inconsistent with their initial preferences, and divergent or creative thinking is stimulated. This does not necessarily mean that mental models are abandoned or compromised, just that they become more comprehensive. Huber and Lewis (2010, p. 11) note the case of legislators with different ideologies who do not share the same mental model but who are better able to work together through cross-understanding. To some extent, professions might be compared to different political parties. Finally, integration is improved by cross-understanding through its effects on behaviors. Members are better able to predict the effect of their actions on others and make adjustments to their behavior in advance. They are more likely to "fill in the blanks" proactively and inform others when necessary, because they realize what information is needed by the other members. Members with cross-understanding are more likely to solicit information that others hold. For example, physicians who are familiar with the mental health counseling competencies of social workers will be more likely to ask the social workers about patients' mental health needs or ask them to provide mental health services. Synergistic outcomes (outcomes not possible from the individual efforts of members) are more likely to emerge when members have cross-understanding.

Recent research on how perceptions of teamwork differ by profession underscores the need for improvement in cross-understanding. For example, 2 studies of the quality of communication and collaboration between nurses and physicians (one in general medical units of hospitals, one in operating rooms) found that nurses rated quality of communication and collaboration lower than physicians did (Carney et al, 2010; O'Leary et al, 2010). In both studies, physicians perceived that the quality of collaboration and communication was higher than nurses perceived it to be. Another study that included registered nurses, nurse practitioners, pharmacists, and physicians revealed that each profession rated its own collaborative behavior higher than members of other professions rated that profession's collaborative behavior (Holden et al, 2010). The *egoistic bias* of individuals (the tendency to rate ourselves higher than others do) seems to be reflected in professions as well.

In summary, teams comprised of different professionals are highly differentiated by profession, which produces attitudes and behaviors that differ among team members. To produce high quality processes and outcomes, integration must be achieved. Cross-understanding is a means to create that integration.

HEALTHCARE OCCUPATIONS OR HEALTHCARE PROFESSIONS?

The reader will note that the term *profession* is used widely in this chapter and book. We refer to workers in healthcare delivery organizations as members of healthcare professions, rather than healthcare occupations. We find it unproductive for most purposes to distinguish between healthcare occupations and healthcare professions—although there are some exceptions.

These exceptions include, for example, discussing the historical evolution of nursing later in this chapter and explaining the weaker power of healthcare administrators compared to many healthcare professionals, in Chapter 5. For those purposes where a distinction is important, the basis for distinguishing professions from occupations usually is the characteristics of the occupation's knowledge base and the attendant formal entry barriers to acquiring the knowledge base (Begun and Lippincott, 1993, pp. 40-41; Freidson, 2001, p. 127). Accordingly, Abbott (1988, p. 8) defines professions as "exclusive occupational groups applying somewhat abstract knowledge to particular cases." Professions typically create exclusivity by controlling entry to the occupation. Entry to a profession requires advanced formal education in a specialized knowledge base, and education often is followed by required certification or licensure.

However, in general, the line between professions and occupations is highly arbitrary. Registered nurses (RNs) are required to have a specialized diploma or degree to qualify for a licensure examination. The specialized diploma or degree can take 2, 3, or 4 years beyond high school to complete. Common usage refers to RNs as healthcare *professionals*. Licensed practical nurses (LPNs) receive formal education of 1-2 years beyond high school and pass a licensure examination. Are LPNs *professionals*? Is the length of formal education the primary determinant of whether individuals in the field are professionals, or are other features associated with professions, such as the degree to which the knowledge base is abstract, equally important to consider? Such questions illustrate that the term *profession* is "an intrinsically ambiguous, multifaceted folk concept" that varies in meaning across cultures and indeed does not exist in some cultures (Freidson, 1994, p. 25). Among individuals working in healthcare teams, focus on the term can create distance in conversations and negotiations if one team member is referred to as a professional, and another team member is not. Avoiding making the distinction between *professional* and *non-professional* is appropriate for most purposes in discussing and providing team-based health care.

WHO'S A "DOCTOR"?

Marta Daingerfield had recently completed her Doctor of Nursing Practice (DNP) degree and was anxious to start off on the right foot in building professional relationships with her associates. Tomorrow she is due to meet her new colleagues on the hospital-wide infection control committee. Will she be introduced as "Doctor" Daingerfield? If not, should she correct the speaker? Should she introduce herself to others as "Doctor"? That certainly was her expectation when she enrolled in the DNP Program, one that was reinforced in her education. How would the "real" doctors respond to that? What if they ask her where she attended medical school?

An issue related to the use of the term *profession* is the use of the term *doctor.* Both terms vary in meaning over time and across settings. Historically in the United States, *doctor* has been used to refer to physicians (in healthcare usage) and to those attaining a "doctoral" or "doctorate" degree from a university (in general usage). Over time, several health professions have elevated their educational preparation to a level defined by that profession as a "doctoral" level, as described in the earlier vignette about 2 pharmacists. Recently, for example, the doctorate of nursing practice has been initiated as the most advanced degree for clinical nurses. Pharmacy and physical therapy, among other health professions, issue practice degrees labeled *doctorate* by the profession. Despite that, many pharmacists and physical therapists holding the doctorate degree often do not refer to themselves as doctor.

Individual administrators and clinicians will evolve different positions on use of the appellation, both as it applies to themselves (if they hold a doctorate degree) and to others. Many physicians use the term *doctor* only to refer to other physicians. One administrator who is a colleague of the authors only uses first names in talking to clinicians and to other administrators, to imply that "we are all equals." Part of relating to other professionals effectively is to understand how the other professional prefers to use the term "doctor," and to consciously make the decision to respect that individual's decision or not. Often, the decision will have implications for the extent to which the other professional feels valued as a team member.

ROLES, EDUCATION, AND VALUES OF FIVE HEALTH PROFESSIONS

The gray areas discussed above—sensitivity over whom to label *professional* and whom to call *doctor*—illustrate the importance of knowing the recent history and intra-professional norms of other professions. In support of practitioners learning about each other's professions, we next present a rudimentary knowledge base for cross-understanding among health professions. Key differentiators among professionals that are relevant to teamwork are the typical roles, education, and values of the professions. We compare 5 healthcare professions or categories of healthcare professions. The 5 professions—medicine, nursing, pharmacy, social work, and healthcare administration—are the largest in number of the healthcare professionals involved in interprofessional teamwork in healthcare delivery. Literally, over 100 other professions participate in interprofessional teamwork in healthcare, and we make reference to several professions in addition to those we focus on primarily. Recent changes in the 5 professions that affect their involvement in interprofessional teams also are presented.

Values of individuals refer to their preferences regarding appropriate courses of action or outcomes. Professional values are inculcated through education and socialization into the professions. In healthcare professional education, the values generally are assumed rather than explored or challenged (Sharpe and Curran, 2011, p. 76). Below, we comment on the primary values of the 5 professions. In addition, we present information on a category of characteristics of occupations labeled *interests* by the Occupational Information Network program (O*NET) of the US Department of Labor (US Department of Labor, 2010). The O*NET program compiles information on US occupations and professions by randomly sampling incumbent workers in different occupational categories and surveying them with a standardized questionnaire. A benefit of the O*NET program is that it provides a common set of categories and an empirical basis for observations about the similarities and differences among health professions. The O*NET Program defines *interests* as preferences in a work environment, and the 6 preferences or interests derive from a history of research that relates personality types to work environments (Holland, 1997). The research established that certain personality types are attracted to and thrive in certain types of occupations and professions. The 6 interests are: Realistic, Investigative, Artistic, Social, Enterprising, and Conventional. *Realistic* interests are quite practical and hands-on. *Investigative* ones require thinking and solving problems. A preference for self-expression, often without strict rules, is labeled *Artistic. Social* interests involve working with others and helping them. *Enterprising* interests entail leading and making decision and, often, taking risks. *Conventional* interests reflect a preference for following set procedures and rules. Table 3–1 displays more detailed definitions of the 6 interests.

Occupations are assigned a profile of interests, with the primary interest listed first. The fairly elaborate methodology for constructing the profiles is described by researchers (Rounds et al, 1999; Rounds et al, 2008). Occupations were categorized by a combination of empirical analyses and judgment by trained raters,

Table 3-1. Occupational interests: definitions from the O*NET program

Realistic—Realistic occupations frequently involve work activities that include practical, hands-on problems and solutions. They often deal with plants, animals, and real-world materials like wood, tools, and machinery. Many of the occupations require working outside, and do not involve a lot of paperwork or working closely with others.
Investigative—Investigative occupations frequently involve working with ideas, and require an extensive amount of thinking. These occupations can involve searching for facts and solving problems mentally.
Artistic—Artistic occupations frequently involve working with forms, designs, and patterns. They often require self-expression, and the work can be done without following a clear set of rules.
Social—Social occupations frequently involve working with, communicating with, and teaching people. These occupations often involve helping or providing service to others.
Enterprising—Enterprising occupations frequently involve starting up and carrying out projects. These occupations can involve leading people and making many decisions. Sometimes they require risk taking and often deal with business.
Conventional—Conventional occupations frequently involve following set procedures and routines. These occupations can include working with data and details more than with ideas. Usually there is a clear line of authority to follow.

Source: US Department of Labor, 2010.

resulting in each occupation being characterized by a profile of 1-3 interests. A 3-interest profile, which is assigned in most cases, means that the first interest is most descriptive of the occupation, the second interest is less descriptive but salient, and the third interest is even less descriptive but still salient. A 2-interest classification (the case for social work below) means that the first interest is most descriptive, the second interest is less descriptive but salient, and none of the other interests is salient.

The following descriptions of professions include generalizations that may not apply to particular individuals in the professional roles. Many of the generalizations have an empirical anchoring in occupational research, such as the Department of Labor survey program, which is cited. Other generalizations are based on experiences of the authors or others. To avoid stereotyping (assigning characteristics to all members of a category that apply only to some members), there is no substitute for learning about the particular individuals on one's team. The individuals may differ quite substantially from the generalized depictions presented here.

PHYSICIANS

Every weekday at 8 a.m., Jane Daggett, MD, begins seeing patients in her clinic. Dr. Daggett is a general internist. Her patients are all adults. Patients are scheduled for 15-minute or 30-minute visits or, occasionally, for a 45-minute visit. The standard time slot is 15 minutes, but Dr. Daggett requests longer visits for patients with greater need, for example, older patients and patients who have several complicated medical problems. The patients are brought to one of Dr. Daggett's 2 examination rooms by Cindy Wolff, CMA (Certified Medical Assistant), who confirms the patient's reason for seeing Dr. Daggett, measures the patient's weight, takes his or her blood pressure, and updates the patient's medication list in the electronic health record. Dr. Daggett then sees the patient, taking his or her medical history, doing a physical examination as relevant to the patient's symptoms or disease, and planning treatment or changes in treatment such as changes in medication doses. Sometimes she performs a joint injection (for example, injecting medication into a patient's knee), but, as a general internist, she does not do many procedures.

Dr. Daggett finishes her morning schedule officially at 11:30 a.m. However, her last patient for the morning usually leaves 15-20 minutes after this time. If she has not already finished writing notes in the electronic records of the patients she has seen, she completes her notes then. She also answers telephone calls from patients, responds to secure e-mail messages sent by patients, and reviews laboratory results that are delivered to her in the electronic record, where they are flagged so that she is alerted to the arrival of the results.

She usually eats lunch with other physicians in the cafeteria from about 12:30 to 1:00, then returning to the clinic to continue answering telephone messages, writing referral requests for patients who need specialist consultation, and doing other tasks generated by her interactions with patients that morning or during the previous few days.

Sometimes there is a midday meeting to attend, perhaps an Internal Medicine Department meeting or a quality improvement (QI) project meeting. Dr. Daggett has a particular interest in the management of diabetes and participates in a long-term project to improve the processes used in the clinic for managing patients with diabetes. Other members of the QI project team are a nurse practitioner (NP) who specializes in diabetes care, 2 CMAs, a family physician, and a staff person from the QI office, who manages the project and collects and analyzes data for the team.

In the afternoon, from 1:30 to 4:30 p.m., Dr. Daggett again sees scheduled patients. Occasionally an NP in the department will knock on Dr. Daggett's door and ask a question or ask Dr. Daggett to see a patient for a quick consultation. At the end of the day, Dr. Daggett returns to writing notes in the electronic record, filling in disability forms or other forms requested by patients, and carrying out other work that flows from her direct contacts with patients.

In total, Dr. Daggett sees about 20 patients each day or about 100 per week. Earlier in her career, she began each day in the hospital, rounding on 2-6 patients whom she had admitted to the hospital. She then would drive to the clinic to see scheduled patients. Her hours in the clinic were fewer then. In recent years, she has stopped doing hospital work. In contrast, some of her internal medicine colleagues have stopped doing work in the clinic and see patients only in the hospital, that is, they have become hospitalists.

Roles

As illustrated by the vignette about Dr. Daggett, physicians diagnose illnesses, and prescribe and administer treatment for people suffering from injury or disease. They examine patients, obtain medical histories, order and interpret diagnostic tests, prescribe drugs, perform surgery, and manage chronic disease. They also counsel patients on diet, hygiene, preventive health care, and mental health problems. There are 2 types of physicians: those with a Doctor of Medicine (MD) degree and those with a Doctor of Osteopathy (DO) degree, with MDs being the vast majority (over 90% of physicians in the United States). MDs attend medical school; DOs attend osteopathic schools. In osteopathy there is a historical preference for understanding and using manual therapy, or manipulation, but similarities between the training of MDs and DOs far outweigh the differences (Bodenheimer and Grumbach, 2012, p. 75).

In 2007, there were about 941,000 physicians in the United States, of which 67% were graduates from a US school of medicine (conferring the MD degree), 7% were graduates from US school of osteopathy (conferring DO degrees), and 26% were graduates of foreign medical schools (American Medical Association, 2010; American Osteopathic Association, 2010). Thus, a large number of physicians in the United States were trained outside the United States. Foreign-trained physicians must pass the US medical licensing board examinations, and complete internships and residencies in the United States before being licensed to practice medicine.

Physicians are highly specialized. The American Board of Medical Specialties (ABMS) encompasses 24 major specialties with certification in 145 specialties and subspecialties (ABMS, 2012). The 5 largest specialties are internal medicine, family medicine, pediatrics, obstetrics and gynecology, and anesthesiology (US Census Bureau, 2011, p. 115). The continued development of biomedical knowledge as well as new specializations and new arenas for care giving, such as hospitalist care, spawn more and more specialization and subspecialization. For example, internal medicine approved 4 new subspecialties in the 2006-2010 period—transplant hepatology, sleep medicine, hospital and palliative medicine, and advanced heart failure and transplant cardiology (Cassel and Reuben, 2011). As noted below in a comparison of internal medicine and surgery, specific specialties in medicine attract different personality types, creating differences by specialty not only in knowledge base and approach to medical problems but also in contributions to team processes.

Many physicians—chiefly family physicians, general internists, pediatricians, obstetrician/gynecologists, and psychiatrists—work in small private offices or clinics, assisted by a small staff of nurses, certified medical assistants, and administrative personnel. Increasingly, though, physicians are practicing in groups or are employed by large healthcare organizations. Physicians working in group practices or as employees of a healthcare organization often work with other physicians, nurses, and other professionals to coordinate care for a number of patients. They are less independent than solo practitioners, whose numbers are steadily decreasing. Surgeons and anesthesiologists usually work in hospitals or in surgical outpatient centers;

they also conduct office visits to evaluate patients for surgery and do follow-up surgical visits. Many physicians work long, irregular hours. Physicians often travel between office and hospital to care for their patients, although this is rapidly decreasing with the strong growth of hospital-based medicine. While on call (available at short notice), a physician will deal with many patients' concerns over the phone and make emergency visits to hospitals or nursing homes.

Some 60,000 physician assistants (PAs) work in the United States, practicing medicine under the direct supervision of physicians. Studies conclude that the work domain of PAs overlaps with approximately 80% of the scope of work of primary care physicians (Bodenheimer and Grumbach, 2012, p. 77).

Education

Physicians go through an extended period of formal education and training. In the United States, physicians typically complete a bachelor's (undergraduate) degree followed by 4 years of medical school and then residency training in a particular specialty for 3-7 years. Residency training is sometimes followed by a fellowship of 1-3 years in a subspecialty. Radiologists, for example, typically have 5 years of training beyond medical school, general surgeons have 5 years, cardiac surgeons have 7 years, and family physicians have 3 years of training.

Physicians apply for licensure at the state level in the United States, with requirements determined by each state. Requirements that are common across the states include passing the United States Medical Licensing Examination (USMLE) and training beyond medical school of at least 1 year. As mentioned above, foreign-trained physicians wanting to practice in the United States must pass the USMLE and then must complete residency training at a US institution, regardless of their years of experience abroad. Those wanting to specialize also must repeat specialty training such as fellowships. For many foreign-trained physicians, the path to practice in the United States is long and difficult.

An additional credential held by most physicians is specialty board certification. About 75% of physicians are board-certified (Young et al, 2011). Board certification is not required for state licensure, but many hospital medical staffs require board certification for medical staff membership and privileges to admit patients to the hospital. A physician becomes board-certified by passing an examination conducted by a certifying organization, such as the American Board of Surgery.

Physician assistant education averages 27 months, with most programs requiring a baccalaureate degree as a prerequisite and granting a master's degree. To be eligible for licensure in most states, PAs must graduate from an accredited program and pass a national certifying examination (Bodenheimer and Grumbach, 2012, p. 77).

Values

Department of Labor sources (US Department of Labor, 2012) state that people who wish to become physicians should be detail oriented, have good communication skills, and have patience to work with those who need special attention. Empathy for patients and their families is important for compassionate care. Dexterity with their hands and physical stamina also are noted as important qualities for clinical care. Leadership and organizational skills help with practice management. Finally, problem-solving skills are important in making diagnoses and administering appropriate treatment. Medical education has been described by many as rigorous and competitive. Thus, the "prototypical medical school student is extremely bright and achievement-oriented, and astute at adapting to the environmental cues necessary to achieve success" (Garman et al, 2006, p. 832). Prospective physicians must be willing to study throughout their careers to keep up with medical advances.

In practicing health care, physicians value excellence in diagnosis and treatment, including drug treatment and surgery, and achieving cure of the patient's disease (or minimizing symptoms). The focus on cure and a push for excellence underlie some of the behavior that other professionals may find intimidating or too forceful. Other key distinguishing values and interests of physicians that affect healthcare teamwork include the following:

1. Physicians are ordinarily concerned about costs of their services only as a secondary issue. Accurate diagnosis and cure for the patient are to be pursued regardless of cost, within reason as judged by the physician and patient, not an insurance company employee or healthcare administrator.
2. Physicians are very independent. They expect to have clinical decision-making autonomy. They do not automatically follow hierarchical commands.

3. Physicians expect problems to have solutions. Problems are not to be discussed *ad nauseam*. Work is expected to proceed at a fast pace.
4. Physicians expect high social status. They aspire to achieve the esteem of patients, peers, and the local community.
5. Physicians respect scientific evidence. They look for objective evidence to make patient-related decisions.

Another perspective on physicians' values is provided by the occupational database, O*NET, described earlier. Consistent with the long educational stint served by physicians, the top-ranked interest of physicians is labeled as *Investigative*. People with investigative interests enjoy working with ideas and thinking more than performing physical activity. They like to search for facts and solve problems mentally rather than to persuade or lead people (US Department of Labor, 2012).

Different medical specialties attract different personality types. Comparing 2 specialties with quite different work responsibilities, surgery and internal medicine, illustrates the point. Both surgeons and internists have the same trio of top interests: Investigative, Realistic, and Social. Both have Investigative as their top interest. For surgeons, the second-ranked interest is Realistic. Individuals with realistic interest enjoy practical, hands-on problems and solutions. For internists, on the other hand, the second-ranked interest is Social. Social occupations involve working with, communicating with, and teaching people. Table 3–2 displays the interest profile of internists and surgeons, along with the other professions examined in the following sections of this chapter.

Teamwork Implications

Physicians often are suited to lead or play a central role on teams based on their expertise or, in some cases, their legal obligation to oversee care. It is appropriate for physicians to have central roles on many teams, but not on all teams and not on all issues. There are many teams that can be led by others and many that should be led by others. Physicians may have a difficult time ceding control of teams to others, or playing a limited role on some teams, such as management project teams formed to improve quality. They may have impatience with the time required to accommodate to and learn about the work of other professions. Physicians can be the most difficult of the professions to meld into team-based health care.

When physicians are team leaders, they need to be good leaders. This means performing as described in Chapter 8. Among other things, good leadership includes creating unity in the team, drawing the best from all team members, attending to the social health of the team, treating all members with respect, and pursuing improvement of the team's performance.

NURSES

Tamara Montoris, BSN, RN, arrived at the hospital on Thursday about 6:30 a.m. She worked in one of the adult "med-surg" (medical-surgical) wards of Carlisle Memorial Medical Center.

Table 3–2. Occupational interest profiles of seven health professions

Profession	Primary Interest	Secondary Interest	Tertiary Interest
Internists	Investigative	Social	Realistic
Surgeons	Investigative	Realistic	Social
Registered nurses	Social	Investigative	Conventional
Nurse practitioners	Social	Investigative	Realistic
Pharmacists	Investigative	Conventional	Social
Social workers	Social	Investigative	(none specified)
Healthcare administrators	Enterprising	Conventional	Social

Source: US Department of Labor, 2010.

She worked the day shift, that is, from 7 a.m. to 3 p.m. most weekdays. She also worked some shifts on weekends and holidays. These shifts were distributed across all of the RNs working in the med-surg wards as fairly as possible, although there were always complaints from some of the nurses about how the schedules were managed. When Ms. Montoris was younger, she often had worked evenings (3 p.m. to 11 p.m.) and nights (11 p.m. to 7 a.m.). When she accumulated enough seniority to work days—with occasional exceptions—she was quite pleased.

On this particular Thursday, she began her day as usual by receiving reports on her patients from a nurse who was ending his shift. Ms. Montoris cared for 7 patients that day. She was briefed by one of the night-shift nurses about each of the 7. Each briefing included information about the patient's diagnosis, any surgery that had been performed during the hospital stay, the pain medications the patient was receiving, how the patient had fared during the night, any discharge plans, and other matters.

Ms. Montoris' day consisted primarily of caring for her patients, performing many tasks. One patient required careful swabbing of his mouth because of a viral infection that caused painful sores in the lining of his mouth. Another patient needed a new intravenous line inserted because the old one had become blocked where the needle entered the vein. Late in the morning, another patient needed to have fluid withdrawn from her abdomen by a physician. Ms Montoris assisted in the procedure. She also went on rounds with one of the hospitalists, who was the physician for 5 of her 7 patients. The other 2 patients were cared for by the surgeons who had operated on them during the past few days.

Nursing assistants also provided many services for Ms. Montoris' patients. They measured patients' temperatures, blood pressures, and pulse rates. Ms. Montoris reviewed this information every 3-4 hours except when one of the assistants brought an unexpected reading to her attention. The assistants also helped patients with bathing and using the restrooms, sometimes helping them to use bedpans.

Ms. Montoris ate a brown bag lunch with 3 other nurses in the break room of the ward next to hers. As it happened, she had only 20 minutes for lunch that day.

In the early afternoon, Ms. Montoris had a discussion with Fiona Bevan, a 76-year-old patient. Mrs. Bevan's daughter and Susan Hale, MSW, also participated in the conversation. Ms. Hale was one of hospital's social workers. Mrs. Bevan had suffered a stroke and was not able to care for herself—at least not yet. Ms. Hale and Ms. Montoris were helping Mrs. Bevan and her daughter to talk through their options for Mrs. Bevan's care immediately after her hospital stay. Ms. Hale had identified 3 facilities where Mrs. Bevan could receive convalescent care. Her daughter had visited all 3 of the facilities and favored one of them. The conversation consisted mainly of descriptions of the 3 facilities given by Ms. Hale and Mrs. Bevan's daughter, followed by Mrs. Bevan's reactions. Of course, the underlying issue was Mrs. Bevan's need to come to terms with the fact that she could not go directly home. Ms. Montoris participated in the conversation mainly to help Mrs. Bevan to accept this turn of events and not to feel so distressed about it.

About 2 p.m. Ms. Montoris had a brief conversation with the nurse manager of the ward and 2 other nurses about a proposed change in the way the ward's supply room would be organized and how frequently it would be re-stocked with surgical dressings, procedure kits, urinary catheters, and other items.

Ms. Montoris finished her shift by reporting on her 7 patients to the nurse who would care for them in the evening shift. She finished her report about 3:15 p.m. Occasionally she had a meeting to attend after her shift was completed—sometimes an educational session to acquaint her with newly purchased equipment, sometimes a meeting of the nurses' union at the union headquarters. But on this day, there was no meeting to attend, and she headed for home.

Roles

Nursing is the largest healthcare profession, with 2.7 million employed registered nurses (RNs), 750,000 licensed practical nurses (LPNs) and licensed vocational nurses (LVNs), and 1.5 million nursing aids, orderlies and attendants (US Department of Labor, 2012). Healthcare teams frequently include RNs with advanced education, such as nurse practitioners, numbering about 180,000 (Kaiser Family Foundation, 2012), or clinical nurse specialists, numbering some 75,000 (National Association of Clinical Nurse Specialists, 2012). Registered nurses care for patients, educate patients, and the public about various medical conditions, and provide advice and emotional support to patients' family members. RNs record patients' medical histories and symptoms, help perform diagnostic tests and analyze results, operate medical machinery, administer treatment and medications, change surgical dressings, and help with patient follow-up and rehabilitation. RNs teach patients and their families the management of their illnesses or injuries, explaining post-treatment home care needs; diet, nutrition, and exercise programs; and self-administration of medication and physical therapy. RNs also might run general health screening or immunization clinics, blood drives, and public seminars on various conditions (US Department of Labor, 2012).

About 3 in 5 nurses work in hospitals. Many others work in physician's offices. They help with medical tests, give medicines, and dress wounds. Some also do laboratory and office work. Home health and public health nurses travel to patients' homes, schools, community centers, and other sites. Patients in hospitals and nursing care facilities require 24-hour care; consequently, nurses in these institutions may work nights, weekends, and holidays. Nurses who work in offices, schools, and other settings that do not provide 24-hour care are more likely to work regular business hours. Many nurses work part-time—approximately 20% of RNs worked part time in 2010 (US Department of Labor, 2012).

Education

Different levels of nursing require different levels of education spanning a wide range. Table 3–3 displays educational requirements for several levels of nursing. Nursing assistants or nurse technicians receive certificates for in-hospital training programs, usually of length under 1 year. LPNs or LVNs are usually trained for 1 year in a technical school or community college. RNs have 3 educational pathways to licensure: associate's degree,

Table 3–3. Educational requirements of nurses

Nursing Role	Typical Educational Credentials
Nursing assistants	Postsecondary certificate (most training programs last under 1 year and are offered by hospitals, nursing homes, community colleges, vocational and technical schools). State licensure requires examination that varies by state.
Licensed practical nurse, licensed vocational nurse	Postsecondary certificate or associate's degree (most training programs last about 1 year and are offered by community colleges, vocational and technical schools). State licensure requires national examination.
Registered nurse	• Diploma (2-3 years, typically offered by hospitals) • Associate's degree in nursing (2-3 years, typically offered by community and junior colleges) • Bachelor's degree in nursing (4 years) State licensure requires national examination.
Nurse anesthetist	Master's degree in nursing (transitioning to Doctor of Nurse Anesthesia Practice). Certification required as well.
Nurse practitioner	Master's degree in nursing (transitioning to Doctor of Nursing Practice [DNP]). Certification required as well.
Nurse midwife	Master's degree in nursing (transitioning to DNP). Certification required as well.
Clinical nurse specialist	Master's degree in nursing (transitioning to DNP). Certification required as well.
Nurse doctorate—practice focus	DNP
Nurse doctorate—research focus	PhD

diploma, or bachelor's degree. Nursing has long struggled internally over proposals to require the bachelor's degree as the minimum requirement for the RN license. Common usage of the term *professional nursing* refers to RNs (excluding LPNs, LVNs, and assistants) and above in educational level. However, some use the term to refer only to those RNs who hold the bachelor's degree and above. *Advanced practice nurses*, who train 1-2 years beyond the baccalaureate level and attain a master's degree, include nurse anesthetists, NPs, nurse midwives, and clinical nurse specialists. NPs and clinical nurse specialists are further differentiated by specialty. NPs can specialize in family health, pediatrics, acute care, adult care, adult psychiatric care, family psychiatric care, school health, and a number of other fields. Clinical nurse specialists have similar specializations.

The number of nurses who hold a clinical nurse doctorate is growing rapidly. The American Association of Colleges of Nursing (AACN) recommends that all entry-level nurse practitioner educational programs be transitioned from the Master of Science in Nursing (MSN) degree to the DNP degree by the year 2015 (AACN, 2004). Previously, nurses with PhD degrees in nursing or related fields were alone at the pinnacle of the educational hierarchy of nursing.

In all states in the United States, to become licensed RNs, students must graduate from an approved nursing program and pass a national licensing examination, known as the National Council Licensure Examination, or NCLEX-RN. Other eligibility requirements for licensure vary by state (US Department of Labor, 2012). Generally, a graduate degree and national board certification are required for state licensure of advanced practice nurses.

Values

The key identifying principle of nursing is patient care and advocacy for the patient (Garman et al, 2006). Nurses seek to optimize the patient's experience of illness and health care. They value attention to the whole person, including the social and emotional dimensions of the illness experience (Clark, 1997). The focus on *care* sometimes is contrasted to the focus of physicians on *cure*. Among qualities of nurses, a detail orientation, compassion, critical thinking skills, patience, compassion, and speaking skills are desirable (US Department of Labor, 2012).

The O*NET classification reflects important differences between physicians and nurses. Interests of nurses are classified as Social-Investigative-Conventional (for RNs) or Social-Investigative-Realistic (for NPs) (see Table 3-2). Contrasting physicians and nurses, Garman and colleagues (2006, p. 834) conclude that "while physicians embody the *Investigative* component of the Holland model, nurses most closely embody the *Social* component. The distinction has parallels in the professional roles; while medicine tends toward a primary focus on healing *interventions*, the primary focus of nursing tends to be the healing *relationship*" [italics in original]. Comparing 2 types of roles in nursing, RNs and NPs, the different third interest (Realistic for NPs, Conventional for RNs) likely reflects the fact that RN work involves more routine procedures, precise standards, and clear lines of authority than does NP work.

For many nurses, the field is a calling with a principled and noble heritage. Nursing heroines dating from Florence Nightingale have exemplified the selflessness and patient care values promoted by the profession. Many nurses think that it is important to continue to professionalize nursing so that it is more similar in status and power to medicine, by continuing to raise educational standards and codifying its knowledge base. Nursing also carries a heritage of victimization at the hands of more powerful physicians and administrators, making some nurses sensitive to being disrespected by other professionals (Begun and White, 1999). Over 90% of nurses in the United States are female, which adds to a heightened sensitivity to disrespect or inequity (because of their gender, in addition to their profession) on the part of some nurses.

Teamwork Implications

Many nurses are used to performing supportive roles, but most are proud of the differentiation of their roles, education, and values from physicians and other professionals, considering nursing to be a separate and equal profession rather than a supportive profession. Nurses are a key element of most healthcare teams and in fact often take on leadership functions previously performed mostly by physicians. Related to their "underdog" heritage and struggle to professionalize, many nurses are sensitive to equity issues on healthcare teams.

PHARMACISTS

Rapidaman General Hospital is a suburban hospital with 150 beds. It employs 16 pharmacists, 9 of whom hold a PharmD degree and 7 of whom are more experienced and hold a BSPharm degree.

Richard Okafor, PharmD, is one of the 16 pharmacists. His day usually begins at 8 a.m. with a brief meeting, held in the central pharmacy and led by the Director of Pharmacy. These morning meetings last for about 10 minutes and consist of announcements about pharmacy operations and broader hospital issues, followed by an opportunity for the pharmacists and pharmacy technicians to ask questions. After the meeting, Dr. Okafor spends most of his morning overseeing the filling of medication orders coming from the hospital wards and intensive care units (ICUs). The actual filling of the orders—counting tablets or capsules and mixing intravenous drug preparations—is handled by the pharmacy technicians, who ask for direction from Dr. Okafor from time to time.

Occasionally, a medication is ordered that is incompatible with another medication the patient is already receiving. Sometimes a physician orders a medication to which the patient is allergic, according to the pharmacy's records. In the case of medication incompatibility or allergy, Dr. Okafor decides whether to contact the nursing station from which the order has come or to contact the physician who wrote the order. If the issue is a straightforward allergy that apparently has been overlooked, Dr. Okafor usually contacts the nursing station and leaves the matter for the nurses to resolve by contacting the physician. In essentially all of these cases, the physician cancels the first order and orders a different drug. In the cases of drug incompatibility, Dr. Okafor typically telephones the physician directly and talks the issue through. Some drug incompatibilities are absolute, and a different drug is needed regardless of any other consideration. Sometimes, however, there might be a problem if the 2 drugs are administered together, but it is not certain that the patient would be adversely affected. In those cases, judgment must be used in deciding whether the chance of reduced drug effectiveness or some other problem is justified by the patient's needs. In these cases, Dr. Okafor and the ordering physician review the issues and make a decision. Rarely, he and a physician disagree and the physician insists on ordering the drug that might generate a problem. And, very rarely, Dr. Okafor declines to fill the order because he believes it is his professional responsibility to decline.

The central pharmacy fills hospital discharge medication orders as well as orders for medications to be administered in the hospital. Many patients bring the discharge prescriptions written for them to the hospital pharmacy. The technicians fill the prescriptions and let the patients know that they can speak with a pharmacist if they wish to receive advice. Dr. Okafor and the other pharmacists often meet with these patients to explain how the medications should be taken and what side effects might occur. Occasionally, for certain medications (for example, those with a high likelihood of distressing side effects), the pharmacy staff tactfully insist on a pharmacy consultation before providing the medication to the patient.

Dr. Okafor normally has lunch with other pharmacists and hospital staff in the hospital cafeteria. Sometimes he spends part of his lunch break in the hospital library, checking an article needed to settle some pharmaceutical issue that has arisen during the morning.

His afternoons are ordinarily similar to his mornings although sometimes there are management meetings involving all or most of the pharmacists and, occasionally, including the Vice President for Support Services, to whom the Director of Pharmacy reports.

Two of Dr. Okafor's colleagues spend most of their time in the wards and ICUs of the hospital, rounding with physicians and nurses, offering guidance on pharmacy issues and answering the other clinicians' questions. These 2 pharmacists have done pharmacy residencies and are specialists, one in oncology pharmacy and one in pharmacotherapy. The demand for direct participation by pharmacists in clinical teams is high at Rapidaman, and Dr. Okafor has made known his interest in doing this kind of work for part of his time. At this point, however, the pharmacy is not adequately staffed with pharmacists to be able to spare another pharmacist to join clinical teams on the wards.

Dr. Okafor finishes his work days about 5:00 or 5:30 p.m. He also works nights and weekends about twice a month, participating in a rotation that includes all of the pharmacists. A pharmacist is always on call through the night, but Dr. Okafor and his colleagues do not work night shifts in the hospital.

Roles

Pharmacists distribute prescription drugs to individuals for the treatment of disease in response to the prescription of a physician, nurse practitioner, or other provider with prescription privileges. In small pharmacies, pharmacists distribute drugs directly. In large pharmacies, like the one in the vignette about Dr. Okafor, pharmacists oversee the distribution process and provide their expertise to technicians as required. Pharmacists also advise their patients, physicians, and other healthcare practitioners on the selection, dosages, interactions, and side effects of medications, as well as monitor the health and progress of those patients to ensure that they are using their medications safely and effectively.

There are about 275,000 employed pharmacists in the United States. Most pharmacists work in a community setting, such as a retail drugstore, or in a healthcare facility, such as a hospital (US Department of Labor, 2012). Often pharmacists are assisted by pharmacy technicians or aides.

Education

Historically, pharmacy education was baccalaureate-level, requiring the Bachelor of Pharmacy degree (BSPharm or BPharm). The Doctor of Pharmacy (PharmD) degree has replaced the Bachelor of Pharmacy degree, which is no longer being awarded, though many pharmacists now in practice are graduates of the older baccalaureate programs. To be admitted to a PharmD program, an applicant must have completed at least 2 years of specific postsecondary study including chemistry, biology, and anatomy, after which the PharmD generally takes 4 years to complete. Some PharmD graduates obtain further training through 1-year or 2-year residency programs or fellowships in a specialty field, such as ambulatory care pharmacy, nuclear pharmacy, nutrition support pharmacy, oncology pharmacy, pharmacotherapy, psychiatric pharmacy (US Department of Labor, 2012). After completing a PharmD degree, pharmacists must pass 2 examinations to attain state licensure—one in pharmacy skills and knowledge, another in pharmacy law in the state issuing the pharmacy license.

For pharmacy technicians a high school degree is typically required, and some states require formal training programs and passage of a licensure examination. Formal postsecondary training programs generally last 1 year or less, and there are some 335,000 pharmacy technicians in the United States (US Department of Labor, 2012).

Values

Pharmacists value excellence in the choice and dosing of drugs used for treating disease, as well as achieving cure of the patient's disease (or decrease in symptoms). Prospective pharmacists should have several relevant qualities: analytical skills to evaluate patients' needs and prescribers' orders; communication skills to deal with patients, other clinicians, and staff; an orientation to detail, to ensure attention to exact and accurate filling of prescriptions; and managerial skills to oversee a staff and manage inventory (US Department of Labor, 2012).

The O*NET profile of pharmacists' interests classifies them as Investigative-Conventional-Social, with the primary interest (Investigative) the same as physicians, reflecting the scientific basis of pharmacy's knowledge base (see Table 3-2). The second interest, Conventional, illustrates the more predictable or routine nature of the work roles of pharmacists, as well as the need for caution and conscientiousness in dispensing potentially dangerous medications. Like surgeons, pharmacists register a Social interest in the third rank.

Teamwork Implications

Pharmacists typically work in a hierarchical organization, which gives them experience with delegation and accountability. The recent requirement of the PharmD degree has given many pharmacists the knowledge base to expand the boundaries of their contributions to healthcare teams, and many are interested in expanding the scope of pharmacy practice. Pharmacists' knowledge is often greater than other team members may realize. Their education and training have been upgraded in recent years. Physicians and other team members may need tactful prompting to assure that patients get full benefit from the pharmacists. As a result of pharmacists' broader knowledge base, they and physicians now have substantial overlapping turf. They are at risk of conflict, adding to the importance of team building and team training for teams that include pharmacists and physicians.

SOCIAL WORKERS

Penny Starling, MSW, LICSW, is a social worker in a large, urban hospital. She and 2 other social workers cover the adult ICUs, working principally with the nurses, physicians, and surgeons who have patients in those units.

On Wednesday, she began her day at 7:30 a.m. on rounds in the surgical ICU. The others in the team were a trauma surgeon, a respiratory therapist, 2 surgical residents, and the nurse caring for each of the patients seen on rounds. Ms. Starling happened to know that the first patient the rounding team would see that morning was Ms. Jorgenson, a female patient with severe head trauma caused by an automobile accident. The plan for the patient's post-ICU care was not yet settled. Ms. Starling needed to know more about the patient's anticipated medical needs and to know the surgeon's and nurse's impressions of how the patient's family was coping with the patient's disabilities. In the discussion outside of the patient's room, Ms. Starling asked questions about the patient's prognosis and about her family. The answers about the family were provided mainly by the nurse. The patient did not participate; she was unconscious. Ms. Starling did not round on all ICU patients; only some of them needed her help. She left the rounding team after they visited that first patient.

Later that morning she met with the patient's husband and 2 of the daughters in the family, who had flown in from out of town. Ms. Starling asked questions to learn obliquely whether the husband understood the severity of his wife's injuries. It became clear that either he did not understand or was in a state of denial. Ms. Starling asked the husband whether he had given any thought to identifying a long-term care facility in the event that his wife needed long-term care. The husband and daughters all looked shocked. Ms. Starling wished she had worded her question differently. She continued by saying that it would not hurt to consider even very unlikely possibilities since arranging for suitable care is often difficult and time-consuming. The husband then looked relieved. Ms. Starling set aside the topic for another day. She asked the husband and daughters a few questions about how they were faring in the wake of Ms. Jorgenson's accident and injuries. They answered in a way that showed their gratitude for Ms. Starling's concern for them and for Ms. Jorgenson.

Ms. Starling spent part of her morning on the telephone with a medical director for an insurance company in another state. The insurance company wanted one of their policy holders, an ICU patient who had undergone emergency surgery for an intestinal obstruction, to be transferred by air ambulance back to her home city, where the insurance company was located. Ms. Starling was able to persuade the medical director that transferring the patient at that time would not be safe. She told the insurance company medical director that he could talk to the trauma surgeon if he wished, but the medical director said that this was not necessary.

Ms. Starling had a quick lunch in the cafeteria with a friend who was a nurse in one of the ICUs. She then went to her office to answer various telephone calls. Her afternoon was spent meeting with both patients and families, talking about arrangements for care after discharge from the ICU or discharge from the hospital. Some of the patients she saw were no longer in the ICU, but she continued to follow them anyway because she had interacted with them and their families extensively in the ICU. She, the patients, and the families did not want to switch to new social workers after their relationships had been established.

Occasionally Ms. Starling participated in a care conference focused on a particular patient, usually a patient who had been hospitalized at length following a stroke, trauma, or an orthopedic surgical procedure accompanied by postoperative pneumonia or some other complication. These care conferences were attended by nurses, physicians (usually rehabilitation specialists), speech therapists, physical therapists, and occupational therapists. However, on that particular Wednesday, there was no care conference to attend.

Ms. Starling finished her day at 5:30 p.m. The work day had been a bit long but otherwise was not unusual.

Roles

Of approximately 650,000 social workers in the United States, 43% work in health care, with almost half of those in mental health and substance abuse (US Department of Labor, 2012). In addition to mental health and substance abuse, other specialties for healthcare social workers include gerontological social work and hospice and palliative care social work. Healthcare social workers provide individuals, families, and groups with the psychosocial support needed to cope with chronic, acute, or terminal illnesses. Services include advising family care givers, providing patient education and counseling, and making referrals for other services. Healthcare social workers help patients and families with payment arrangements and with locating long-term care or residential placements for people with disabilities and elderly patients. They may also provide care and case management or interventions designed to promote health, prevent disease, and address barriers to access to healthcare. Some social workers go into private practice. Most private practitioners provide psychotherapy, usually paid for through health insurance or by the clients themselves.

Social work, while satisfying, can be challenging. Understaffing and large caseloads add to the pressure in some agencies. Full-time social workers usually work a standard 40-hour week, but some occasionally work evenings and weekends to meet with clients, attend community meetings, and handle emergencies (US Department of Labor, 2012).

Education

A bachelor's degree in social work (BSW) is the most common minimum requirement for a job as a social worker. Bachelor's degree programs prepare graduates for service positions, such as caseworker, mental health assistant, group home worker, and residential counselor. Although a bachelor's degree is sufficient for entry into the field, a master's degree in social work (MSW) is typically required for positions in many health and school settings and is required for clinical social workers, who diagnose and treat mental, behavioral, and emotional issues. Master's degree programs prepare graduates for work in their chosen field of concentration and continue to develop the skills required to perform clinical assessments, manage large caseloads, take on supervisory roles, and explore new ways of drawing upon social services to meet the needs of clients. Formal university education training often includes or is followed by additional training and structured supervision leading to licensure, whose forms vary from state to state (US Department of Labor, 2012). Common licensure designations are LICSW (Licensed Independent Clinical Social Worker) and LCSW (Licensed Clinical Social Worker). Supervisory, administrative, and staff training positions usually require an advanced degree. College and university teaching positions and most research appointments normally require a doctorate in social work (DSW or PhD). While some sources argue there is little if any difference between the DSW and PhD in social work, others claim a practice orientation to be more prevalent with the DSW and an academic orientation with the PhD.

Values

Social workers value attention to psychological response to illness and to the social context of illness (Clark, 1997). They also emphasize improving the mental health of the patient. Social workers are attentive to the experience of illness on the part of the patient and the family, especially the prospect of behavioral changes due to mental disorders and the responses of families to those changes. They are also mindful of the place of the patient and family in a nexus of societal, legal, and governmental rules and institutions. Social workers are well positioned to help with all of these connections. The US Department of Labor (2012) lists important qualities of prospective social workers as compassion, listening skills, people skills, and problem-solving skills, underscoring the importance of human interaction in social work. Time-management and organizational skills are also listed as important, due to the need to balance demands from multiple clients.

The O*NET interest profile of social workers is described as Social-Investigative (see Table 3–2). The Social interest validates the primary work of the profession as working with people in need, and the Investigative interest reflects the fact that social workers are problem solvers.

Teamwork Implications

The professional scope of social workers overlaps with nurses. At times both may see themselves as the best advocates for the patient, family, or both. This sometimes leads to rivalries or conflicts.

Some healthcare professionals, especially physicians and pharmacists, are not well acquainted with the capabilities of social workers and tend to see them only as connectors with agencies. Administrators often are not aware of social workers' knowledge of organizational behavior and so, in dealing with organizational problems, do not avail themselves of help nearby.

HEALTHCARE ADMINISTRATORS

Bob Martin, MBA, MHA, is the administrator of Summit Maple Community Hospital, a highly regarded rural hospital serving a 15-county area. Summit Maple has 132 beds and employs 800 nurses, pharmacists, and other staff. The medical staff consists of 175 physicians in all specialties except for cardiac surgery. The physicians have hospital privileges but are not employed by the hospital.

Mr. Martin's days have no regular pattern. On one Tuesday last month, he spent most of the morning working through options for financing a renovation of the obstetrical unit in the hospital. He met with the Director of Patient Care (a nurse manager), the Chief Financial Officer, and a representative of the local county government, which owns the hospital and would issue any bonds that might be needed. An obstetrician on the medical staff joined the meeting for 30 minutes or so. At midday, Mr. Martin made a presentation to the Rotary Club in town, describing the changing role of the hospital as healthcare organizations in the state grow larger and larger through mergers and as communication technology changes how hospital care can be delivered. In the evening, he met with the leaders of the orthopedic medical group in town. He discussed with them a plan for upgrading the hospital's facilities for doing both outpatient and inpatient orthopedic procedures. The group was interested in partnering with the hospital in the creation of a new outpatient surgical facility.

That Tuesday was not a typical day because there are no typical days. Mr. Martin handles medical staff relations, business strategy for the hospital, financial planning, media relations, leadership of the senior administrative staff at the hospital, and many other matters. He represents the hospital to the state hospital association and sometimes testifies at the legislature on rural health issues.

Unlike many of his administrative colleagues in other institutions, Mr. Martin takes pains to stay in close contact with clinical care. For example, he visits the medical staff lounge frequently, often without any particular agenda in mind. When he enters the lounge on one of these unstructured visits, he looks to see which physicians are present and resumes conversations on topics that they had discussed several days or weeks ago. He also goes on "safety rounds" with physicians, surgeons, and nurses whom he knows particularly well. On these rounds, he and the clinicians visit patients and discuss (out of earshot of the patients) safety concerns and how they might be addressed by changing procedures or using new equipment. The Director of Patient Care is always present with him on these rounds.

Mr. Martin works about 55 hours per week although this number varies considerably from week to week. He often has meetings in the evening and on Saturdays. He does not work at night although an extreme emergency (for example, a hospital-wide computer failure) might some day require his participation.

Roles

Healthcare administrators lead and manage healthcare organizations. Medical and health services managers held about 303,000 jobs in 2010. About 39% worked in hospitals, and another 9% worked in offices of physicians. Many of the others worked in nursing care facilities, home healthcare services, and outpatient care centers (US Department of Labor, 2012).

Administrators are responsible for setting and monitoring organizational strategy, monitoring performance of the organization, and implementing the business functions of finance, human resource management, information management, marketing, and environmental management (maintenance of physical facilities). In complex settings like hospitals, administrators work with professionals in clinical support services, nursing, and the medical staff to monitor quality of care and customer service. Overall, Garman and colleagues (2006, p. 840) argue that "The administrators' role in sustaining the financial health of the organization sits in starkest contrast to the other professions." Administrators have an adage, "no margin, no mission," that asserts the importance of fiscal health as one of the goals of healthcare organizations. No other profession shoulders that responsibility to the extent that healthcare administration does.

Education

A master's degree in health administration (MHA), public health (MPH), or business administration (MBA) is the standard credential for most generalist positions in this field. Any of these may be followed by a fellowship of 1-2 years in a hospital or other healthcare institution.

However, a bachelor's degree is sufficient for some entry-level positions in smaller facilities, at the departmental level within hospitals, and in health information management. Physicians' offices and some other facilities often hire candidates with on-the-job experience instead of specified formal education. For people seeking to become heads of clinical departments, a degree in the appropriate clinical field (for example, a nursing degree) and work experience may be sufficient early in their careers. However, a master's degree in health administration, nursing administration, or a related field often is required to advance.

There is no requirement that healthcare administrators be licensed, except in the nursing home sector, and the educational requirement for nursing home administrator licensure typically is the bachelor's degree. As a result, the body of knowledge attained by healthcare administrators is apt to vary substantially depending on the level and source of their education. Those with public health degrees, for example, may have less extensive coursework in financial management than those with business administration degrees, and more extensive coursework in healthcare policy.

Values

Healthcare administrators generally have a *systems* view of their work. They draw attention to the effect of micro-level decisions (decisions at the patient-clinician level, for example) on the larger unit and organization, in terms of impact, precedence, and equity. They are loyal to their organizations and are favorably disposed toward its growth and success. Administrators are comfortable working in a chain of command, and they value interpersonal skill and organizational political skill. Having a practical orientation, administrators look for solutions that will work, as opposed to those that sound good in theory. *Evidence-based management* is a relatively new development in their field, relative to the clinical professions, promoting the increased use of research evidence on management decision making.

Administrators manage organizational performance on multiple dimensions, including but not limited to quality of care to patients. In particular, as noted earlier, fiscal performance is viewed as fundamental to the ability of the organization to continue to thrive in the long run.

The O*NET classification for administrators reflects the different values of administrators relative to clinical professionals. The interest profile of healthcare administrators is reported as Enterprising-Conventional-Social (see Table 3-2). The Enterprising category fits none of the other professions reviewed here as a primary interest. The Enterprising type commonly is associated with business careers and is described as having an orientation toward controlling others (Garman et al, 2006). The Conventional element of the profile is shared with pharmacists, and reflects an interest in following set procedures and routines. The Social element of the profile also appears in the profiles of all of the other professions we have examined earlier (though in various ranked positions), reflecting that all of the professions are "people" professions, with service to others as a shared value.

Teamwork Implications

Healthcare administrators tend to be comfortable working in teams. They understand that complex decisions are best made by effective teams—and effective teams are those whose members are comfortable with disagreement and trust that the team can work through conflict. Managers generally are more accepting of conflict and negotiation than are clinical professionals, recognizing that the best strategy for negotiation is *win-win* rather than *win-lose* (Smith, 2003, p. 611). Administrators' lack of professional status and understanding of clinical care (discussed in more detail in Chapter 5) can be a hindrance to their being fully accepted as members of healthcare teams.

OTHER PROFESSIONALS IN HEALTHCARE TEAMS

A wide variety of other professions are represented in interprofessional teams, more than can be mentioned. One cluster of these professions is sometimes referred to as *allied health professions*, although that term is not particularly informative and can be construed as labeling those professions as secondary in status to the referent professions to whom they are *allied*. The American Medical Association lists 18 allied health professions, including respiratory therapy, kinesiotherapy, and cardiovascular technology, for example, as well as more than 60 other professions that provide specialized care directly or indirectly to patients, sometimes practicing under medical supervision (American Medical Association, 2012). Among those distinct professions are audiology and speech-language pathology; dentistry and the related roles of dental assistant, dental hygienist, and dental laboratory technician; podiatrists; expressive or creative arts therapies including art therapy, dance/movement therapy, and music therapy; 11 professions within laboratory science; physical therapy and physical therapy assistants; occupational therapy and occupational therapy assistants; and veterinarians and veterinary technologists and technicians. Seven vision-related professions are listed in addition to ophthalmology (MDs or DOs), including optometrists, ophthalmic medical technicians, ophthalmic dispensing opticians, orientation and mobility specialists, orthoptists, and vision rehabilitation therapists. Public health workers are another category of healthcare team members, which includes epidemiologists, biostatisticians, environmental health and occupational health experts, nutritionists, health educators, community health workers, and many more specialties. The degree of specialization is staggering. Most of these professions are eligible for licensure or certification of some type.

The wide range of work activities and roles attract different personality types to each profession. The O*NET classification of interests, for example, lists Investigative as the top interest for medical technology, whose second and third rank interests are Realistic and Conventional. This profile is similar to that of surgeons, who have Social rather than Conventional in the third rank. Occupational therapy is classified as Social and Investigative, the same as social work. The interests of optometrists, Investigative-Social-Realistic, are the same as those of internists, while the profile for chiropractors, Social-Investigative-Realistic, mirrors the profile of NPs.

Health professions also can be clustered by the types of illnesses they strive to treat and prevent. One substantial and diverse cluster of such professions is the mental health professions. Some of these professionals, specializing in the care of patients with mental health problems, are psychiatrists (who hold MD or DO degrees), psychologists (PhD or PsyD), licensed professional counselors (MA or MS in psychology, counseling, or a similar discipline), marriage and family therapists (MA), and expressive therapy (MA). Many other health professions have a specialty in mental health. Social workers, nurses, pharmacists, physician assistants, and occupational therapists, for example, can all specialize in care for patients with mental illness or other mental health problems. The diversity of professions serving mental health patients makes it even more important that members of mental health care teams be familiar with the education and certification backgrounds of their colleagues.

Mental health professionals often function separately from general and other specialty healthcare, whether they practice alone or in mental health care teams. However, the depth of knowledge created by specialization in mental health enables these specialists to make valuable contributions to teams providing other forms of health care, especially primary care. Various initiatives are under way to integrate mental health care and primary care (Sanchez et al, 2010).

RECENT CHANGES IN ROLES AND EDUCATION

Of particular importance for teamwork in health care are several recent developments mentioned in the preceding portrayals of 3 of the professions—medicine, nursing, and pharmacy. The roles and education of healthcare social workers and healthcare administrators have remained relatively stable in recent decades, although that may change in future years, of course.

Physicians

Historically physicians have had a dominant role in healthcare delivery in the United States. This dominance has been manifest in almost all settings in which they participate, including teams. More recently this dominance has been challenged, especially by nursing and pharmacy. The upgraded educational credentials of nurses and pharmacists create a new dynamic in many healthcare teams, which requires adjustment by many physicians, especially those who have been in practice for many years.

Nurses

The educational requirements for many nursing roles are increasing and will continue to increase. In addition, the scope of practice of advanced practice nurses is broadening, particularly for NPs. NPs have prescription privileges, of varying degrees, in most states, and several states allow independent practice for NPs, some not requiring any physician involvement and some requiring a collaborative agreement with a physician. Several nurse-managed health centers offer health services directed by advanced practice nurses, primarily nurse practitioners (www.nncc.us). Teams can expect that nurses will take more assertive roles and leadership roles as this trend continues.

Pharmacists

The scope of pharmacy is expanding in the area of medication therapy management (MTM), with pharmacists carrying out functions that previously were performed only by physicians (Schommer et al, 2012). There is some resistance to this expansion within the profession of pharmacy. Those with misgivings cite lack of consensus regarding the profession's goals in this new arena, work environments that provide little or no opportunity for patient-centered practice, lack of reimbursement for pharmacists' clinical services, and underdevelopment of practitioners' interpersonal skills (American College of Clinical Pharmacy, 2000). Factors that appear likely to promote expansion of the pharmacist's role include expanded use of technology and technicians in the dispensing of medications, new opportunities for pharmacists in community, ambulatory, long-term care, and home care settings, pressure from managed care organizations to control pharmaceutical expenses, and the huge increase in the numbers of drugs used in patient care in recent decades. Many physicians and NPs welcome the input of pharmacists particularly regarding drugs they rarely prescribe and regarding interactions among drugs.

COMMON ALLIANCES AND CONFLICTS

The different education, roles, and values of health professions create some common patterns in healthcare team dynamics. A number of typical alliances and conflicts emerge on teams, even among just the 5 professions emphasized in this chapter. We note 4 examples of alliances and 4 examples of conflicts below. They are summarized in Tables 3–4 and 3–5. We generalize, of course, and all conflicts and alliances do not exhibit these patterns. The general point is that teams should expect alliances and conflicts to emerge and should be prepared to understand and manage those conflicts.

Nurses and physicians commonly unite on the primacy of patient care relative to cost considerations. In

Table 3–4. Common alliances among five health professions

Alliance	Issue
Nurses and physicians vs. social workers, pharmacists and administrators	Emphasis on patient care considerations (nurses and physicians) vs. cost considerations (social workers, pharmacists and administrators)
Nurses and social workers vs. physicans, pharmacists and administrators	Attend to person rather than disease (physicians), medications (pharmacists) or process of treatment (administrators)
Pharmacists and physicians vs. nurses and social workers	Greater importance of timely administration of drugs (pharmacists and physicians)
Social workers and administrators vs. nurses, physicians and pharmacists	Greater emphasis on community or population health concerns and resources (social workers and administrators)

Table 3-5. Common conflicts among five health professions

Conflicting Professions	Issue
Nurses vs. physicians	Focus on patient experience (nurses) vs. focus on disease (physicians)
Physicians vs. pharmacists	Who has greater expertise in prescribing drugs
Social workers vs. nurses	Greater breadth of community interventions (social workers)
Administrators vs. physicians and nurses	Greater focus on resource constraints (administrators)

contrast, pharmacists are attuned to cost issues from their education and their training as retail dispensers of pharmaceuticals. Both social workers as well as healthcare administrators are trained to be aware of the context in which health care is provided, including cost considerations. Thus nurses and physicians may be more likely to insist that patient care considerations trump cost considerations.

Nurses and social workers frequently ally on attending to the person as opposed to the disease. In contrast, physicians may focus on curing a specific disease; pharmacists on aspects of illness that can be affected by medication; and administrators on the efficiency of the *process* of attending to the person or the disease.

Pharmacists and physicians may unite on the importance of timely administration of drugs. Nurses and social workers may (relatively) downplay the potential importance of medication therapy in the overall health of the patient. Administrators will add the issue of cost to the discussion.

Social workers and administrators sometimes unite on the importance of considering health care in the larger social context, raising community or population concerns in addition to the interests of individual patients. In some settings, the potential strength of this alliance is vitiated because some administrators rank community and population health issues as less important than promoting the interests of their specific organizations.

In addition to common alliances, there are some common conflicts that emerge from differences among the 5 professions. First, nurses and physicians may disagree over whether to focus on the experience of the patient (nurses) or the disease (physicians). The conflict is based on the different definition of the problem held by the 2 professions.

Physicians and pharmacists sometimes have disputes about who is expert in prescribing drugs and who should perform the prescribing function. The opening vignette in this chapter, concerning a newly graduated pharmacist, illustrates the historical dominance of medicine in medication expertise, which is now being complemented by pharmacy's expertise.

Social workers and nurses sometimes vie over helping the patient psychologically, with social workers drawing on a wider range of community interventions than nursing. Again, this distinction is based on the underlying community systems perspective of social work and the greater familiarity of social workers with the wide range of community resources and the living conditions of their clients.

Physicians and nurses often have conflicts with administrators over how organizational funds should be used. As noted earlier, the work of administrators involves setting limits on organizational expenditures and setting priorities among competing organizational needs for funds and resources such as staff and equipment. Administrators often can be cast as the adversary by physicians, nurses, and other clinicians who are less constrained by their roles in advocating for more funding and more resources for particular components of patient care. The clinicians typically will present as stronger advocates of patients and patient care quality.

CONCLUSION

Most healthcare professionals identify passionately with their professions, a passion engendered by years of study, training, and socialization. Each healthcare profession has a rich and unique history, a distinctive work domain, and its own educational pathways, professional journals, professional associations, rituals, heroes, and heroines. The differentiation that results from these professional identities makes cross-understanding a vital component of successful interprofessional teamwork.

The common roles, education, and values of different health professions give each profession a distinctive character on teams. It is useful for team members to know and expect distinctive contributions from those in other professions. For example, physicians' actions frequently reflect their scientific background and focus on finding an evidence-based cure. Nurses may focus on understanding the patient's perspective and treating the whole person as opposed to the disease. Pharmacists hone in on the pharmaceutical needs of patients. Social workers commonly interpret patients' situations in light of their socioeconomic position and their connection to family, social, and community resources. Administrators remind teams of the need to be well organized and fiscally prudent. All of the 5 professions emphasized in this chapter and the multitude of other health professions have valuable contributions to make to team decisions and team outcomes.

In the next chapter, we consider those team members who are central to healthcare teams but are not healthcare professionals, that is, patients and their families.

REFERENCES

Abbott A. *The System of Professions: An Essay on the Division of Expert Labor*. Chicago, IL: University of Chicago Press; 1988.

American Association of Colleges of Nursing. *AACN Position Statement on the Practice Doctorate in Nursing.* October 2004. http://www.aacn.nche.edu/DNP/pdf/DNP.pdf. Accessed March 23, 2012.

American Board of Medical Specialties (ABMS). *About ABMS Medical Boards.* 2012. http://www.abms.org/about_abms/member_boards.aspx. Accessed March 23, 2012.

American College of Clinical Pharmacy. A vision of pharmacy's future roles, responsibilities, and manpower needs in the United States. *Pharmacotherapy.* 2000;20:991-1020.

American Medical Association. *Careers in Health Care.* Chicago, IL: American Medical Association; 2012. http://www.ama-assn.org/ama/pub/education-careers/careers-health-care/directory.page? Accessed March 23, 2012.

American Medical Association. *International Medical Graduates in American Medicine: Contemporary Challenges and Opportunities.* Chicago, IL: American Medical Association; 2010. http://www.ama-assn.org/resources/doc/img/img-workforce-paper.pdf. Accessed October 27, 2012.

American Osteopathic Association. *2010 Osteopathic Medical Profession Report.* Chicago, IL: American Osteopathic Association. http://www.osteopathic.org/inside-aoa/about/who-we-are/Documents/Osteopathic-Medical-Profession-Report-2010.pdf. Accessed October 27, 2012.

Begun JW, Lippincott RC. *Strategic Adaptation in the Health Professions: Meeting the Challenges of Change.* San Francisco, CA: Jossey-Bass; 1993.

Begun JW, White KR. The profession of nursing as a complex adaptive system: strategies for change. In: Kronenfeld JJ, ed. *Research in the Sociology of Health Care.* Vol 16. Greenwich, CT: JAI Press; 1999:189-203.

Bodenheimer T, Grumbach K. *Understanding Health Policy: A Clinical Approach.* 6th ed. New York, NY: McGraw-Hill; 2012.

Carney BT, West P, Neily J, et al. Differences in nurse and surgeon perceptions of teamwork: implications for use of a briefing checklist in the OR. *AORN J.* 2010;91:722-729.

Cassel CK, Reuben DB. Specialization, subspecialization, and subsubspecialization in internal medicine. *N Engl J Med.* 2011;364(12):1169-1173.

Clark PG. Values in health care professional socialization: implications for geriatric education in interdisciplinary teamwork. *Gerontologist.* 1997;37:441-451.

Freidson E. *Professionalism Reborn.* Chicago, IL: University of Chicago Press; 1994.

Freidson E. *Professionalism: The Third Logic.* Chicago, IL: University of Chicago Press; 2001.

Garman AN, Leach DC, Spector N. Worldviews in collision: conflict and collaboration across professional lines. *J Organ Behav.* 2006;27:829-849.

Hofstede G, Hofstede GJ. *Cultures and Organizations.* 2nd ed. New York, NY: McGraw-Hill; 2004.

Holden LM, Watt DD, Walker PH. Communication and collaboration: it's about the pharmacists, as well as the physicians and nurses. *BMJ Qual Saf.* 2010;19:169-172.

Holland JL. *Making Vocational Choices: A Theory of Vocational Personalities and Work Environments.* 3rd ed. Odessa, FL: Psychological Assessment Resources; 1997.

Huber GP, Lewis K. Cross-understanding: implications for group cognition and performance. *Acad Manage Rev.* 2010;35:6-26.

Kaiser Family Foundation. *statehealthfacts.org.* 2012. www.statehealthfacts.org. Accessed November 2, 2012.

Lawrence PR, Lorsch JW. Differentiation and integration in complex organizations. *Adm Sci Q.* 1967;12:1-47.

National Association of Clinical Nurse Specialists. *Advanced Practice Registered Nurses: The Clinical Nurse Specialists (CNS).* 2012. http://www.nacns.org/docs/APRN-Factsheet.pdf. Accessed November 2, 2012.

O'Leary KJ, Ritter CD, Wheeler H, et al. Teamwork on inpatient medical units: assessing attitudes and barriers. *BMJ Qual Saf.* 2010;19:117-121.

Rounds J, Armstrong PI, Liao, H, et al. *Second Generation Occupational Interest Profiles for the O*Net System: Summary.* Raleigh, NC: National Center for O*Net Development; 2008. www.onetcenter.org/dl_files/SecondOIP_Summary.pdf. Accessed November 4, 2012.

Rounds J, Smith T, Hubert L, et al. *Development of Occupational Interest Profiles for O*Net.* Raleigh, NC: National Center for O*Net Development; 1999. www.onetcenter.org/dl_files/OIP.pdf. Accessed November 4, 2012.

Sanchez K, Thompson S, Alexander L. Current strategies and barriers to integrated health care: a survey of publicly funded providers in Texas. *Gen Hosp Psychiatry.* 2010;32:26-32.

Schommer JC, Doucette WR, Johnson KA, et al. Positioning and integrating medication therapy management. *J Am Pharm Assoc.* 2012;52:12-24.

Sharpe D, Curran V. In: Kitto S, Chesters J, Thistlethwaite J, et al, eds. *Sociology of Interprofessional Health Care Practice: Critical Reflections and Concrete Solutions.* New York, NY: Nova Science Publishers; 2011:69-85.

Smith R. What doctors and managers can learn from each other. *BMJ.* 2003;326:610-611.

US Census Bureau. *Statistical Abstract of the United States: 2012 (131st Edition).* Washington, DC; 2011. http://www.census.gov/compendia/statab/. Accessed October 1, 2012.

US Department of Labor. O*Net Online Resource Center. 2010. http://www.onetcenter.org/overview.html. Accessed September 29, 2012.

US Department of Labor. *Occupational Outlook Handbook, 2012-13 Edition.* 2012. http://www.bls.gov/ooh/home.htm. Accessed November 2, 2012.

Young A, Chaudhry JH, Rhyne J, et al. 2011. A census of actively licensed physicians in the United States, 2010. *Journal of Medical Regulation.* 2011;96(4):10-20.

Patients and Families in Healthcare Teams

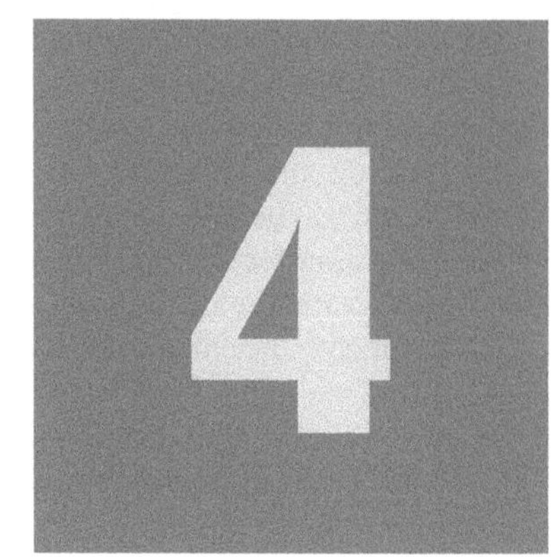

The previous chapter deals with the healthcare professionals who are found in healthcare teams. Now we turn to the person at the center of each team, namely, the patient. Patients sometimes are referred to as *clients* by some healthcare professionals, especially social workers. By using the word *patient* we do not mean to suggest any disagreement with those who prefer to use the word *client.* Specifically, we do not mean to imply that all patients are or should be passive or dependent. Of course, sometimes patients *are* dependent—for example, when they are acutely ill and cannot think and act normally, say, because of severe chest pain or the effects of a life-threatening infection. But these examples of dependency are unusual. Most of the time patients are fully capable of making decisions about their care. Nurses, physicians, pharmacists, and most other healthcare professionals ordinarily use the word *patient* when referring to a person who is receiving health care. Since these professionals comprise most of the readership for this book, we use the word *patient* too.

Others may refer to patients as *consumers* or *customers.* If we were thinking of people who are choosing health insurance or choosing which clinic to select for care—especially if they have no immediate need for health care—these terms might be appropriate. But this is a book for people who are providing care, not a book for people who are marketing or selling health insurance or health services. We have more to say about consumers and consumerism below.

PATIENT-CENTERED CARE

In 2001, the Institute of Medicine (IOM) published *Crossing the Quality Chasm* (Institute of Medicine, 2001). This book changed how the quality of health care is conceptualized in the healthcare professions in the United States. Echoes from its pages are still heard today and probably will continue to be heard for many more years. Among other innovations, the IOM report provided a functional definition of quality that has become the standard starting point for endeavors to measure healthcare quality and improve it.

Prior to the publication of *Crossing the Quality Chasm*, the most commonly quoted definition of quality in health care came from an IOM report issued 11 years earlier. That report defined quality as "the degree to which health services for individuals and populations increase the likelihood of desired health outcomes and are consistent with current professional knowledge" (Institute of Medicine, 1990, p. 21). While the 1990 definition was an improvement on earlier definitions and served its purposes, in hindsight the definition is remarkable for what it leaves out, namely, any reference to patients and to the goals that patients have in seeking health care. The 1990 definition is crafted from the viewpoint of healthcare professionals. It implies, without directly stating so, that defining healthcare quality is a task appropriate for individuals who can judge whether health services "are consistent with professional knowledge" and that their proper central concern is whether health services achieve "desired health outcomes." In other words, the assumed touchstone for quality is whether health care cures disease or, if cure is not possible, alleviates symptoms. There is no mention of how patients experience their care, whether they receive comfort and emotional support, whether their questions are answered, or whether they play any role in the process of care.

The definition offered in *Crossing the Quality Chasm* in 2001 was not a refinement of the earlier definition. The newer definition represented a major shift in understanding the elements of good health care (Berwick, 2009). The 2001 report framed its definition in terms of 6 aims for the improvement of care, stating that "health care should be safe, effective, patient-centered, timely, efficient, and equitable" (IOM, 2001, p. 40). There are 4 new elements in this definition as contrasted with the 1990 definition. Safety and effectiveness are implied by the earlier definition, but patient-centeredness, timeliness, efficiency, and equity are all new. Although all of these aims are important, the purpose of this chapter is to explain the role of the patient in healthcare teams; and so we focus on the concept of patient-centeredness. The other 5 aims are discussed in Chapter 6.

In advocating that care be patient-centered, the authors of *Crossing the Quality Chasm* might have meant that care should be more tightly focused on treating diseases as they appear in different forms or presentations in particular individuals. In that case, the IOM definition would have continued the professional orientation of the 1990 definition. However, it is clear that the authors of the report meant to propose a different and much broader notion of patient-centeredness. The report highlighted the need to eliminate patients' frustrations with being blocked from participating in decision making and their frustrations in obtaining information about their own situations and about health care generally (IOM, 2001, pp. 48-51). The report also called for "respect for patients' values, preferences, and expressed needs." In other words, patient-centeredness means satisfying not only patients' needs, which might be determined by the professionals using their views of what is needed, but also patients' wants, which can be known only if patients state what their wants are or are asked about them (Berwick, 2009, pp. w558-w559). Alternatively, one could say that patient-centeredness means fashioning care so that it serves the patients' interests *as defined by them*, not by the professionals who provide their health care.

The essence of patient-centered care is recognition of the autonomy, dignity, sensibility, and self-awareness of the individual patient. It stands in contrast to what is usually called *paternalistic care*, in which patients are regarded essentially as children who do not have the ability or the right to make good decisions about their own health care. It also stands in contrast to a degraded form of paternalism in which the thoughts and feelings of patients are neglected and patients are treated essentially as mammals in need of repair.

Although *Crossing the Quality Chasm* brought patient-centeredness to the forefront of discussions about healthcare quality, it actually has a history of many decades. An early expression of this value in the United States came from William J. Mayo, co-founder of Mayo Clinic, who said in a 1910 medical school commencement address, "The best interest of the patient is the only interest to be considered" (Mayo, 2000, p. 554). Dr. Mayo's statement is not entirely unambiguous in that he does not say who is expected to determine the patient's interest. It is possible that he meant for the patient's interest to be determined by the physician, who has special knowledge that the patient does not have. But even if this was his meaning, his statement foreshadowed the future by asserting that the proper aim of health care is advancing the patient's interest instead of making best use of professional knowledge. As the 20th century progressed, the role of science in health care expanded, and medicine placed increasing emphasis on identifying and repairing defects in human bodies seen as biological machines. By about 1950, a growing number of nurses, physicians, and others began to confront the limitations of health care conceived primarily as biological investigation and repair. The term *patient-centered approach* first appeared in the nursing literature about 1960 (Martin, 1960). In Britain, Michael Balint, a physician and psychoanalyst, created study groups in which general practitioners could improve their abilities to understand their patients' experiences of illness and medical care (Balint, 1964). In the United States, George Engel, an internist and psychiatrist, promoted medical practice that integrates knowledge of a patient's physiological function with an understanding of the patient's psychological and social life (Engel, 1977). Later, Susan Edgman-Levitan and her colleagues in the Picker/Commonwealth Program for Patient-Centered Care developed the concept of patient-centeredness and devised criteria for measuring whether care is patient-centered (Gerteis et al, 1993). Similar inquiries led to the development of narrative medicine, which emphasizes the value of understanding the patient's story of his or her illness, including his or her experience of health care (Greenhalgh and Hurwitz, 1999). Over the past 35 years, Moira Stewart and others, located mainly in Canada, have developed the *patient-centered clinical method*, which emphasizes understanding the patient's experience of illness, life history, and social context as the basis for finding common ground on which the clinician and patient establish goals for working together to improve the patient's health (Stewart et al, 2003). Patient-centered care has remained an important concept in nursing education and nursing practice in the decades since discussion of the concept first appeared in print in 1960. Alleviating vulnerability, whether physiological or psychological, has been a central component of the concept as it has been interpreted in nursing (Hobbs, 2009). The people mentioned here and many others have contributed to changing the focus of clinical care from repairing the machine to regarding the whole person with respect as an autonomous, dignified human being.

The authors of *Crossing the Quality Chasm* drew on all of these developments. They did, however, also add something new and important. Patient-centered medicine, narrative medicine, and the other approaches noted above are all concerned with improving the way that individual clinicians go about doing their work in diagnosing and caring for one patient at a time. In these approaches, patient-centeredness, whether or not this term is used explicitly, is conceived as a property of individual clinical practice. In *Crossing the Quality Chasm*, patient-centeredness is presented not only as a characteristic of the work of individual healthcare professionals but also as a characteristic of the operations of health systems. In other words, the authors of the IOM report urged whole healthcare institutions to be patient-centered. This broadening of the concept leads immediately to questions about teamwork in institutions, the physical appearance and function of healthcare facilities, billing procedures, reward systems for employees of hospitals, and so on. Expanded in this way, patient-centeredness brings together systems thinking and the concept of the patient as person (instead of the patient as biological machine). This combination sets the stage for understanding how patients can and should participate in healthcare teams—if they choose to do so.

CONSUMERISM

We noted earlier that some individuals refer to patients as consumers. Many clinicians, especially physicians, bristle at the notion of patient-centeredness because they think it signals consumerism insinuating itself into health care. Some object because they do not believe that patients should be in charge. We offer no defense for that viewpoint. Other clinicians object even though they do believe that patients should be in charge if they want to be.

Does the IOM concept of patient-centeredness imply that patients should be regarded as consumers? Maybe. It depends on what the word *consumer* is taken to imply.

If health care is to serve patients' interests as defined by them, then the patients are in charge—just as someone buying a refrigerator or purchasing a lawn mowing service is in charge. If patients are in charge, they remain dependent on healthcare professionals for information about their diseases and treatment options, but they are no longer dependent on the professionals to make decisions about their care. Instead the dependency for decisions is reversed, and the professionals must take their cues from the patients. With this reversal, patients are no longer the passive recipients of health care deemed appropriate for them by the professionals. Patients decide what they will receive—and how and when. Evidently, they become consumers. As described in one influential book on doctor-patient communication, consumerism is one legitimate prototype for interactions between patients and healthcare professionals. (In that account, the other legitimate prototypes are paternalism and mutuality.) And consumerism has sweeping implications:

> *Caveat emptor, "let the buyer beware," rules the transaction, with power resting in the buyer (patient) who can make the decision to buy (seek care) or not, as the patient sees fit. The physician's role is limited to that of a technical consultant who has the obligation to provide information and services that are contingent on the patient's preferences (and within professional norms). (Roter and Hall, 2006, p. 27)*

But this line of reasoning overreaches. Labeling patients as consumers suggests that the relationships between a patient and those who provide his or her health care are commercial relationships. If patients and healthcare professionals relate to one another fundamentally as buyers and sellers, then apparently both the patients and the professionals may engage in frankly commercial behavior. For example, the seller apparently is permitted or even expected to exaggerate claims of effectiveness, contrive to hide ignorance, and stimulate demand artificially. Cautioning the buyer to beware implies that there is something to beware of, something that the healthcare professionals may deliberately not disclose. The warning *caveat emptor* makes sense only if misrepresentation and evasion are real possibilities—as they are in some commercial dealings.

Incidentally, Dr. Mayo would have been dismayed if he could have foreseen that in the 21st century patients might become consumers who need to beware. At the time of Dr. Mayo's commencement address mentioned earlier, patients were emerging from a time when they did indeed need to beware. In his speech, he applauded the end of the pre-scientific era in medicine, when physicians had "stage properties," "charlatanism," and "commercial instincts" (Mayo, 2000).

Labeling patients as consumers also suggests that various limits on the behavior of patients no longer apply because the customer (or consumer) is always right and is not bound by evidence about the effectiveness of various treatments. Apparently, patients as consumers may request and receive treatments for which evidence of effectiveness is lacking and treatments for which there is evidence of ineffectiveness. Perhaps they will demand and receive treatments that are actually harmful. Perhaps they will demand unlimited time from physicians, nurses, and others. Perhaps they will, in general, behave like some demanding customers when they are buying television sets or airline tickets to Paris.

In fact, the writers of *Crossing the Quality Chasm* did not use the terms *consumer* or *consumerism* and did not intend to encourage a return of unrestrained commercialism in health care. Patient-centeredness *does* imply an end to unqualified professional authority. However, an end to unqualified authority does not mean the end of professionalism. A profession is not simply a conspiracy to maintain status and control. Members of a profession have responsibilities to put the interests of those whom they serve ahead of their own interests, to maintain their professional knowledge and skills, and to use their knowledge and skills with integrity—hiding nothing and being forthcoming and truthful in providing any information that is requested and any information that would be useful to those whom the professionals serve, even if those who are served do not know enough to ask for the information. Society has every reason to maintain these aspects of healthcare professionalism even though the patients have the last word. Patients do not expect or want to have commercial relationships with their nurses, physicians, and pharmacists. They want the professionals to remain professional. Conflating patients with consumers generates undesirable suggestions for professionals and for what patients can expect from professionals.

If labeling patients as consumers is meant to mark the principle that patients have final say in their own health care, well and good. However, if consumerism in health care were to mean that patients must beware because healthcare professionals are released from their obligations as professionals and have entered the commercial world, then both patients and society as a whole would be harmed. If consumerism were to mean that patients are now marketplace consumers, the consequences would also be undesirable. Patients then would no longer be expected to attend either to evidence about healthcare effectiveness or to the fact that ordinarily most of the costs are paid by someone other than the patients—a situation sharply different from that of real consumers. These understandable interpretations of consumerism, taken from our understanding of consumerism in other economic sectors and imported into health care, are both unwelcome and unnecessary. Moreover, they are unwanted by both patients and healthcare professionals.

In the end, the undesirable implications of consumerism in health care are probably the result of a simple confusion, invited by the word *consumer*. Perhaps we need a new term to label the relationship between patients-in-charge and healthcare professionals who retain professional obligations. Instead of *consumerism*, it could be called *clientism*. In any case, embracing patient-centeredness as an aim in health care does not require embracing consumerism as that concept is usually understood. A healthcare team that provides patient-centered care does not need to regard its patients as consumers. As Dr. Mayo said in 1921, "Commercialism in medicine never leads to true satisfaction, and to maintain our self-respect is more precious than gold" (Camilleri et al, 2005, p. 1341). The same could be said of commercialism among patients.

ENABLING PATIENTS TO PARTICIPATE IN DECISION MAKING

Patient-centeredness is a desirable feature of team-based health care, and the concept provides a touchstone or reference point for understanding the different roles that patients (and their families) can have in the decision making that occurs in healthcare teams. Patient-centered care raises both opportunities and problems that do not arise with paternalistic care, and these will be considered below. But let us first use the touchstone to differentiate 3 stories about patients participating in teams.

Asking Someone Else to Make Decisions

Adam Trudell was a 54-year-old writer and political activist, living in Rapid City, South Dakota. Mr. Trudell had a long history in literature and in politics, having published 4 novels and having served in the federal Bureau of Indian Affairs and in Congress. His education included a bachelor's degree and a master's degree in public administration. However, he had no education in the natural sciences beyond an introductory geology course in college.

Mr. Trudell had known for several years that he had heart disease, specifically, narrowed passages in the arteries supplying blood to his heart (coronary artery disease). His first symptom was chest pain that occurred while he was running. Once he began using medication, he was able to exercise again, but occasionally he still had chest pain with exertion.

One evening while eating dinner, Mr. Trudell experienced crushing chest pain that did not relent when he tried using nitroglycerin under his tongue. Mary Trudell, his wife, telephoned 911, and he was transported to the hospital. Linda Hill, RN, an emergency department (ED) nurse, greeted him, took a brief history, measured his blood pressure, and attached electrocardiographic monitor wires to his chest with small adhesive pads. James Dudik, MD, the ED physician, then took a longer history, did a physical examination, and ordered several tests. He then advised Mr. Trudell that he recommended immediate x-ray investigation of Mr. Trudell's coronary arteries (angiography), to be followed by opening of any arterial blockage that might be found (angioplasty). Mr. Trudell asked 2 or 3 questions about what the procedure would involve. Dr. Dudik then asked Mr. Trudell whether he wished to go ahead with the procedure or be transferred to the Coronary Care Unit, where he would be treated without angiography or angioplasty.

Mr. Trudell paused for a moment, still in pain. He looked at Ms. Hill and then looked back to Dr. Dudik, but he said nothing. Then he asked Dr. Dudik to do as he thought best. Dr. Dudik asked whether he should explain the situation to Ms. Trudell and ask her to make the decision. Mr Trudell responded by repeating that he wanted Dr. Dudik to do as he thought best. A cardiologist was called, and Mr. Trudell was transferred to the catheterization laboratory for angiography.

At first glance, it might appear that Mr. Trudell's care was paternalistic rather than patient-centered. Mr. Trudell behaved passively, and Dr. Dudik made the important decision about angiography. But passivity on the part of the patient does not by itself mean that the patient is receiving paternalistic care. Whether care is patient-centered depends on the attitude and behavior of the care giver or the healthcare team.

Mr. Trudell's care was patient-centered because Dr. Dudik respected Mr. Trudell's autonomy and dignity. Dr. Dudik began with the assumption that Mr. Trudell would make the decision about angiography. When Mr. Trudell said that he did not want to make the decision, Dr. Dudik again showed that he was treating Mr. Trudell as a person by asking him whether he wanted Ms. Trudell to serve as his agent in making the decision. The vignette does not make clear why Mr. Trudell declined to take this pathway. Perhaps he had good reason to think that his wife would also defer to Dr. Dudik. In any case, Mr. Trudell had every opportunity to be in charge. His thoughts, feelings, values, and goals were respected. He exercised his self-determination by choosing not to be the one to make an important decision about his care. This is one role open to patients as members of healthcare teams.

There is another issue to clarify here. Mr. Trudell was in pain when he made his decision not to make a decision about his care. Did he make that decision competently, or did Dr. Dudik do him a disservice by accepting his statement that he wanted Dr. Dudik to make the decision? This question often arises. Sometimes pain diminishes a patient's capacity to think clearly and make a decision. Sometimes emotional turmoil interferes with clear thinking. Sometimes the patient has a decreased level of consciousness due to serious illness or injury. Clinicians must always be attentive to the possibility that the patient is not able to make a valid decision, and, if so, must engage a surrogate, usually a family member, to act on behalf of the patient when that is practical. In this case, Dr. Dudik might have tactfully insisted on engaging Ms. Trudell in the process if he believed that Mr. Trudell was sufficiently incapacitated. This could have taken the form of Dr. Dudik speaking separately with Ms. Trudell; but a gentler approach, more attentive to Mr. Trudell's expressed wishes, would have been for Dr. Dudik simply to draw Ms. Trudell into the conversation that Dr. Dudik and Mr. Trudell were having. If a patient is not able to make decisions for herself or himself, making sure that the decisions are being made by a person who can truly speak for the patient—because that person knows the patient's values and beliefs—is part of providing patient-centered care. Attending to the patient's capacity for decision making is quite obviously appropriate when she or he is making decisions about what actions will be taken in the process of care, that is, what tests will be done and what treatments will be used. Attending to the patient's ability to make decisions is also necessary when the patient is deciding what role she or he will have in the healthcare team.

Partnering on Decision Making

Rheumatoid arthritis is a chronic, highly variable disease, sometimes no more than a serious nuisance for people who have it, sometimes a serious disability for them. Many treatments are available. Some of the treatments have no significant side effects; some of them carry substantial risk.

Isabella Belmonte, age 62, was married with 2 adult children and 4 grandchildren. She worked as an executive assistant in a financial services firm in New York. For 30 years, she had had rheumatoid arthritis. The disease first affected her knees and later also affected her wrists and hands.

Ms. Belmonte received care for her arthritis from a rheumatologist whom she had been seeing for 16 years. She also had a family physician, but she had no significant health problems except for the arthritis, and so she saw her family physician only for preventive care and minor, short-term health problems.

Ms. Belmonte and Dr. Mancuso, her rheumatologist, had an excellent relationship. Ms. Belmonte had been referred to Dr. Mancuso by her family physician, who thought they would get along well. In fact, they got along magnificently. Ms. Belmonte felt that Dr. Mancuso understood her very well. He understood the central place of family in her life, the importance of her work to her, her need to maintain a good income to contribute to her family's well-being, and her delight in interacting with her grandchildren.

Ms. Belmonte had been through many treatments for her arthritis over 30 years. She began with ibuprofen and later used steroids intermittently, both prescribed by her family physician. When these drugs no longer provided adequate relief, her family physician referred her to Dr. Mancuso for more aggressive treatment. Dr. Mancuso discussed with her the use of methotrexate, immunosuppressants, and other drugs, including the drugs' prospects for success and their risks, for example, risk of liver damage and risk of infection. Together they decided whether she would use these more potent drugs. Over the years she had used 4 different drug combinations. Each time a change was made, she and Dr. Mancuso discussed what might lie ahead, how likely it was that an improvement would be achieved with the new regimen, and how her family and work lives might be disrupted if she experienced adverse effects of the drugs.

Dr. Mancuso practiced with 2 other rheumatologists. The office also included a clinical nurse specialist and a physical therapist. Ms. Belmonte had frequent interactions with both of them and learned a great deal from them about how to reduce her symptoms and cope with her disease.

Ms. Belmonte saw herself as a member of her healthcare team. In particular, she viewed herself and Dr. Mancuso as partners in managing her disease. She regarded their decision making about her treatment as shared decision making.

Ms. Belmonte received patient-centered care from Dr. Mancuso's team, but her role in her own health care was quite different from the role chosen by Mr. Trudell in the earlier vignette. Ms. Belmonte's choice for how she interacted with her care providers exemplifies a second option for the role of a patient in his or her healthcare team. She was not passive, but neither was she straightforwardly in charge. She did not want to be the supervisor of her own care; she wanted to be a partner.

She did not regard Dr. Mancuso with suspicion. She did not think that he might be inclined to force her into treatments that he favored but that she might not want. She did not think that he might be exaggerating the effectiveness of new medications or minimizing the prospect of side effects. Ms. Belmonte did not think that she was a buyer who needed to beware, and Dr. Mancuso did not regard her as a consumer.

The question of who was in charge of her care never came up explicitly. From the questions she asked and from her responses to the various treatment options he discussed, Dr. Mancuso could see how Ms. Belmonte wanted to participate in her care. He found it easy to understand her values and goals in life. He presented treatment options that he thought were consistent with her values and likely to serve her goals. Sometimes they discussed her goals as part of making shared decisions. For example, at one point, they delayed beginning a new medication because of the chance that a side effect might prevent her from attending her granddaughter's confirmation. During the delay, she continued to experience pain that was later relieved by the new medication without any side effects. But before she began taking the new medication, there was no way to know what might happen, and Ms. Belmonte did not want to risk missing the confirmation. This choice made sense to her and to Dr. Mancuso. Very little discussion was needed.

Ms. Belmonte felt understood and respected. She knew that her experience of her illness and her health care were important to Dr. Mancuso and to the nurse and the physical therapist in Dr. Mancuso's office. Her questions were always answered as fully as she wished. She had no doubt that her values and goals governed the treatment choices that she made with Dr. Mancuso. The whole process worked very smoothly.

Making Decisions for One's Self

Dorothy Montgomery, age 36, was a high school teacher in St. Louis. She was married and had children aged 10 and 8. As was her custom roughly once a year, she saw Jane Bartnik, her gynecological nurse practitioner (NP) for a health check-up shortly before Thanksgiving. To Ms. Montgomery's dismay, Ms. Bartnik found a lump in Ms. Montgomery's left breast. A mammogram and several other tests were done, confirming the presence of a solid lump in the left breast, but there were no indications that there might be cancer elsewhere. Ms. Bartnik referred Ms. Montgomery to Wanda Richmond, MD, a surgeon in the same medical group. Dr. Richmond obtained tissue samples by inserting a needle through Ms. Montgomery's skin into the lump (core needle biopsy). Examination of the tissue under a microscope revealed invasive ductal carcinoma, that is, breast cancer.

Even before the mammogram was done, Ms. Montgomery began gathering information about breast cancer. First, she spoke with 2 friends who had undergone treatment for breast cancer within the past few years. She then asked her NP for suggestions of websites and consulted several of them: the BJC HealthCare website, the National Cancer Institute website, and others.

After the biopsy showed that the lump was cancerous, Ms. Montgomery and her husband returned to Dr. Richmond to discuss treatment options. Ms. Montgomery was well aware that the breast cancer represented a threat to her life. She had many questions. Although she was agitated and sometimes had difficulty maintaining her concentration, for the most part she directed the conversation. At times her husband reminded her to ask questions that the 2 of them had discussed in advance. Dr. Richmond answered her first few questions in detail but then the answers became shorter, and eventually Dr. Richmond said that she thought Ms. Montgomery should have the lump removed along with lymph nodes from the armpit adjacent to the breast with the lump. The tumor tissue would then be tested, and further treatment would depend upon the results of the surgery and tests. Ms. Montgomery tried to ask some additional hypothetical questions about choices to be made once the results were known. She was already well informed about most of the tests and what they might show. Dr. Richmond indicated tactfully but firmly that she thought further exploration of hypothetical possibilities was not appropriate until the lump was removed and tested.

Ms. Montgomery left Dr. Richmond's office disappointed. She was anxious. To cope with the situation and to make the necessary decisions, she felt she needed to understand fully what might lay ahead. She discussed her views with her husband and decided to seek another surgeon, one who would answer her questions.

Ms. Montgomery did not receive patient-centered care. The role she sought—but was not permitted—is a third option for patients participating in their own healthcare teams, a role different from the one chosen by Mr. Trudell and different from the one chosen by Ms. Belmonte. Ms. Montgomery wanted more than partnership in making decisions about her care. She wanted to make the decisions herself. She wanted to discuss the situation thoroughly with her surgeon, other physicians, and her husband, but she did not want her surgeon (or anyone else) to make the final decisions. Nor was she interested in shared decision making.

Dr. Richmond was polite but did not accept Ms. Montgomery's concept of her role as a patient. Dr. Richmond appeared to believe that she knew best and that it served no useful purpose to discuss a long list of questions—and possibly that a long discussion would cause harm by adding to Ms. Montgomery's distress. The surgeon intended to discuss matters further with Ms. Montgomery and her husband after testing provided more information about the cancer, information that would narrow the range of possible courses of action and thus simplify the discussion. There was a mismatch between Ms. Montgomery's choice of role in her health care and the role that her surgeon was willing to permit her to have. The surgeon's care of her was not centered on Ms. Montgomery's wants and needs. The failure of Dr. Richmond to provide what Ms. Montgomery wanted highlights the nature of the role that Ms. Montgomery sought and the gap between patient-centered care and the care that Dr. Richmond thought was appropriate. Ms. Montgomery had a clear notion of how she wanted to participate in her own healthcare team. It was also clear to her that it was time to move on to some other surgeon and team.

Models of the Patient-Team Relationship

The roles of Mr. Trudell and Ms. Belmonte, and the role that Ms. Montgomery sought (but was not permitted to exercise), can be drawn together in a framework for understanding the roles that patients can have in healthcare teams. These roles represent variants of patient-centered care, each variant flowing from a different choice available to the patient.

Table 4–1 summarizes different models of the patient-team relationship. For the health care of small

Table 4–1. Models of the patient-team relationship

	Model		
Feature of the Model	Paternalism-by-Permission	Partnership	Patient-in-Charge
Patient selects model?	Yes	Yes	Yes
Decision maker	Healthcare professional (or the professionals in the team)	Both the patient (or a surrogate) and the healthcare professional (or professionals in the team) decide jointly	Patient (or, rarely, a surrogate)
Source of information about the patient's values and goals	Patient (or a surrogate, usually a family member)	Patient (or a surrogate, usually a family member)	Patient (or a surrogate, usually a family member)
Source of healthcare information (about disease, options for diagnosis, options for treatment, prognosis)	Healthcare professional (or professionals in the team)	Usually the healthcare professional (or professionals in the team), but sometimes both the patient and healthcare professionals	Often both the patient and the healthcare professional (or professionals in the team)
Weighing of options	Healthcare professional (or professionals in the team)	Both the patient and the healthcare professional (or professionals in the team)	Patient, but often including the healthcare professional (or professionals in the team)
Does the patient have a veto?	Yes	Yes	Yes
Does the healthcare professional (or team) have a veto?	Yes	Yes	Yes

children, the models are models of the parent-team relationship. Although the models do apply to doctor-patient relationships they are not limited to patients and physicians. They apply to the relationships between the patient and each of the members of the healthcare team and the team as whole. If, at a given point in time, the patient is interacting with only one healthcare professional, then the relationship is the patient-doctor relationship, or the patient-nurse relationship, and so on.

The relationship models pertain to the roles of patients in true teams, template teams, and knotworks, as described in Chapter 2. Patients participate only very rarely in clinical networks, which are not genuine teams in any case. The relationship models do not apply to certain template teams because some template teams are assembled and complete their tasks so quickly that there is no opportunity for the patient (or a surrogate decision maker) to participate in any decision making. Examples of these short-lived template teams are emergency resuscitation teams ("code blue" teams) and emergency room teams operating under conditions of extreme urgency.

Paternalism-by-Permission

Three models are shown in Table 4–1. The first is called *paternalism-by-permission*. Mr. Trudell chose to relate to his healthcare team in accordance with this model. The relationship between the patient and team in this model results from the patient deciding that he or she wants decisions to be made by a healthcare professional (or professionals) and not by himself or herself. For fundamental decisions about actions to be taken for diagnosis or treatment, the healthcare professional will usually be a physician. But in some situations, the professional could be a nurse practitioner, a pharmacist, a social worker, or some other professional, depending upon the issue to be decided. Sometimes 2 or more professionals will collaborate to make the decision. For example, an orthopedist and a physical therapist might decide together on the sequence of physical therapy for a patient who has undergone a joint replacement procedure.

Paternalism-by-permission is importantly different from the paternalism mentioned above in explaining patient-centeredness. For clarity's sake, we call that form of paternalism as *simple paternalism*. In paternalism-by-permission, the patient makes a choice to delegate authority and then steps back from making decisions. In simple paternalism, the choice of the relationship model is made by the healthcare professional and is either imposed on the patient or passively accepted by the patient. Simple paternalism is not included in Table 4-1 because it is not a form of patient-centered care. Once the patient elects paternalism-by-permission, however, the behavior of the professionals and the patient are just the same as they would have been under simple paternalism. Of course, with paternalism-by-permission, the patient retains the right to reverse the decision at any point, that is, to withdraw the permission.

In medicine, paternalism-by-permission is sometimes called the *physician-as-agent* model (Charles et al, 1999, p. 652). This model is often chosen by patients, more frequently by older patients than younger ones. When it is used, it is frequently adopted with minimal discussion, often because a physician interprets a patient's pattern of questions and expressed expectations to mean that the patient prefers to defer to the physician to make the decisions. The risk, of course, is that the physician's interpretation may be incorrect, leading to the imposition of simple paternalism because the patient does not feel free to object.

When paternalism-by-permission is working well, the patient provides information on her or his values and goals, usually by answering questions posed by the physician or some other clinician. The clinician or clinicians contribute scientific information pertinent to the choices to be made, but this information is normally not conveyed to the patient unless the patient asks for it. The deliberation about the best course of action is handled by the clinician or clinicians working by themselves. And, of course, the decisions are made by the clinician or clinicians. The patient retains veto power over whatever is decided.

Partnership

The second relationship model is called *partnership*. This is the model illustrated in the interactions of Ms. Belmonte with her rheumatologist, clinical nurse specialist, and physical therapist. With this model, the patient genuinely works along with his or her care givers in making decisions. The patient does not defer to the professionals. Neither does she or he ever simply take charge, overruling the professionals. All issues are talked through until agreement is reached. The patient conveys information about his or her values and goals to the care givers. The physician and other clinicians provide medical and other scientific information to the patient. Different action options are weighed and sorted by both parties jointly. Decisions are made by common agreement. The patient retains veto power, which may be used if the patient changes his or her mind at any point. The health professional (or team) also retains a veto, as is discussed below in connection with the model called *patient-in-charge.*

Partnership is even more commonly used than paternalism-by-permission. In practice, however, the model has many variations. Some of these variations obscure the fact that the patient and professional are actually using this model. Some patients want a great deal of scientific information before moving on to confer with the professionals about which treatment option to choose, and so it may appear that the patient is headed toward making the decisions alone. Some patients ask for limited information from the professional and then want to do their own homework, returning for further discussion of what they have learned. Some patients ask for very little scientific information, quickly requesting the professional's recommendations and then following up with questions to test whether the patient's values and goals have been adequately taken into account by the professional in arriving at the recommendations. And some patients wish to have discussions about their values and goals before bringing these considerations together with the scientific ones.

In another variant of the partnership model, a surrogate, for example, a spouse or close friend of the patient, is designated by the patient to partner with the healthcare team or a single professional in making the decisions. When this variant is chosen by the patient, he or she may be present for all of the interactions between the surrogate and the team or healthcare professional, but the patient does not actively participate

Table 4–1 could be elaborated to distinguish different sub-types of partnership, resulting in more than one model clustered under the heading of partnership. In particular, some authors distinguish different kinds of partnership by distinguishing among different roles that the healthcare professional can have in the partnership (Emanuel and Emanuel, 1992). With this approach, in one kind of partnership, the professional provides information about the disease and treatment options and counsels the patient about values and goals, seeking to help the patient clarify his or her own values and goals and resolve any inconsistencies. In a second version of partnership, one with more intense interaction, the professional not only provides healthcare information but also acts as a teacher in dealing with values and goals, seeking to persuade the patient to improve his or her values and goals so that he or she makes the most admirable choice possible, using only persuasion and avoiding coercion. Few professionals and patients nowadays would choose this second type of partnering, which borders on simple paternalism.

The partnership model is often called *shared decision making.* This term is well established in the literature (Charles et al, 1999, pp. 652, 655-656), but it carries a misleading suggestion. Because the label has been associated for many years with the work of organizations that develop decision aids to convey healthcare information to the patient, the label suggests to many healthcare professionals that decision aids are part of the model. These aids include interactive videos, audio tapes, and flip charts, among others (Flood et al, 1996). The aids can certainly help in making the model work smoothly, but they are not defining features of the model, which can be used even if the patient and professional simply talk—as did Ms. Belmonte and her rheumatologist.

Patient-in-Charge

The third relationship model is called *patient-in-charge.* This is the model that Ms. Montgomery sought to use although she was thwarted in her attempt because her surgeon did not accept the model. Sometimes this model is called the *informed* model because the patient, once properly informed, makes the decisions (Charles et al, 1999, p. 653). The defining feature of the model is that the patient makes the decisions, not the healthcare professional alone and not the patient and professional proceeding as partners. The healthcare professional provides the patient with information about the disease, diagnostic options, and treatment options. The patient may reflect on his or her values and goals but does not discuss them with the professional. Deliberations are carried out by the patient, combining the healthcare information with his or her values and goals to arrive at a decision. In a variant of the patient-in-charge model, not often used, the patient designates a surrogate, for example, a family member, to make the decisions alone.

Does this mean, then, that the professional must do whatever the patient dictates? No. The healthcare professional retains a veto in the sense that no physician, nurse, administrator, or other professional is obliged to take action that he or she believes will seriously harm the patient—regardless of whether the patient believes that harm will be done. The health care received by a patient who chooses to be in charge is always subject to this constraint. Of course, the team or professional is not entitled to take action contrary to the patient's wishes. If the patient and the team or professional reach a point of disagreement because the patient's chosen course of action is regarded by the professionals as likely to be harmful, the team or professional is entitled to decline to participate further. The same can be said of patients' choices to take action that would be utterly wasteful. We elaborate on these limits below.

In its extreme version, the patient-in-charge model provides that the healthcare professional or team has "no legitimate role to play in the discussion or recommendation of treatments" because he or she might "harm the patient by inadvertently steering her (or him) in a certain direction which reflects the physician's (or other healthcare professional's) own bias" (Charles et al, 1999, p. 654). This version of the model seeks to protect the patient's autonomy at almost any cost. It seems to be a theoretical option that has few or no takers. In other words, it seems unlikely that any patient would completely rule out any discussion of treatment options with his or her healthcare professional to avoid the risk of being influenced by the values and goals of the healthcare professional.

The distinction between the partnership model and the patient-in-charge model is probably best understood as a matter of degree rather than as a sharp distinction. Patients who choose either of these 2 models can be represented on a spectrum that runs continuously across both of the models taken together. Some patients are highly dependent on the healthcare professional and want extensive discussion of options, including consideration of scientific matters as well as some teaching or advice about how to make treatment decisions. Other patients, like Ms. Montgomery in the last vignette, want to make the decisions themselves, seeking only very little discussion with the healthcare professional for the purpose of validating their thinking. Still other patients seek a middle ground of joint deliberation. Those who make their decisions by themselves and seek absolutely no input on their choices from their healthcare professionals—beyond scientific facts—are rare. One can imagine a patient who is a physician, nurse, or other healthcare professional—once well informed about the scientific and healthcare facts at issue—making a decision entirely on her or his own. But this is not the only type of patient who is very near the extreme end of the spectrum spanning the partnership and patient-in-charge models. Consider the following real (but disguised) case.

> *In 1980, Carl Ulmanis was a 34-year-old attorney in Louisville. He practiced business law and was in great demand throughout the United States for representing clients in certain types of real estate contract negotiations. He was accustomed to being in charge and quietly reveled in his skill and his repeated successes.*
>
> *Mr. Ulmanis and his wife took a vacation in Arizona, where they attended a rodeo in a hot and dusty desert area. After returning to Louisville 2 weeks later, he developed severe pneumonia and was hospitalized. Tests of his blood and phlegm revealed that he had coccidioidomycosis, an unusual infection caused by a fungus found in the southwestern United States. Intravenous antifungal medication was started, but within 2 or 3 days he began to have severe headaches and fatigue. A sample of spinal fluid was obtained through a needle inserted into his spinal canal at the level of his low back (lumbar puncture). It showed white blood cells (lymphocytes) and a low level of sugar (glucose). He was diagnosed as having meningitis caused by the fungus, a condition which is fatal if untreated.*
>
> *At this point, he and his wife asked an internist friend whether he had any advice. The internist recommended that Mr. Ulmanis seek care from a physician who had extensive experience in treating this rare type of meningitis. There were no such experienced physicians in Louisville. In fact, there were very few outside of California. Mr. Ulmanis was transferred at his request to a hospital in San Diego. Treatment was begun with antifungal medication injected into his spinal canal.*
>
> *Mr. Ulmanis began to have extended discussions with his physicians, who found him to be an engaging patient because of his curiosity about the disease and his high intelligence. Soon he was reading medical textbooks and articles in obscure journals on infectious diseases and neurology.*

He continued with treatment, and his blood and spinal fluid were repeatedly tested. He kept detailed records of the events in his health care, including all of the test results.

Mr. Ulmanis's principal physician in San Diego recommended that he move to San Diego to continue receiving treatment that he could not receive in Louisville. After all, the stakes were high. Almost no one with coccidioidal meningitis had ever survived. His treatment required frequent testing and interpretation of the results. More importantly, for technical reasons, the medication had to be administered by cisternal puncture, that is, by injection into his spinal canal at the base of his skull. This is a high-risk procedure in itself. It is performed by only a few physicians.

Mr. Ulmanis remained confident and optimistic. He wanted to return to his law practice in Louisville, his life-long home. While still in San Diego, he identified a radiologist in Louisville who was skilled in performing cisternal puncture because he used the procedure frequently to carry out certain x-ray examinations unrelated to coccidioidomycosis. Mr. Ulmanis persuaded the radiologist to consider administering the antifungal medication by cisternal puncture, at the same time withdrawing spinal fluid for testing. The radiologist had not previously used cisternal puncture to administer medication. He conferred with the San Diego physician by telephone and decided that Mr. Ulmanis's suggestion was feasible and safe.

Mr. Ulmanis returned to Louisville and continued his treatment there. For several years, he underwent antifungal treatment by cisternal puncture, administered initially 3 times weekly but with decreasing frequency over time. He maintained records of his spinal fluid and blood test results. He communicated with his physician in San Diego by telephone and fax, conveying his symptoms, test results, and the events of his care in Louisville. From time to time, the physician altered the dose and frequency of antifungal drug administration. Mr. Ulmanis relayed these changes to the radiologist who was administering the drug. He traveled to San Diego once annually to see his physician in person. Eventually, the physician advised that treatment was no longer necessary although testing of spinal fluid did continue for some months after the drug was stopped.

Several years after Mr. Ulmanis first met the "cocci" expert in San Diego, the physician invited him to deliver a paper at a national meeting of infectious disease specialists. Mr. Ulmanis spoke about his experience with coccidioidomycosis and about how he organized and oversaw his own care. His paper was published in an infectious disease journal. Meanwhile, he continued to practice law, and he continues to practice law today.

Mr. Ulmanis was in charge of his own health care. Within 2 years or so after the time of his diagnosis, he knew almost as much about coccidioidal meningitis as did his physician in San Diego. And he certainly understood his own values and goals. He conferred with his San Diego physician about the technical aspects of his treatment. But he discussed his values and goals with his physician only once, when he wanted to return from San Diego to Louisville. Even then he did not seek counsel from his physician to clarify his values or resolve inconsistencies. There was nothing to clarify or resolve. Mr. Ulmanis probably represents the extreme autonomous end of the spectrum encompassed by the partnership and patient-in-charge models.

Lack of Superiority of One Model Over Another

The partnership model is commonly touted as the most desirable model (Barry and Edgman-Levitan, 2012). Nowadays many nurses, physicians, and healthcare teams proudly report that they partner with their patients. Without doubt, the partnership model is superior to simple paternalism, which is coercive. But is it superior to paternalism-by-permission or the patient-in-charge model?

There is nothing substandard about paternalism if it has been chosen by the patient. When Mr. Trudell told his physician in the emergency room that he wanted the physician to decide on the next step in his care, he made a legitimate choice, not a defective one. Sometimes healthcare professionals' encouragement of decision-making partnership is a subtle means of criticizing patients for timidity—sometimes used, for example, when patients are contemplating choosing paternalism. Such criticism, if apparent to the patient, cannot be helpful for the patient's experience of care.

And one wonders what a healthcare professional proud of partnering would do with a patient like

Mr. Ulmanis. Mr. Ulmanis did not want a partner. He wanted to be in charge of his own fate. Again, his choice was legitimate. Consider the analogy between a patient seeking health care and a car owner seeking repairs for her car. If the car owner were to encounter a master mechanic who said that he pledged to partner with her in repairing her car, she would be quite surprised if not annoyed. If accustomed to speaking bluntly, she might say that she would be making the decisions about repairs on her car and that he should not presume to be her partner. Of course, normally mechanics do not presume partnership. They investigate the problems reported by the car owner and then present options to the owner, who decides what will be done, what will be deferred, and what will be left undone. So too, healthcare professionals should not presume to be partners of their patients. Partnership is comically inappropriate in car repair, but it does make sense in health care—if the patient wants it. If the patient wants a partner, then she should be accorded partnership. If the patient wants to be in charge, then she should be in charge. Sometimes healthcare professionals' talk of partnering is a means for trying to hold onto some of the power that professionals, especially physicians, used to have—a means used, for example, when dealing with patients like Ms. Montgomery and Mr. Ulmanis, who are trying to make it clear that they do not want to share the decision making.

The point to keep in mind is that the choice of model is and should be in the hands of the patient, as emphasized in Table 4–1 in the first row, where the question "Patient selects model?" is answered with "Yes" for all 3 models. The objective of those on the healthcare team should not be the promotion of one or another of the models shown in Table 4–1. Instead the objective should be to achieve the best match possible between the model preferred by the patient and the way that the team members interact with him or her. Unfortunately, investigations into whether patients receive care in accordance with their choices of models—delegation of treatment choice to the professional, collaborative decision making, or deciding for themselves—have shown that a good match between patient choices and the care actually received is reported by patients to have been achieved only about half of the time (Degner et al, 1997).

Managing the process of affording genuine choice to the patient is complicated by the fact that it is not always easy to know what the patient's choice is. Sometimes it is quite difficult. Any one of several obstacles may arise. For example, some patients (as well as some physicians, nurses, and social workers, and other professionals) think that choosing paternalism-by-permission is timid or perhaps even that it demonstrates a character flaw, marking the patient as less than a full person. For a patient with this belief, choosing paternalism-by-permission is an occasion for shame although the patient may realize only dimly that she or he has this view. In a new healthcare situation, patients with this view will usually appear at first to want to relate to healthcare professionals as partners, but as time passes the professionals observe that the patients' questions are few and that they defer to the professionals to make treatment decisions. The patients will not want to discuss their choice to defer, and to force them to deal openly with the choice serves only to damage their self-esteem. (Low-key reassurance about the legitimacy of paternalism-by-permission is helpful; this requires substantial tact and skill in communication.) In contrast, some patients do not realize or even understand when they are told that they have a choice about how to relate to members of the healthcare team. In these cases, most commonly encountered in older patients, usually the presumed relationship model is simple paternalism—perhaps with the patient asking more questions than patients did some decades ago. Also, some patients who would prefer to be in charge hide this preference because they think that it will be unwelcome to healthcare professionals, especially physicians. And finally, over time patients often change their preferences for how they want to relate to professionals in the healthcare team. For example, Mr. Trudell chose paternalism-by-permission in the emergency room when he was having chest pain. Later on he might well want to partner with his healthcare providers or even to be in charge.

Healthcare professionals need to be alert to clues about what role patients want to have in their healthcare teams—passive recipient, partner, or director. The most straightforward method for getting the answer, of course, is to ask the question at appropriate junctures in the course of care. However, as just noted, being straightforward is sometimes ineffective and sometimes even psychologically harmful. To answer the question by interpreting the patient's words and actions takes some skill. Although questionnaires for determining patient decision-making preferences do exist, they are used in research settings and would be interpersonally awkward or simply impractical to use in ordinary clinical care, at least currently (Chewning, 2012). All healthcare professionals who have direct contact with patients need to value and develop their abilities to detect the clues that patients provide about how they want to relate to their care givers, including clues that point to a mismatch between what patients want and the manner in which they are being treated. These clues include, of course, facial expressions and body postures as well as tone of voice and what patients actually say. If clinicians lack the abilities to detect the clues and act upon them, patient-centered care cannot be achieved. It is also appropriate and helpful for team members to point out these clues to other team members who may not have noticed them. Achieving patient-centered care is a team endeavor.

The Feasibility of Patients Being in Charge

The framework in Table 4–1 provides a means for understanding the different roles that patients can have in healthcare teams and for helping patients to make their choices. It is an elaboration on the notion of patient-centered care, which has been widely praised and embraced since the publication of *Crossing the Quality Chasm* (IOM, 2001).

At the same time, some professionals believe there will be problems with the choices that patients make (Bardes, 2012; Berwick, 2009). The objections to the framework shown in Table 4–1 are the objections that have been made to patient-centeredness. Most of the objections are focused on the perceived undesirability of consumerism in health care. More specifically, most of the objections center on the idea that patients could be in charge and at the same time not be financially responsible (because most health care is insured) and therefore not be subject to marketplace discipline. Under these circumstances, as predicted by some critics, patients will demand and be entitled to health care that is wasteful and to care that is, on the evidence, ineffective or harmful.

A commonly offered case in point is the demand by patients for needless diagnostic imaging. Examples include high-technology imaging—magnetic resonance imaging (MRI) scans or computed tomography scans—for recent-onset back pain with no other symptoms or abnormalities on physical examination or for knee pain of short duration with no other symptoms or findings. Professionals retain their rights to try to persuade patients that unnecessary high-technology scans are indeed unnecessary. Some emboldened patients will not be persuaded. To deal with these situations the healthcare system in which the professional works, or the insurance company (or government) paying the bill or the government as regulator can make the rules. Sometimes a physician, nurse practitioner, or physician assistant will in the end order a pointless MRI scan in order to avoid rupturing his or her relationship with the patient. This is a small price to pay for putting the patients-in-charge if they want to be in charge. And occasionally a patient may insist on a course of action that is so egregiously wasteful that the professional or team will need to decide whether to part company with the patient.

Unrestrained demands for care that would harm the patient are a different matter. Healthcare professionals actually have an obligation not to take action that will harm the patient. Thus, for example, if a patient were to insist on chelation therapy for her coronary heart disease (blockage of arteries supplying blood to the heart), a physician, nurse, or pharmacist would be obliged to refuse—not merely entitled to refuse—to order or participate in the treatment because chelation promises no benefit for heart disease, as judged by the evidence, and can cause health problems (Mitka, 2008).

In addition, critics are concerned that patients-in-charge or patients who are partnering will demand large amounts of time from healthcare professionals, who will need to answer their questions and engage in extended discussions about decisions to be made. Critics contend that this would be another form of waste and that it would have ill effects on the practice of nursing, medicine, and other professions because it would exhaust the already overly busy practitioners. This would be a problem, so it is said, especially in primary care. No doubt it is true that more time will be required if many more patients choose to partner with their healthcare teams or to be in charge. But the time spent will improve patients' experience of care and lead to more professional satisfaction for many healthcare professionals. And professionals always have the option of ending the discussion on any given day, although they may find it difficult to do so. In any case, there is no doubt that more family physicians, nurse practitioners, and others are needed in primary care—regardless of whether patients were to begin to require more time to discuss their treatment choices (Bodenheimer and Pham, 2010).

Finally, some clinicians anticipate that large numbers of patients participating more fully in decision making will change the character of professional practice. This is an issue specifically for medicine and perhaps for pharmacy. These patients' demands, so it is said, will change professional practice so that it is no longer sharply focused on clear-headed diagnosis, treatment planning, management of disease, and surgery. Murky assessment and discussion of patients' concerns will be introduced, some of these concerns being psychological and some of them being simply ill-informed. The objectivity, rationality, and scientific character of medicine will be blurred. In other words, it will make medicine more like nursing or social work. This is true, and this is the point. Patient-centered care will change medicine—for the better. Some physicians went to medical school solely to be able to apply science to alleviating symptoms and curing disease. They may not welcome patient-centered medical practice, which is an expansion of their responsibilities as physicians. They may simply not want to practice patient-centered medicine. This potential problem marks an otherwise beneficial change, that is, beneficial in the sense that the shift to patient-centered care serves the interests of patients.

HELPING PATIENTS TO IMPROVE THEIR OWN HEALTH

The previous several sections of this chapter deal with one important aspect of patient-centeredness, namely, the roles of patients in decision making about their own health care. Once it is established how a patient will participate in these decisions about goals and means for achieving the goals, the next question is how the patient will participate in action to carry out the decisions made.

These 2 questions are separate. Many patients who choose to be in charge of their own decision making also choose to be active in improving their health, but other patients who make the same choice about their role in decision making are not active in their own health care at the level of day-to-day details. Many patients who delegate all decision making to clinicians play a passive role in day-to-day management, but others become active managers of their care. Bodenheimer and colleagues (2002), characterizing chronic illness care, mark this distinction by positing 2 components of health care for people with chronic conditions: collaborative care and self-management education. Collaborative care is a partnership paradigm for decision making, and self-management education enables patients to solve problems in their own day-to-day care. One can generalize this 2-part conception by acknowledging that the decision-making component may not be one of partnership but instead may be based on the paternalism-by-permission model or the patient-in-charge model. Regardless of which of the 3 decision-making models is adopted, the patient may choose to be more or less active in managing the details of her or his care. For a patient-in-charge, sometimes there is little decision making to be done day-to-day. For example, Mr. Ulmanis, the young lawyer with chronic meningitis, described earlier, was a patient-in-charge; he made the principal decisions about whether to receive care and who would provide it. However, the administration of the antifungal drug, the amount of drug used, and frequency of dosing all required decisions that only his physicians could make safely. Sometimes, a patient evaluates the treatment choices actively, makes a decision as a patient-in-charge, and then chooses a very traditional approach to receiving care. For example, a patient with high blood pressure might choose to be treated with medication and then have her blood pressure measured and her medications adjusted only at the time of physician or NP visits, declining to measure her own blood pressure or to make any changes in medication doses by herself. In contrast, a diabetic patient might leave the decision about when to begin to use insulin (instead of oral medication) entirely to his physician or NP but then actively participate in making choices about insulin dosage, diet and exercise, learning how to adjust his doses of insulin in response to blood sugar measurements, his plans for exercise for the day, and other factors. Of course, some patients choose not to participate in any significant way in their care, leaving to their clinicians all or nearly all decisions about goals and treatment and choosing not to learn about their diseases and not to take on the day-to-day tasks of caring for their diseases. Sometimes a patient makes this choice because of other concerns in her life, for example, the needs of a mentally ill husband or child, require her attention and are more important to her.

Healthcare team members need to be able to accept the role decisions made by patients—although attempts to persuade patients to be more active in improving their health are justified. As discussed below, there is evidence (a) that patients who are more active have better health outcomes, and (b) that many patients who state that they do not want to be active change their minds if their healthcare professionals interact with them using the techniques of motivational interviewing.

For those patients who choose to self-manage their health care, healthcare teams can provide help in many ways. The options for encouraging and assisting patients have expanded dramatically in the past 20 years.

Shared Decision Making

In recent years, shared decision making, mentioned earlier, has taken on an important place in discussions of decision making in health care (Elwyn et al, 2012). Shared decision making is an approach to aiding patients' decision making by systematically providing them with evidence relevant to their decisions and, as needed or requested, supporting them as they consider the evidence and their own goals and values in the process of arriving at choices. Various tools are used in delivering information about the evidence, including written materials and visual aids, sometimes including very elaborate aids such as interactive videos.

Shared decision making is, of course, a means for involving patients as participants in their own health care. Strictly speaking, however, it is not a means for enabling patients to improve their own health. Keeping in mind the 2-part framework described in the last section, shared decision making pertains to the decision making portion of the framework rather than the self-management portion. Shared decision making could be used by patients who choose either the partnership model or, paradoxically, the patient-in-charge model of decision making. Presuming that the patient does decide to embark on a course of treatment, having participated in making this decision, the patient is more likely to take ownership of the course of action chosen and thus to engage in active self-management.

Group Visits

Group visits are visits to one or more clinicians by groups of patients rather than by one patient at a time (Burke and O'Grady, 2012). Group visits provide the guidance of a healthcare professional as do visits by individuals to individual physicians, NPs, or other clinicians. In addition, group visits provide the support and knowledge available from the other patients attending the visit. It is postulated that peer encouragement and perhaps detailed knowledge obtained from other patients with the same condition will enable more effective self-management and thus improve outcomes. Group visits for patients with type 2 diabetes have shown promise in improving outcomes and lowering costs, but as yet there is no evidence that group visits are superior to traditional office visits (Riley and Marshall, 2010). The effectiveness of group visits has also been studied for a few other chronic medical conditions with similar, promising but inconclusive results (Edelman et al, 2012).

Support Groups for Patients

Support groups are perennially popular for patients with a wide variety of conditions, including breast cancer, osteoarthritis, multiple sclerosis, and many others. These groups consist of peers with the same condition; the groups do not include a healthcare professional. The purposes of the groups vary somewhat, but important aims for any support group are emotional support and information sharing among the members (Davison et al, 2000). The groups usually meet in person but their members can interact by telephone or by use of the Internet (Han et al, 2012). Evaluation of the impact of support groups is difficult because of the variation in purposes, composition, and methods used by different groups; few well-designed evaluations have been done. One study of a support group for people with osteoarthritis showed improvement in pain control and physical function. A support group for people with mental illness reported improved communication abilities and greater confidence among its members. However, one study of a support group for patients with multiple sclerosis showed no benefit and perhaps some deterioration in measures of the patients' quality of mental health (Uccelli et al, 2004). Regardless of whether improved disease outcomes are ever firmly demonstrated, support groups are likely to remain common because the patients who participate value the emotional support they receive.

Health Coaching

Health coaching is one-on-one assistance aimed at providing patients with both information and strengthened motivation so that the patients will be able to manage their own illnesses more effectively (Bennett et al, 2010). Coaching is provided by nurses, medical assistants, community health workers, and other healthcare professionals—but, by definition, not by physicians.

At present, there is no standard definition of the content or methods of health coaching and no agreement on what should be minimal training for coaches (Wolever and Eisenberg, 2011). In many programs, the coaching is provided by telephone, but in other programs coaching is provided in person. Evaluations of the effectiveness of health coaching have produced mixed results, probably reflecting the wide variety of educational backgrounds of coaches and the many different approaches used in coaching.

Motivational Interviewing

Motivational interviewing is a well-defined approach to improving the resolve and ability of patients to make behavioral changes that will benefit their health (Miller and Rollnick, 2012). The technique is based on a 5-stage model of behavior change. The interviewer first seeks to identify the patient's stage of change with respect to stopping smoking, beginning to exercise, or some other behavioral change that would have favorable health consequences. Depending on the stage of change identified, the interviewer then takes action as appropriate to the stage. For example, if a patient is contemplating quitting smoking, the interviewer invites the patient to weigh the pros and cons of making the change. Specific questions are used to engage the patient in becoming clear about how he or she views the benefits and risks of quitting. If the patient is at the stage of preparing to act, then the interviewer makes comments and asks questions aimed at encouraging the patient to make a concrete and realistic plan. Overall, the first step in the method is to identify any discrepancies between what a patient wants and his or her current behavior. Then, if a discrepancy is found, the interviewer seeks to encourage the patient to take action to eliminate the discrepancy. This second step involves encouraging planning and increasing the patient's confidence that he or she can succeed. This sequence is sometimes described as "resolving ambivalence," that is, ambivalence about making change. Motivational interviewing has been shown to be superior to placebo interviewing (and to lack of any discussion of change) in treating alcohol and drug dependency (Hall et al, 2012). It has also been shown to be effective in enabling patients to quit smoking, in diabetes care, and in enabling patients to improve their diets and exercise habits (Martins and McNeil, 2009). At present, the use of motivational interviewing is expanding rapidly, especially in primary care. The Veterans Affairs Palo Alto Health Care System, for example, recently trained 160 of its primary care clinicians in motivational interviewing (Cucciare et al, 2012).

Patient Activation

Patient activation is the process of enhancing patients' activity and effectiveness as managers of their own health care (Greene and Hibbard, 2012). Hibbard and colleagues have devised a valid and reliable measure of patient activation called the *PAM* (Patient Activation Measure). Patients with a low PAM score are passive and do not believe in the need for patients to be active as managers of their own health. Patients with a high PAM score take initiative to improve their health and engage in many health-promoting behaviors. Several studies have found correlations between high PAM scores and desirable health behavior. Correlations have also been found between high PAM scores and a few health outcomes. However, these studies do not necessarily mean that healthcare teams can intervene to improve health by increasing patients' activation levels. A high PAM score might simply be a marker of a patient who is engaged, regardless of anything that any clinicians have done to promote her or his engagement. Some studies have shown that patients' PAM scores can be increased though specific interventions by clinicians. However, evidence has not yet been produced to show that the increases in PAM scores produced by the interventions confer health benefit in the form of improved outcomes. Whether or not these interventions are eventually shown to be beneficial, clinicians may be able to use PAM scores to identify patients who are good candidates for motivational interviewing or self-management education.

Self-Management Education

As noted earlier, the aim of self-management education is to enable patients to identify and solve problems that they encounter in the day-to-day management of their care (Bodenheimer et al, 2002). Self-management education is different from traditional patient education, which provides patients with information and specific skills (for example, to enable diabetic patients to give themselves insulin injections). The objectives of self-management education include providing information and teaching skills, but, in addition, self-management education seeks to enable patients to identify problems—arising from the disease but also from tensions among the patient's own goals—and then to solve these problems. For example, a patient with high blood pressure may normally take a daily morning medication that on rare occasions causes her to be light-headed later in the day. On a given morning, because her schedule that day includes an important business meeting and she does not want to be light-headed during the meeting, she may be faced with a decision about whether to take the medication that morning. Self-management education can equip individuals to recognize problems of this kind, enumerate different courses of action, and make a choice among the available options. Self-management education emphasizes *self-efficacy*, that is, the confidence that one can succeed in taking action that might be daunting. A patient who believes he will fail in pursuing an exercise program is more likely not to try to make the change. With a stronger sense of self-efficacy, the patient is more likely to take action. Self-management education seeks to strengthen a patient's sense of self-efficacy.

Self-management education programs have been designed and provided for patients with asthma, diabetes, arthritis, and chronic disease of any kind. The programs differ with respect to the specific educational components included in the program, making evaluation difficult. Nonetheless, there is evidence for the effectiveness of self-management education for asthma, arthritis, and chronic disease in general.

A prominent contributor to the development of self-management education has been the Stanford Patient Education Research Center, headed by Kate Lorig, RN, DrPH (Stanford Patient Education Research Center, 2012). The Center has developed programs for individuals with arthritis, diabetes, chronic pain, and other conditions. Of particular interest is the Chronic Disease Self-Management Program (CDSMP), which enables individuals with any chronic disease to manage their diseases more effectively. The program teaches problem-solving skills and coping skills, and it enhances patients' self-efficacy. Six weekly sessions are conducted by trained facilitators, who have chronic diseases themselves and are not healthcare professionals. They follow a prescribed agenda and use scripts. The program has been rigorously evaluated (Lorig et al, 1999). When compared with a control group in a randomized trial, participants had fewer symptoms, improved physical activity levels, improved health behavior, and fewer hospital days. The program is now delivered throughout the United States by a wide variety of organizations, including hospitals, other kinds of healthcare delivery organizations, state and county health departments, and healthcare professional schools and colleges. Groups attending these programs are commonly called *Lorig groups*.

Patient-Centered Medical Homes

In recent years, many observers have noted that US health care is fragmented and that primary care is under great pressure due to shortages of primary care physicians, NPs, and physician assistants (Bodenheimer and Pham, 2010). In response to these problems, The American Academy of Family Physicians (AAFP) and several other national professional bodies have developed and promoted the concept of a patient-centered medical home (PCMH). A PCMH provides (a) first-contact care, (b) coordinated care, (c) comprehensive care, and (d) sustained personal relationships (Nutting et al, 2011). The National Committee for Quality Assurance (NCQA) offers formal recognition for medical practices that wish to be acknowledged as PCMHs (National Committee for Quality Assurance, 2012). By the end of 2010, 1500 medical practices in the United States had been awarded formal recognition. The NCQA recognition process scores medical practices on 27 criteria or "elements," including 6 "must-pass" elements. The "must-pass" elements are (1) access during office hours, (2) use of data for population management, (3) systematic planning and management of patients' health care, (4) support for self-care by patients, (5) tracking and follow-up of referrals, and (6) implementation of continuous quality improvement. The federal Patient Protection and Affordable Care Act (PPACA) of 2010 contains provisions that explicitly encourage the development of PCMHs, as do statutes passed recently in many states. The PCMH is a broad concept for redesigning and strengthening primary care; it is not aimed specifically at encouraging and assisting patients to self-manage their health care. However, as the concept has been interpreted by AAFP, NCQA, and other organizations, one of the components of the PCMH is support for self-management.

FAMILIES AND OTHER CARE GIVERS IN CLINICAL TEAMS

Besides healthcare professionals and the patient, the families of patients also participate in teams—as well as others who have close ties to the patient, for example, a close friend or a life partner who is not married to the patient and has no legally assured access to information about the patient. The roles for these additional people vary a great deal and are affected by laws concerning privacy of health information, which also vary state to state.

Setting these variations aside for the sake of simplicity, one can say that the general rule is that family members, friends, and others can and should be included in the team if the patient wants them to be included. What exactly family and friends do also depends on the patient's preferences as well as on some practical considerations. It is workable to include a patient's husband, son, and daughter in all information sessions and deliberations about treatment—if this is the patient's choice. It is not feasible to include 25 members of an extended family. Sometimes it is necessary for a professional in the healthcare team to have a discussion with the patient about how many family members can be included directly in the discussions. If not all can be included directly because they are too numerous (or too numerous and located far away), arrangements can be made for designated family members to keep other specifically identified family members informed and, sometimes, to relay the questions and concerns of these other family members back to the team. Again, the wishes of the patient should govern how these arrangements are handled.

Similarly, decision-making authority can be delegated from the patient to a family member or to another surrogate as noted earlier in the discussion of models of the patient-team relationship. The surrogate can interact with the healthcare professionals in accordance with the partnership model of decision making or with the patient-in-charge model—which, in this situation, becomes a surrogate-in-charge model. If there are legal concerns about the validity of delegation, as long as the patient is mentally competent, these concerns can be satisfied by asking the patient to affirm what the chosen decision maker has decided.

The question of surrogate decision making is more complex if the patient is not mentally competent, because of a neurological disorder, a psychiatric disorder, or the effects of severe injury or illness. Some patients have *healthcare directives* or *advance directives*, which specify a particular person to be the surrogate (Annas, 1991). In other cases, the provisions of state law need to be taken into account. In general, when the patient is not competent to make decisions, healthcare teams can turn to a spouse or, in the case of elderly patients without a spouse, to a son or daughter. Whenever possible, it is important that a surrogate be engaged and that the surrogate be someone who knows the patient's values and goals. The surrogate then can enable the care team to come as close as possible to patient-centered care. The surrogate should be asked how the patient would have wanted decisions to be made if he or she were able to participate in the decision making. The answer may be that the patient would have chosen paternalism-by-permission. In that case, the professionals can move ahead as they would with any other patient who makes the same choice. If the approach chosen for decision making is partnership or patient-in-charge, then the surrogate stands in for the patient in deliberations about treatment decisions. The surrogate should address the issues *as if he or she were the patient* instead of making decisions based on what the surrogate would want in the same situation. Sometimes surrogate decision makers need to be reminded of this distinction. These situations are often ones of high emotion and distress. Healthcare teams should have a clear picture in advance of how to handle surrogate decision making in order to avoid yet more distress, as well as mistakes that cause care to be less than patient-centered.

PATIENTS AND FAMILIES IN MANAGEMENT TEAMS

Finally, it is important to note that patients and families have legitimate roles in management teams as well as clinical teams. The IOM concept of patient-centeredness includes institutional patient-centeredness as well as patient-centeredness in the delivery of care by specific healthcare teams to individual patients. To achieve institutional patient-centeredness, patients and families need to be included in the committees and other groups that design and oversee how the hospital, medical clinic, or other institution operates.

Boards of directors are not management teams as that type of team is defined in Chapter 2. Still, it is convenient to note here that hospitals now commonly include on their boards people who have received care at the hospital and are not healthcare professionals. Medical clinics include patients on their boards only rarely although they are doing so more frequently than they did, say, 20 years ago.

Patients and family members also have valuable roles to play in various healthcare delivery committees and other groups. Including them in management teams makes sense whenever the perspective of a patient or a family member promises (1) to heighten awareness of patients' experience of health care in the other management team members, or (2) to generate ideas that are more likely to come from patients or family members than from healthcare professionals. For example, patients are more likely to make suggestions about how their experience might be improved by changes in care processes, organizational structure and role definitions, and the architecture and interior design of healthcare facilities.

Patients are suitable members of project teams and consultative teams as these team types are explained in Chapter 2. It is less likely that patients will be able to contribute as regular members of operational teams or leadership teams although it is valuable for these teams to consult patients and family members directly on particular issues. For example, an operational team in a hospital might meet with the family of a patient who received inadequate care in the portion of the hospital managed by the team. From such a meeting the team could learn the details of how the healthcare delivery team did or did not interact helpfully with the family.

There are many examples of patients and family members on project and consultative teams. In Chapter 2, one vignette tells the story of an emergency department expansion team. This was a project team. No patients were included on that team, and it is easy to imagine that a patient's perspective would have been useful, especially in designing the new space and the traffic flow for patients and families. Alternatively, the team could have consulted with patients and family members, and it did so in a limited way by soliciting input from the hospital's patient advisory council. The patient and family advisory council described in another vignette in Chapter 2 was a consultative team. It consisted principally of former patients or family members of former patients. Many hospitals now use advisory councils of this kind as do some medical groups.

There are many more examples of patients and families participating in management teams across the United States. Cincinnati Children's Hospital has been a leader in integrating the viewpoints of family members and older pediatric patients into their work to improve both patient experience and the technical processes of care delivery (Britto, 2006). At this hospital, family members are included on every performance improvement team. Family members are also included on advisory councils attached to specific in-patient units, and the hospital safety committee and hospice care committee include family members. The Medical College of Georgia Hospitals and Clinics also has been a leader in including patients and families in advisory councils, facility planning committees, and care process improvement project teams (Hobbs and Sodomka, 2000).

Caution needs to be exercised in choosing patients or family members to participate in management teams. Ideally the patients and family members should be people who can challenge the healthcare professionals' thinking without disrupting the team's function. Patients or family members whose behavior is driven by anger about past experiences of health care should be avoided as regular team members although they could be usefully consulted separately from team meetings. Participants need to be reasonably articulate and able to function well in a group setting. They also need to have the confidence to speak up in a setting dominated by professionals who may have more formal education and more experience in committee work. On the other hand, it is *not* important that they have medical, nursing, or other knowledge that the healthcare professionals have. In fact, it is probably a disadvantage for participants to have this knowledge because it may lead to their adopting the professionals' viewpoint instead of representing the viewpoint of patients and families.

Both management teams and clinical teams might consider including patients in team training and team building activities. Such training potentially could broaden the possibilities for inclusion of more patients on healthcare teams and improve their effectiveness as team members.

MEASURING PATIENT-CENTEREDNESS

At present there is no commonly agreed method for measuring patient-centeredness (Lin and Dudley, 2009). The relevant considerations are those discussed earlier: (1) whether the patient's dignity, autonomy, values, and sensitivities have been respected, (2) whether clinicians have ascertained the patient's preference for his or her role in decision making, (3) whether there is a match between the patient's role preference and the actions taken by the clinicians, (4) whether the clinicians have performed well in conveying relevant information and assisting the patient in making decisions about care, and (5) whether the patient has been provided with high-quality assistance in self-management—assuming that the patient wants this assistance. If one were to combine these considerations into a single measure, using the measure would probably turn out to be unworkable; it may be necessary to measure different dimensions of patient-centered care and accept that they are not amenable to being combined.

In any case, it is clear that patient-centeredness is not well measured by measuring patient satisfaction (Kupfer and Bond, 2012). Patient satisfaction measurements are measurements of whether the health care that was received by a patient met or exceeded the patient's expectations. Even when the quality of care is low, levels of satisfaction can be high if the patient's expectations are low. In other words, if a patient does not expect health care to meet the standards for patient-centered care listed in the last paragraph, he or she may be entirely satisfied even if he or she received care that was far from patient-centered. Conversely, a patient's expectations may be so high that he or she will never regard the expectations as having been met even if patient-centered care as defined earlier is actually delivered. Patient-centeredness can be measured only by asking the patients about how his or her care was delivered. The appropriate question to ask is not simply whether the patient was satisfied. Instead one must ask whether the patient's dignity and values were respected, whether he or she was permitted to participate in decision making as desired, and so on. Measuring patient satisfaction is important and has an important role in determining whether care possesses certain aspects of patient-centeredness, for example, respect for patients' values and sensitivities. However, measuring patient-centeredness is not accomplished by measuring satisfaction alone.

CONCLUSION

The roles of patients in healthcare teams are highly varied but can be understood by using the concept of patient-centeredness, specifically, the IOM concept of patient-centeredness, which includes attention to patients' dignity and self-determination as well as patients' experience of care. The options for decision-making roles for patients are summarized in Table 4–1. There are 3 models of effective patient participation: paternalism-by-permission, partnership, and patient-in-charge. The patient should be in charge if she or he wants to be in charge, that is, if she or he wants to be the final decision maker about what health care will be provided. However, this does not mean that patients have become consumers. The relationships between patients and their healthcare professionals have not become commercial relationships. Healthcare professionals retain their obligations to be professional, and patients should not need to beware of being misled or pressured to receive unnecessary services. For patients who wish to manage their own care, healthcare teams have several means for providing assistance. For patients who are ambivalent about self-management, means are available for boosting their resolve and confidence. Patients and family members have appropriate roles in management teams as well as their own clinical teams. Finally, although there is not yet a consensus about how to measure patient-centeredness, it is clear that an adequate method will not be the same as measuring patient satisfaction alone.

We have defined and explained the roles of patients, who do not have training as clinicians but are nonetheless members of healthcare teams. The topic of Chapter 5, the next chapter, is another group of team members who typically do not have clinical training, namely, healthcare administrators. Some clinicians will be surprised by the idea that administrators are healthcare team members. We explain why and how administrators should participate in teams and, more generally, why and how they should have closer working relationships with clinicians for the sake of protecting and advancing the welfare of patients and families.

REFERENCES

Annas GJ. The health care proxy and the living will. *N Engl J Med.* 1991;324:1210-1213.

Balint M. *The Doctor, His Patient, and The Illness.* Revised and enlarged 2nd ed. London, UK: Pitman Medical Publishing; 1964.

Bardes CL. Defining "patient-centered medicine." *N Engl J Med.* 2012;366:782-783.

Barry MJ, Edgman-Levitan S. Shared decision making—the pinnacle of patient-centered care. *N Engl J Med.* 2012;366:780-781.

Bennett HD, Coleman EA, Parry C, et al. Health coaching for patients. *Fam Pract Manag.* 2010;17(5):24-29.

Berwick DM. What 'patient-centered' should mean: confessions of an extremist. *Health Aff (Millwood).* 2009;28: w555-w565.

Bodenheimer T, Lorig K, Holman H, et al. Patient self-management of chronic disease in primary care. *JAMA.* 2002;288:2469-2475.

Bodenheimer T, Pham HH. Primary care: current problems and proposed solutions. *Health Aff (Millwood).* 2010;29:799-805.

Britto MT, Anderson JM, Kent WM, et al. Cincinati Children's Hospital Medical Center: transforming care for children and families. *Jt Comm J Qual Patient Saf.* 2006;32:541-548.

Burke RE, O'Grady ET. Group visits hold great potential for improving diabetes care and outcomes, but best practices must be developed. *Health Aff (Millwood).* 2012;31: 103-109.

Camilleri M, Gamble GL, Kopecky SL, et al. Principles and process in the development of the Mayo Clinic's individual and institutional conflict of interest policy. *Mayo Clin Proc.* 2005;80:1340-1346.

Charles C, Gafni A, Whelan T. Decision-making in the physician-patient encounter: revisiting the shared treatment decision-making model. *Soc Sci Med.* 1999;49:651-661.

Chewning B, Bylund CL, Shah B, et al. Patient preferences for shared decisions: a systematic review. *Patient Educ Couns.* 2012;86:9-18.

Cucciare MA, Ketroser N, Wilbourne P, et al. Teaching motivational interviewing to primary care staff in the Veterans Health Administration. *J Gen Intern Med.* 2012;27: 953-961.

Davison KP, Pennebaker JW, Dickerson SS. Who talks? The social psychology of illness support groups. *Am Psychol.* 2000;55:205-217.

Degner LF, Krisjanson LJ, Bowman D, et al. Information needs and decisional preferences in women with breast cancer. *JAMA.* 1997;277:1485-1492.

Edelman D, McDuffie JR, Odone E, et al. *Shared Medical Appointments for Chronic Medical Conditions: a Systematic Review.* VA-ESP Project #09-010. Washington, DC: Dept. of Veterans Affairs; 2012. http://www.ncbi.nlm.nih.gov/pubmedhealth/PMH0048765/pdf/TOC.pdf. Accessed November 1, 2012.

Elwyn G, Frosch D, Thomson RT, et al. Shared decision making: a model for clinical practice. *J Gen Intern Med.* 2012;27:1361-1367.

Emanuel EJ, Emanuel LL. Four models of the physician-patient relationship. *JAMA.* 1992;267:2221-2226.

Engel GL. The need for a new medical model: a challenge for biomedicine. *Science.* 1977;196:129-136.

Flood AB, Wennberg JE, Nease RF, et al. The importance of patient preference in the decision to screen for prostate cancer. *J Gen Intern Med.* 1996:11:342-349.

Gerteis M, Edgman-Levitan S, Daley J, et al. *Through the Patient's Eyes.* San Francisco, CA: Jossey-Bass; 1993.

Greene J, Hibbard JH. Why does patient activation matter? An examination of the relationships between patient activation and health-related outcomes. *J Gen Intern Med.* 2012:27:520-526.

Greenhalgh T, Hurwitz B. Narrative based medicine: why study narrative? *BMJ.* 1999;318:48-50.

Hall K, Gibbie T, Lubman DI. Motivational interviewing techniques: facilitating behavior change in the general practice setting. *Aust Fam Physician.* 2012;41:660-667.

Han JY, Kim J-H, Hye JY, et al. Social and psychological determinants of levels of engagement with an online breast cancer support group: posters, lurkers, and nonusers. *J Health Commun.* 2012:17:356-371.

Hobbs JL. A dimensional analysis of patient-centered care. *Nurs Res.* 2009;58:52-62.

Hobbs SE, Sodomka PF. Developing partnerships among patients, families, and staff at the Medical College of Georgia Hospital and Clinics. *Jt Comm J Qual Improv.* 2000;26:268-276.

Institute of Medicine. *Crossing the Quality Chasm: A New Health System for the 21st Century.* Washington, DC: National Academy Press; 2001.

Institute of Medicine. In: Lohr KN, ed. *Medicare: A Strategy for Quality Assurance.* Volume I. Washington, DC: National Academy Press; 1990.

Kupfer JM, Bond EU. Patient satisfaction and patient-centered care. *JAMA.* 2012;308:139-140.

Lin GA, Dudley RA. Patient-centered care: what is the best measuring stick? *Arch Intern Med.* 2009;169:1551-1553.

Lorig K, Sobel D, Stewart AL, et al. Evidence suggesting that a chronic disease self-management program can improve health status while reducing hospitalization: a randomized trial. *Med Care.* 1999;37:5-14.

Martin AB. On a patient-centered approach. *Am J Nurs.* 1960:60:1472-1474.

Martins RK, McNeil DW. Review of motivational interviewing in promoting health behaviors. *Clin Psychol Rev.* 2009;29:283-293.

Mayo WJ. The necessity of cooperation in medicine. *Mayo Clin Proc.* 2000;75:553-556.

Miller W, Rollnick S. *Motivational Interviewing: Helping People Change.* 3rd ed. New York, NY: Guilford Press, 2012.

Mitka M. Chelation therapy trials halted. *JAMA.* 2008;300:2236.

National Committee for Quality Assurance. Patient-Centered Medical Home Web site. http://www.ncqa.org/Programs/Recognition/PatientCenteredMedicalHomePCMH.aspx. Accessed November 2, 2012.

Nutting PA, Crabtree BF, Miller WL, et al. Transforming physician practices to patient-centered medical homes: lessons from the national demonstration project. *Health Aff (Millwood).* 2011;30:439-445.

Riley SB, Marshall ES. Group visits in diabetes care: a systematic review. *Diabetes Educ.* 2010;36:936-944.

Roter DL, Hall JA. *Doctors Talking with Patients/Patients Talking with Doctors.* 2nd ed. Westport, CT: Praeger Publishers; 2006.

Stanford Patient Education Research Center. Chronic Disease Self-Management Program Web site. http://patienteducation.stanford.edu/programs/cdsmp.html. Accessed November 2, 2012.

Stewart M, Brown JB, Weston WW, et al. *Patient-Centered Medicine: Transforming the Clinical Method.* 2nd ed. Abingdon, UK: Radcliffe Medical Press Ltd; 2003.

Uccelli MM, Mohr LM, Battaglia MA, et al. Peer support groups in multiple sclerosis: current effectiveness and future directions. *Mult Scler.* 2004;10:80-84.

Wolever RQ, Eisenberg DM. What is health coaching anyway? *Arch Intern Med.* 2011;171:2017-2018.

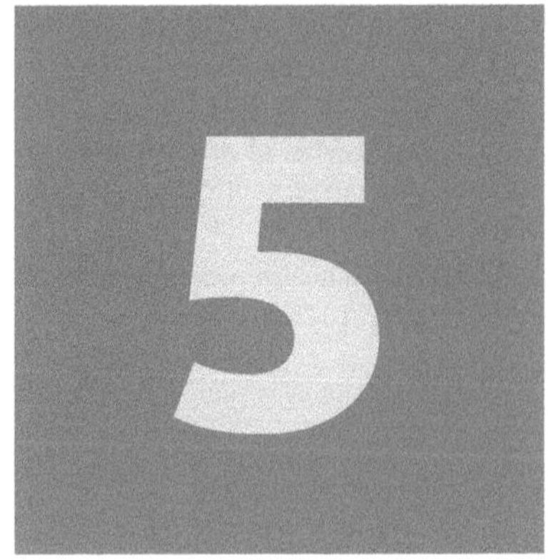

Healthcare Administrators in Healthcare Teams

For the past several years, Claire Peace, MD, an ophthalmologist, has performed eye surgery at 2 different hospitals in the Washington, DC, area—one in Washington (Capitol Eye Hospital) and one in Arlington, VA (Baroness Eye Center). In addition to the difference in physical facilities, Dr. Peace has noticed clear differences in the way that the operating room teams function at the 2 hospitals, both daily and over the years that she has worked at both hospitals. At the Capitol Eye Hospital, operating room staff turnover is high, and team members frequently need time to learn each other's roles and styles. Nurses rarely speak to Dr. Peace, interacting primarily with the other nurses. The anesthesiologist at Capitol Eye, Dr. Curmodian, sometimes seems distant and preoccupied.

In contrast, the Baroness Eye Center operating room staff seems fully invested in the surgical process, bantering with each other but focused on the patient. Very few of the staff members leave for better jobs. Dr. Peace also has heard other surgeons at Baroness speak enthusiastically about their own operating room experiences. On her drive from her office to the Baroness Eye Center, Dr. Peace was feeling upbeat. She wondered to herself if Baroness was just luckier to recruit the staff members they have, or if maybe hospital administration had something to do with how the teams functioned at Baroness.

Experienced clinicians like Dr. Peace learn through experience that some healthcare teams function better than others, and indeed, studies show wide variation in teamwork among different healthcare organizations (Schwendimann et al, 2012; Sexton et al, 2006). In the vignette, Dr. Peace wonders if administrators, while not present in her operating room during surgery, may be a "root cause" of such differences. The answer, of course, is "yes." Administrators play a critical role in team-based care delivery. Administrators bring knowledge and skills in leading and working in teams, managing people, project management, workflow design, and a host of other areas relevant to the work of clinical and management teams. In the vignette, the operating room teams at the Arlington Baroness Eye Center appeared to benefit from strong organization-wide promotion of teamwork resources and competencies by hospital administration.

In this chapter, we argue that administrators should play a more prominent role in clinical healthcare delivery teams. By the same token, however, clinicians should play a more prominent role in many healthcare administration teams. Such developments will help surmount a historical barrier between the administrative and clinical functions of healthcare delivery organizations, for the benefit of patients.

THE PROFESSIONAL BUREAUCRACY

Virtually all team-based health care is conducted by teams that operate within a larger organization. Often, those organizations are hospitals, outpatient clinics, or physicians' offices. Those settings can range in scale from a single-clinician practice to a 1000-bed hospital or a much larger system of multiple hospitals and clinics. The management and leadership of those organizations require strategic planning, financial planning and control, marketing, human resource management, information systems, quality control and improvement, environmental services, and a host of other administrative functions. In large organizations, full-time healthcare administrators typically perform those functions. In smaller organizations, such as a small dental practice, one or more clinicians may perform those functions on a part-time basis, often maintaining their clinical practice as well.

It is possible to visualize the administrative functions of healthcare delivery as quite separate from the clinical functions, as shown in the simplified hospital structure depicted in Figure 5–1. Indeed, hospitals have long been conceptualized as *schizophrenic* or *2-part* structures, split between the administration and the medical staff (Harris, 1977). The typical hospital has a governing board as its ultimate authority. The governing board delegates operating responsibility to administration, but clinical quality is delegated largely to the medical staff. The affiliated medical staff is a separate entity with its own bylaws, responsible for ensuring quality care, patient safety, and a sound medical staff. In some states in the United States, the medical staff is recognized as a legal entity with the right to sue the hospital; in most states it is not. The administration and the medical staff form the 2 parts of the split structure, both responsible to the governing board. The medical staff often is seen as more powerful than administration. Hospital administrators typically are told in their training that the best way to lose their jobs is to challenge the medical staff.

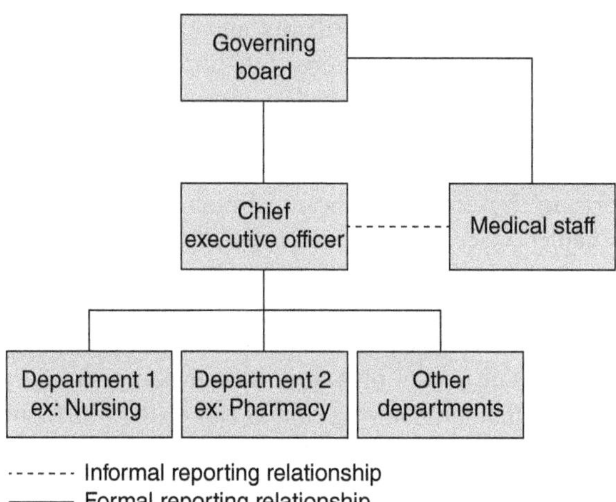

▲ **Figure 5–1.** Conventional hospital structure (simplified).

Nursing staffs in large healthcare delivery settings have a similar, though less pronounced, structure of clinical autonomy, with self-governance mechanisms, nursing union rules, or government regulations insulating certain activities, particularly with regard to healthcare quality, from administrative control. For example, several states have laws that specify a minimum level of nurse staffing or require staffing plans that meet certain criteria. The Magnet Recognition Program, which awards certification to hospitals deemed exceptional places for nurses to work, rewards nurse self-governance and autonomy.

The many clinical professions in complex delivery settings other than medicine and nursing, while not self-governing, are protected from administrative control to a certain degree by their esoteric knowledge bases and specialized training and certification or licensure. A consequence is that healthcare administrators generally shy away from interference in clinical affairs of all clinical health professions.

The concept of a *professional bureaucracy*, first depicted by management scholar Henry Mintzberg (1979), goes far in explaining this state of affairs. The notion of a *bureaucracy* is time-worn and well understood by most people, including health professionals. In the eyes of professionals, bureaucracies are hierarchical organizations with myriad rules and policies and centralized control by those higher up in the hierarchy. Bureaucracies often are perceived as impersonal, slow, and stifling. But the concept of the *professional* bureaucracy is one that most clinicians will find more attractive. The professional bureaucracy is composed of a strategic apex and middle management (the administrators), support and technical staff, and the operating core. Unlike the operating core in the traditional *machine* bureaucracy (for example, a large manufacturing company), the operating core in the professional bureaucracy primarily consists of professional workers. Instead of rules, policies, and central direction emanating from administration, the professional bureaucracy relies for coordination on standardization of skills, training, and socialization within each of the professions. Control over work is entrusted to those professions. The administration does not interfere with the daily operations of the operating core, and the information that administration uses to plan staffing and capacity for technical and support services is comprised largely of information requested from individual clinical professionals. The needs of the operating core, for example, for new technology and staff, are difficult for administrators to assess. Coordination between professionals in the *same* profession or specialty is handled by standardization of skills and knowledge among professional colleagues. (As we argue throughout this book, coordination *between* and *among* professions or specialties is often poorly handled.) The quality and performance standards of the professional bureaucracy, such as practice guidelines and protocols, originate largely from outside the administrative structure. They are developed by external associations of health professionals or by professionals inside the organization. The professional bureaucracy emphasizes the power of expertise, rather than the power of administrative position.

Administrative professionals in a healthcare professional bureaucracy serve important functions—strategic planning, information systems, financial analysis, marketing, human resource management, for example—but they are viewed as facilitators or enhancers of the core work of professionals. In contrast, in a machine bureaucracy, administrators are seen as "directors," not facilitators, of the core work. Former clinicians fill many of the administrative roles in a healthcare professional bureaucracy, reflecting the value of understanding of clinical processes in effective management. For example, managers of clinical service and support service units, such as nursing, pharmacy, and social work, frequently are clinical professionals themselves, who have taken on management responsibilities. Often, clinical professionals perceive the professional bureaucracy, with its associated autonomy for clinicians, to contribute positively to the quality of their work life.

However, there are severe problems with the professional bureaucracy in the delivery of team-based care. Within professions, loyalty to peers within one's profession conflicts with the need for transparency and accountability for patient services that transcend the boundaries of a single profession. Communication, collaboration, and conflict management among different professionals in different clinical departments can be difficult. Patients are forced to give the same information to caregivers of different professions. Patient safety errors are more likely to occur due to shortfalls in communication and collaboration.

The fact that administrators are not full partners on clinical teams is related to their status in the hierarchy of professions. Administrators in the United States in general are not viewed as full professionals, certainly not at the level of physicians or lawyers (Barker, 2010). The competencies of effective administration are too diverse and complex to codify into an exclusive knowledge base that would serve as a basis for requisite entry-level education and certification. In addition, the scientific evidence base of administration, which could anchor and legitimate its body of knowledge, is young and highly limited. Proficient administrators typically require years of on-the-job learning and experience to perform at a high level. To the extent that formal barriers to entry are used to distinguish professions from other occupations, the occupational category *healthcare administration* suffers in comparison to most clinical occupations. There is no requirement for advanced formal education for administrators in any sector of the economy, including health care. While in the healthcare sector many administrators do hold an advanced degree in healthcare management, there is no legal or regulatory requirement for the degree, unlike the requirements for practicing virtually all forms of clinical care. Only administrators of nursing homes are held to educational and licensing requirements, and the education level required is baccalaureate.

Continuation of the separation of the clinical and administrative parts of the professional bureaucracy in healthcare delivery is driven by 5 important forces. First is the need for deep administrative expertise to direct a healthcare delivery organization successfully. Historically, clinical professionals performed most of the administrative functions of such organizations, on a part-time basis. Today, however, the complexity of administration, involving extensive external dealings with payers, vendors, regulators, and partner organizations, for example, requires full-time expertise and attention except in the smallest of organizations. Most clinicians avoid such activities, having chosen professions that are quite different, as reflected in the "enterprising" feature of healthcare administrators noted in Chapter 3. Second, as noted earlier, the work domains of clinical professionals are defined by esoteric technical knowledge that is beyond the reach of administrators. The technical specialization of clinicians is intimidating to administrators. Indeed, many clinicians prefer it this way, viewing clinical care as their turf, out of bounds to administrators. Third, related to their technical specialization, clinicians historically have not been trained to notice and alter system-level factors that affect patient care quality, such as organizational policies and practices. The *person-level* approach to understanding quality seeks change in the direct behavior of the clinician and the patient in order to improve clinical care. The *system-level* approach, which is taught to administrators, identifies conditions under which individuals work and build defenses to avert errors or mitigate their effects (Reason, 2000). A fourth reason that the professional bureaucracy is preserved is that administrators find decision making simpler if clinicians are less involved in the process. Consensus development across professions takes time and requires compromise. Finally, in most large healthcare delivery organizations in the United States, many clinical professionals are less available or interested in administrative decision making because they are not employees of the organization. In particular, most physicians are not employed by hospitals but rather are self-employed or employed by physician group practices. It is more difficult for administrators to call on such clinicians to participate in team-based initiatives in their organizations.

Arguments for maintenance of the division between clinical and administrative domains in healthcare delivery need to be recognized, but maintenance of the division is too constraining, given the need for interprofessional teamwork. Strict separation of the clinical and administrative domains means that no one is in charge of interdependent activities in the whole system (Begun et al, 2011). Administrators can both specialize in their domain and learn enough about clinical care to participate knowledgeably in team-based care. Clinicians can both specialize in their domain and learn enough about administration to participate knowledgeably in interprofessional teams that make administrative decisions. The 2 domains are so interrelated that their bonds need to be tightened, not loosened, in the interests of patient care.

OPPORTUNITIES FOR HEALTHCARE ADMINISTRATORS

Physical therapist Ankur Shukla, MPT, tried to suppress a scowl. He was sitting through another meeting of the Lutheran Rehabilitation Center's quality improvement committee. Today the committee was reviewing diabetes care guidelines. Present were John Ash, the committee chair and Director of Quality Improvement, a recent Master of Health Administration (MHA) graduate with a business background; Melissa Sandusky, RN, a clinical nurse specialist; Alfredo Torres, MD, an endocrinologist brought in specifically for the meeting; and Jean Wyoming, MD, a family physician. Mr. Ash was pushing one of his "lean" quality improvement projects again. He wanted to use an "RPIW" to reduce waste in the provision of care for the Center's patients with diabetes. Only one of the other committee members knew that "RPIW" stands for Rapid Process Improvement Workshop, and none of the committee members knew how an RPIW is conducted. Mr. Ash did not explain. He seemed more interested in adding to his list of cost-cutting projects than in understanding and improving diabetes care. Mr. Ash had never spent time with the rehabilitation center patients who have diabetes or with their caregivers, and he had made no attempt to understand the clinical issues. Mr. Shukla concluded that the only way that Mr. Ash would ever understand diabetes care would be if he had the disease himself.

In this vignette, healthcare administrator John Ash is playing a role as it might be enacted in the professional bureaucracy model, emphasizing his own technical competence to the detriment of collaboration with clinical professionals. His attitude and behavior, while stereotypical and fictional, are all-too-often exhibited by administrators. To add value to team-based care, administrators need to overcome defensiveness about their knowledge base and expertise and to educate and involve those who do not share it. In Chapters 6 and 7, we note the importance of clear and respectful communication among team members. Mr. Ash could communicate much more effectively if he were careful to translate administrative jargon and not to "talk down" to his colleagues on the quality improvement committee.

Increased transparency in public reporting of the quality of healthcare organizations is one trend that supports a more collaborative posture between administrators and clinicians. Patient satisfaction, patient safety, and clinical care quality measures are increasingly available to the public and to payers, who can use these data to reward or punish delivery organizations through changes in reimbursement. Leaders of healthcare organizations increasingly are aware that they must understand and manage patient outcomes as partners with clinical professionals.

At first blush, this new posture may seem improbable. However, consider the position of a chief executive officer (CEO) of a highly technical enterprise (for example, 3M or Exxon), who has spent his or her career in finance before becoming CEO. This CEO is accountable for the performance of the whole organization and needs either to acquire the necessary knowledge of the technical operations (unlikely) or to be able to interact effectively with people who do understand the technical operations. So, too, the administrator of a healthcare delivery organization can be accountable for the whole.

Accountability for the whole organization by the CEO needs to be accompanied by explicit leadership and management of the culture of the organization so that effective team-based care is encouraged and appreciated. The concept of organizational culture and the competencies needed by organizational leaders are discussed in Chapter 18. For the moment, we underscore 2 key competencies that are particularly important for healthcare administrators.

First and foremost is the need to relate effectively to clinicians. While it is more difficult for administrators who do not have clinical backgrounds, this competency can be achieved by all administrators, with education and experience. Educational needs include learning the basic terminology of clinical care, which can be imparted in a typical college-level course, taught either face-to-face or through self-instruction online, then practiced, applied, and supplemented in the particular work setting of the healthcare administrator. Administrators can observe key clinical conditions, processes, and technologies used in the clinical areas for which they are responsible, and do on-the-job learning to attain basic competency in using the relevant terminology. They can note the different healthcare professionals on the teams with which they work and study the histories and cultures of the relevant professions.

It will not be sufficient, by the way, to select administrators who are in fact clinicians. Most clinicians are not interested in or prepared to assume full-time administrative roles. Those who do wish to become administrators often seek advanced training or administration degrees. These administrators with prior clinical experience and credentials may have an easier time dealing with clinicians. However, faced with the need to decide between the interests of their clinical profession and their organization, administrators will side with their employer (the organization). From the clinicians' viewpoint, they are often seen as having "gone over to the dark side," as illustrated in the following vignette:

Michael Storstrand, MD, had practiced medicine in Dale Health System for 18 years. He was a pediatrician with a special interest in children with delayed cognitive development. He was well liked by his physician colleagues, by the nurses at Dale Hospital, and generally by everyone with whom he worked. He had a knack for grasping organizational disagreements quickly and was often able to bring different factions together and facilitate their coming to agreement.

After Dr. Storstrand had been at Dale Health System for 9 years, the Chair of Pediatrics retired, and the Chief Medical Officer (CMO) appointed Dr. Storstrand to be the new Chair. Dr. Storstrand began to deal with administrative issues and found, somewhat to his surprise, that the work was gratifying. He enjoyed thinking about the Pediatrics Department as a whole and guiding it to serve its patients and families while at the same time attending to the financial performance of the Department. During this time, he continued to practice pediatrics half-time.

Within 2 years, Dr. Storstrand was asked by the CEO and CMO to join the Executive Committee of Dale Health System. He became a valued member, relied upon especially for his insights into how to communicate with the whole organization effectively in good times and in strained times. Occasionally, he spoke for the Executive Committee in large meetings, and sometimes he was simply inspiring.

After Dr. Storstrand had served on the Executive Committee for 6 years, the CEO retired. The organization had a tradition of selecting its CEOs from inside the organization, and Dr. Storstrand and 2 others came forward as candidates. The board chose Dr. Storstrand as Dale Health System's new CEO. At this point, he took up the position and decided that he could no longer practice pediatrics. Dale Health System was a large organization with annual revenues of $1.7 billion. The CEO position was a full-time job.

Over the next few months, Dr. Storstrand noticed, not to his surprise, that his relationships with other physicians in the health system were more distant. Personal conversations were less frequent, and he had the sense that some of the other pediatricians avoided him at times. The first 2 annual budgets were tight, and one year he had to explain to the physicians why there were no salary raises for them. From time to time, close colleagues told him that some of the physicians at Dale now regarded him as a "suit," sometimes commenting that he had "gone to the dark side." Dr. Storstrand was not disheartened by these reports, but they did sting. He was well aware that he was now viewed differently than he had been viewed as Chief of Pediatrics, that at times he was now viewed with suspicion. He recalled that the surgeon who was CEO when Dr. Storstrand joined Dale was regarded in the same way.

A second key competency for administrators in team-based organizations is to live and breathe a collaborative leadership style, exemplifying the values of teamwork. "Leadership" as described in the conventional business literature involves one individual, the leader, assuming responsibility for identifying vision, being smarter and tougher than anybody else, and saving the organization through brute will. While such a stereotype may fit a few business organizations, it is of little use in health care. Healthcare leadership involves learning about complex issues from multiple diverse angles, connecting with others to build consensus, and jointly making sense of issues such that decisions are possible (Begun and White, 2008). Learning materials for this leadership style (known variously as collaborative, integrative, adaptive, or complexity leadership) only recently are beginning to permeate the curricula of healthcare administration.

Related competencies for administrators involve shaping the structures, cultures, and resources of organizations so that they support team-based practice and decision making. These conditions include hiring, promoting, and rewarding people for teamwork, managing connections among teams and between teams and external constituencies of the organization, and providing tangible resources for teamwork, from physical meeting space to educational resources to digital technology for sharing of patient information and conducting online meetings.

Healthcare administration educators and program accreditors are showing some recognition of the growing importance of collaborative competencies, but progress is slow. For example, Shewchuk and colleagues (2005, p. 43) include "team building" in their list of 30 competencies, as well as "Knowledge of the physician education process," while not mentioning the clinical professions other than medicine. "Communication and relationship management" is one of the 5 clusters of competencies promoted by a consortium of professional associations, the Healthcare Leadership Alliance (Stefl, 2008). Another widely disseminated competency framework for healthcare administration, developed by the National Center for Healthcare Leadership, notes the importance of collaboration, but the framework conspicuously neglects knowledge of the clinical enterprise (Calhoun et al, 2008). Graduate program accrediting criteria require that healthcare administration programs include opportunities for students to participate in team-based and interprofessional activities (http://www.cahme.org/Resources/Fall2013_Criteria_for_Accreditation.pdf).

Aside from educational preparation, many practicing administrators engage in activities that enhance collaboration with clinicians. *Rounding* for safety is one such example, where administrators and relevant clinicians confer on patient care units about issues that will improve patient care safety and care processes (Campbell and Thompson, 2007). Of course, rounding can be a negative experience for clinicians and administrators alike if poorly performed. Effective rounding requires planning (scouting relevant issues and personnel in advance), representative sampling to assure that all parts of the organization are included, recording of the activity in some format, follow-up to address problems, and dissemination of results, both positive and negative.

Some degree of transformation is exhibited in the educational literature for healthcare administration in the United States. In a leading healthcare administration textbook, for example, patient care teams and aggregates of patient care teams, that is, service lines, are the organizing feature of the well-managed healthcare organization (White and Griffith, 2010). Service lines are defined around patient conditions or types in which the hospital specializes, such as oncology, neuroscience, cardiac services, or women's health. In the most extreme of the service models, employed clinicians report to the director of the service line rather than their clinical department, as they would under the conventional structure. Figure 5–2 depicts one version of service line structure (simplified), a version which

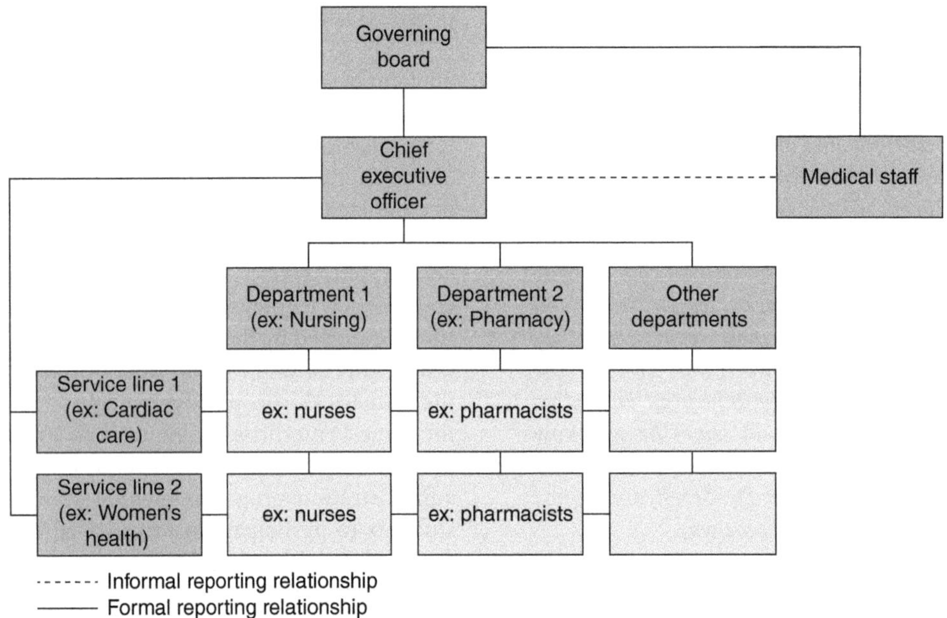

▲ **Figure 5–2.** One version of service line hospital structure (simplified).

retains conventional clinical departments along with service lines. Service lines typically are managed by nurses, physicians, administrators, and pharmacists, sometimes singly but often combined in a team. Interprofessional performance improvement councils, which include both clinicians and administrators, provide coordination across service lines on the quality dimension. The patient care teams, service line management teams, and performance improvement council are interprofessional by design. While administrators are not physically present on every team, particularly patient care teams, those teams are influenced positively if administrators and team members consider administrators to be critical peripheral members.

Service line structures make team-based care easier because direct hierarchical accountability is created for clinical professionals who commonly work together, rather than having accountability split among conventional clinical departments. A new position (a service line manager) is responsible for making sure the pharmacist, nurse, medical social worker, and physician, for example, work together efficiently and effectively in the interests of the patient.

An innovative service line design has been implemented in 3 hospitals in Michigan (Cowen et al, 2008). Collaborative practice teams (CPTs) are the core unit in the hospitals. The authors label the design as an "organizational structure for addressing the attributes of the ideal healthcare delivery system" (Cowen et al, 2008, p. 407). CPTs might be thought of as *mini* service lines. The intent is to have every patient under the advocacy of at least one CPT. CPTs are defined and commissioned by an Interdisciplinary Practice Council. In one application of the model, CPTs were defined for over 30 clinical areas, including surgery, heart failure, glycemic control, obstetrics, pediatrics, pain management, and acute coronary syndromes. CPTs consist of administrators, clinicians, and specialists in information systems, quality improvement, finance, or other areas. The CPT model for organizations reflects 3 management principles: (1) configuration around care-providing clinical microsystems, (2) use of relevant and timely data, and (3) strong connections between the microsystems and administration. Conventional organizational units are retained as well, with both the medical staff and nursing staff having separate units dedicated to issues within those professions, along with conventional clinical support services, such as pharmacy and laboratory. An even more extreme version of the design would do away with such conventional units altogether.

Interestingly, social scientists have observed that economic, technological, and social changes across all sectors of society are driving professionals and administrators to work together more collaboratively. Sociologists posit that the US economy "looks a lot like a professional, collaborative workplace where a premium is paid on teamwork, flexibility, broad training, and drastic reshuffling as people with different competencies are assembled into groups that exist only for the length of specific projects" (Leicht and Fennell, 2001, p. 217). Such arrangements deliver higher quality services more quickly and more cost-effectively. The traditionally "split" structure of healthcare delivery will not deliver the value that consumers and payers demand.

Innovative conceptual models for team-based organizational structures and cultures are being generated in several settings around the world. Scholars in Italy describe the *care-focused* hospital as a global trend, for example (Lega and DePietro, 2005). The care-focused hospital merges management, clinical activity and resources, and engagement of clinicians in management activities, all with patients at the center. One vision for the care-focused hospital aggregates patients into units based on intensity of care, defined as the variable level of services required as a result of clinical instability and care complexity. As envisioned, units for categories of patients such as frail, high-care, recovery, and postacute would exist, all requiring care from multiple clinical specialists and a high degree of team-based care (Lega and Calciolari, 2012).

OPPORTUNITIES FOR CLINICIANS

Returning to her group practice office after doing surgery at Baroness Eye Center, ophthalmologist Dr. Claire Peace reflected on the "root cause" of the superiority of teamwork at Baroness Eye Center compared to Capitol Eye Hospital. She recalled that hospital administrators at Baroness had required teamwork training, as well as simulation exercises, for all of the operating room staff. Administrators seemed to know the staff by name, and they provided regular metrics on operating room performance. They encouraged staff to suggest improvements, and they celebrated successes. Maybe she could get the Capitol Eye Hospital administrator, Jerry Jones, to do more of that at Capitol. After all, he was a trained administrator. Mr. Jones was reluctant to step on any toes, though, so he tended to do whatever the physicians wanted. Maybe he just needed some encouragement to get more ambitious and assertive about team-based care.

Clinical professionals often express concern (or worse) in regard to the contribution of administrators to clinical healthcare delivery. For team-based decision making to work in healthcare delivery organizations, clinical professionals can help by enhancing efforts to enroll administrators in the improvement of delivery, including team-based care. In addition, they can seek to involve themselves in management decisions that influence clinical care, going beyond quality improvement activities—to information systems issues as well as marketing and human resources practices. In the preceding vignette, Dr. Peace seemed likely to engage Capitol Eye Hospital administrator Mr. Jones in such an exchange.

In the same way that an "attitude adjustment" on the part of many administrators is required, the same is true of clinical professionals. Such attitudes are cemented during professional education, which neglects the relationship of administration to clinical care. As one might expect, in the education of clinicians the focus is on developing appropriate clinical expertise, not on understanding the context for care. However, there is no reason that both cannot be done, with education about administration and leadership provided at an introductory level. Clinicians can be introduced to administrators and to administrative functions that affect clinical care. Such education would alert new practitioners to their responsibility to get involved in administrative issues that affect patient care (and almost all do). Arrangements for reimbursement of time, organizational position, and other related issues need to be worked out in collaborative fashion. In the workplace, too, continuing education for clinicians can reinforce their responsibility for involvement in administrative decision making.

CONCLUSION

Administrators of healthcare delivery organizations are notably absent from clinical care teams. Administrators, throughout the organization, from the unit level to the executive suite, are key assets in the delivery of team-based care. They have information, expertise, and access to resources that help teams succeed. In the case of the top leaders, administrators have a view of the whole organization, have relationships with multiple teams, and have linkages with external constituencies, such as payers, the media, and philanthropic organizations that can prove important to patient care teams.

Whether they are physically present in teams or not, administrators should be viewed as partners in every clinical care team effort. Similarly, clinicians (and patients) should infuse management teams with their unique perspectives on management challenges.

REFERENCES

Barker R. No, management is *not* a profession. *Harv Bus Rev.* 2010;88(7/8):52-60.

Begun JW, White KR. The challenge of change: inspiring leadership. In: Lindberg Claire, Nash S, Lindberg Curt, eds. *On the Edge: Nursing in the Age of Complexity.* Bordentown, NJ: Plexus Press; 2008:239-262.

Begun JW, White KR, Mosser G. Interprofessional care teams: the role of the healthcare administrator. *J Interprof Care.* 2011;25:119-123.

Calhoun JG, Dollet L, Sinioris ME, et al. Development of an interprofessional competency model for healthcare leadership. *J Healthc Manag.* 2008;53:375-389.

Campbell DA, Thompson M. Patient safety rounds: description of an inexpensive but important strategy to improve the safety culture. *Am J Med Qual.* 2007;22:26-33.

Cowen ME, Halasyamani LK, McMurtrie D, et al. Organizational structure for addressing the attributes of the ideal healthcare delivery system. *J Healthc Manag.* 2008;53: 407-418.

Harris JE. The internal organization of hospitals: some economic implications. *Bell Journal of Economics.* 1977;8: 467-482.

Lega F, Calciolari S. Coevolution of patients and hospitals: how changing epidemiology and technological advances create challenges and drive organizational innovation. *J Healthc Manag.* 2012;57:17-34.

Lega F, DePietro C. Converging patterns in hospital organization: beyond the professional bureaucracy. *Health Policy.* 2005;74(3):261-281.

Leicht KT, Fennell ML. *Professional Work.* Malden, MA: Blackwell; 2001.

Mintzberg H. *The Structuring of Organizations: A Synthesis of the Research.* Englewood Cliffs, NJ: Prentice-Hall; 1979.

Reason J. Human error: models and management. *BMJ.* 2000;320:768-770.

Schwendimann R, Zimmermann N, Küng K, et al. Variation in safety culture dimensions within and between US and Swiss hospital units: an exploratory study. *BMJ Qual Saf.* 2013; 22:32-41.

Sexton JB, Makary MA, Tersigni AR, et al. Teamwork in the operating room: frontline perspectives among hospitals and operating room personnel. *Anesthesiology.* 2006; 105: 877-884.

Shewchuk R, O'Connor SJ, Fine DJ. Building an understanding of the competencies needed for health administration practice. *J Healthc Manag.* 2005;50:32-47.

Stefl ME. Common competencies for all healthcare managers: the Healthcare Leadership Alliance model. *J Healthc Manag.* 2008;53:360-373.

White KR, Griffith JR. *The Well-Managed Healthcare Organization.* 7th ed. Chicago, IL: Health Administration Press; 2010.

Effective Healthcare Teams

Section I (Chapters 1-5) deals with the concept of a work team, different types of teams, team members in different professions, and the roles of patients and administrators. We have introduced and explained healthcare teams and their members.

In Section II (Chapters 6-12) we cover how healthcare teams function. We begin in this chapter with an account of effective healthcare teams, explaining the characteristics of effective teams and the hazards they must cope with. In Chapters 7-12, we explain what is needed to achieve effectiveness in teams. Chapter 7 covers the competencies that team members need to have. Chapter 8 explains team leadership. Chapters 9-11 deal with decision making, creativity, and managing conflicts—topics that are important for all team members but have special importance for team leaders. Chapter 12 addresses team sponsorship, including the crucial topic of team design.

EFFECTIVE TEAMS

What are the hallmarks of an effective team? How does anyone know that the team she or he belongs to or leads is performing well? The ultimate touchstone of an effective team in any arena is that it achieves the purpose for which it exists. Clinical teams and management teams have different purposes. We consider clinical teams first.

Clinical Teams

The purpose of a clinical team is to deliver excellent health care to its patients, and so an effective clinical team is one that delivers high quality care. As discussed in Chapter 4, in 2001 the Institute of Medicine (IOM) set forth 6 aims for the improvement of health care (Institute of Medicine, 2001, pp. 39-60). The 6 aims are shown in Table 6–1. Taken together, they constitute a definition of quality in health care. An effective clinical team is one that achieves these aims.

Safety

Safe health care is care free of errors that cause injuries to patients (Institute of Medicine, 2000, pp. 18-40). A clinical team is a safe team if it avoids giving patients the wrong medication, failing to diagnose cancer or other diseases at an early stage, performing surgery on the wrong (unintended) body part, and so on. Many medical treatments carry known risk, for example, the risk of infection following high-dose chemotherapy for various cancers. When the risk is justified by the potential benefit for the patient, the occurrence of the unwanted consequence does not mean that the care was unsafe. Unsafe care is care that results from errors, that is, accidents or mistakes. Unsafe care resulting from an accident is either care that includes unintended actions or care from which components are unintentionally omitted, causing or threatening harm. An example of unsafe care due to an accident is surgery during which the surgeon removes the patient's appendix but also unintentionally punctures the nearby small intestine. Unsafe care resulting from a mistake is care that includes actions that are intentional but are improperly chosen, causing or threatening harm. An example of unsafe care due to a mistake is a tonsillectomy

Table 6–1. Six aims for healthcare improvement

Six aims
Safety
Effectiveness
Patient-centeredness
Timeliness
Efficiency
Equity

Source: Institute of Medicine. *Crossing the Quality Chasm: A New Health System for the 21st Century.* Washington, DC: National Academy Press; 2001:41-54.

performed on the wrong child because the child was improperly identified prior to surgery. The surgeon intentionally operated on the child, that is, the removal of the child's tonsils was not an accident; but the identification of the child was mistaken.

Effectiveness

Effective health care is care that can be expected to prevent, cure, or alleviate the symptoms of a disease because the care is known to be successful in achieving one or another of these objectives, ideally on the basis of scientific evidence demonstrating the effectiveness of the diagnostic test or the treatment in question. Effective care achieves its objective of undoing the ill effects of physical or mental disease or of preventing the disease from occurring. At first blush, it may appear tautological and uninformative to define effective clinical teams in part as teams that achieve effectiveness; this would seem to be true by definition. But, of course, the word *effectiveness* is used here in a special sense. Effective clinical teams aim to achieve more than effectiveness in this narrow sense, for example, they aim to achieve patient-centeredness and other objectives noted below. Effective care, in this narrow sense, is care that repairs the biological machine—or repairs the mental machine, or prevents either one from needing repairs.

Patient-Centeredness

Patient-centeredness is discussed in detail in Chapter 4. Patient-centered health care is care that is focused on achieving the patient's goals, is consistent with his or her values and preferences, and is attentive to his or her experience of health care.

Timeliness

Timely health care is care that is free of unnecessary delays. These delays include waits to obtain an appointment to see a clinician in a healthcare team, waits in the emergency room, waits to receive information about test results, waits for surgery to be done, and so on.

Efficiency

Efficient health care is care that uses the fewest resources possible to achieve the desired outcome, whatever it is. The essence of efficient care is absence of waste. Efficient care and low-cost care are not the same. Low cost can usually be achieved by accepting a lesser outcome, in other words, by withholding various services that are necessary to achieve the desired outcome. Under these circumstances, decreasing the cost would not result in high efficiency in achieving the original outcome because that outcome has been set aside. The care might be efficient in achieving the less desirable outcome, but that is a separate question; and this question is commonly of no interest because the lesser outcome is not desired.

Efficient care and high-value care are also not the same. Value is defined as outcome relative to cost as shown in Figure 6–1 (Porter, 2010). High-value health care is care that produces good results—as judged, for example, by the IOM 6 aims—for low cost so that the outcome "numerator" divided by the cost "denominator" yields a value "quotient" that is high. One could improve the value score for an episode of health care either by improving the outcome or lowering the cost. Also, the same value quotient could be achieved by combining a high-outcome numerator with a moderate-cost denominator or by combining a low-outcome numerator with a very low-cost denominator. In other words, high value could be achieved by sacrificing effectiveness as defined above, provided that the cost is low enough. For this reason, it is either incomplete or misleading to say baldly that clinical teams should aim to provide high-value care without saying something about quality and cost as separate considerations. The concept of value encompasses both quality and cost, and it conflates the contributions of the two. Efficiency

$$\text{V(alue)} = \frac{\text{Q(uality)}}{\text{C(ost)}}$$

▲ Figure 6–1. Definition of value in health care.

is a less ambitious concept than value. Any claim of efficiency is made relative to a specified level of achievement of outcomes. Fully efficient care is simply care that is free of waste in achieving whatever outcome is under consideration.

Equity

Equitable health care is care that is delivered without regard to considerations that are irrelevant to health needs, for example, gender, race, ethnic group, or urban versus rural location. Seeking equity in health care means pursuing reductions in disparities across different populations defined by income level and other factors that ought to be irrelevant to the care provided and the quality of care provided. Seeking equity also means providing care at the same level of quality to individuals without regard to these irrelevant factors considered as personal characteristics of the individual.

Assessing a Clinical Team's Effectiveness

Although the burden of measurement would be great, one could in theory determine the effectiveness of a clinical team by measuring its activities and outputs across the 6 IOM aims. Clinical teams vary with respect to the emphasis they place on different IOM aims, but all 6 aims are important for all teams. For example, a team of nurses and social workers staffing a hospital ward typically will be focused heavily on patient-centeredness, but safety, effectiveness, and timeliness also will be important parts of their goal. In measuring team effectiveness, adjustments would be needed to take account of the disease burden in the population of patients served by the assessed team. For some measures, the circumstances under which the team operates would also need to be taken into account, for example, whether a rural hospital has the equipment to handle certain rare emergencies. Making these adjustments would be no small matter. But even without an operational method for measuring effectiveness, the concept of effectiveness—based on the IOM aims—is clear in its application to clinical teams. In other words, clinical teams are effective insofar as they achieve the 6 aims.

Management Teams

All clinical teams are alike in their aims, but different management teams have different aims. All clinical teams aim to provide high-quality health care to their patients. Some management teams aim to devise effective business strategy for healthcare systems; other management teams have a specific time-limited objective, for example, implementation of a new billing system; other management teams provide advice to decision makers but do not take action themselves. Some management teams work to provide good health care in a particular operational unit such as an intensive care unit (ICU), but the operational team for an ICU works only through those who deliver care directly, namely, the clinical ICU team. While the IOM 6 aims define the purpose of the clinical ICU team, they do not define the purpose of the ICU's operational team considered as a separate component of the whole. The IOM aims would not be helpful in determining the operational team's contribution to the success of the entire unit. Other management teams are aimed at more abstract objectives such as financial security or a favorable community reputation for an integrated health system. Again, the IOM aims will not serve to define their purposes. For a management team, as with a clinical team, the touchstone of effectiveness is achievement of its purpose. These purposes can be specified for individual management teams in a way that permits assessment of their effectiveness, but little can be said about how to specify the aims of management teams in general.

CHARACTERISTICS OF EFFECTIVE TEAMS

An effective team is one that achieves its purpose; and when achievement of purpose can be measured, this approach to assessing effectiveness is superior to all others. However, adequate information on achievement of purpose is often difficult to obtain or cannot be obtained within a workable time frame. And so it is useful to have additional measures of effectiveness. Fortunately, many additional measures are available. When achievement of purpose cannot be measured, one can assess the quality of a team by examining characteristics that are conducive to achievement of purpose. This approach is analogous to measuring clinical quality by measuring process measures instead of outcome measures. The approach is sound if the processes measured are known to contribute to achieving the outcomes of interest. In the case of clinical teams, these outcomes are one or more of the IOM 6 aims. In the case of management teams the outcomes depend on the purpose of the team.

Those who come to the topic of teamwork with a background in clinical science, especially pharmacists and physicians, will want empirical evidence for claims that certain team attributes and processes lead to achievement of the team's goals. In medicine, pharmacy, and other clinical fields, best evidence commonly comes from controlled trials, often randomized, controlled trials. But teamwork (including clinical teamwork) is a management topic, not a clinical topic. Unlike evidence-based practice in health care, evidence-based management is in its infancy. Sometimes the desired evidence is available, and some of that evidence is cited in Chapters 1 and 2. For some claims, however, the only evidence available comes from case studies or the experience of managers. Given the usual impracticality (or impossibility) of doing controlled trials, the complexity of organizational systems, and the difficulty of generalizing from one setting to another, we may never reach the level of evidence for management decision making that we already have for making many clinical decisions (Begun, 2009). In the workaday world, one has no choice but to move forward using what is available while pressing for more evidence and sometimes gathering it along the way.

Work Team Defining Characteristics Revisited

In Chapter 1, the defining characteristics of a work team are discussed. In exploring the effectiveness of teams, it is assumed, of course, that these teams are real teams, with all 7 defining characteristics. Some of the characteristics of effective teams are particularly robust or well-developed versions of these defining characteristics, which are listed in Table 1–1 in Chapter 1. Briefly, the characteristics are (1) the presence of a shared goal for the team, (2) shared responsibility for achieving the goal, (3) defined team membership, (4) possession by the team of sufficient authority to achieve its goal, (5) interdependency of team members in accomplishing their tasks, (6) absence of sub-groups that operate without accountability to the whole team, and (7) accountability of the team to the larger organization in which it works (if there is a larger organization).

Effective Team Characteristics

Going beyond these initial 7 characteristics, effective teams can be described with more richness by considering their attributes under 5 categories: (1) structure of the team, (2) focus of the team on the patient, (3) orientation of team members to the team, (4) collaborative work done by the team, and (5) management of the team. The different types of healthcare teams are discussed in Chapter 2. The types of clinical teams are listed in Table 2–1, and the types of management teams are listed in Table 2–9. The characteristics falling under each of the 5 categories of effectiveness apply to true clinical teams and template clinical teams. Only some of the characteristics apply to clinical knotworks. This limitation is not surprising since knotworks do not have all 7 defining characteristics of work teams and are team-like groups rather than full-blown teams. The characteristics under each of the 5 categories also apply to management teams, that is, to operational teams, project teams, consultative teams, and leadership teams. Figure 6–2 depicts the 5 categories, considered as clusters of components of effective team performance.

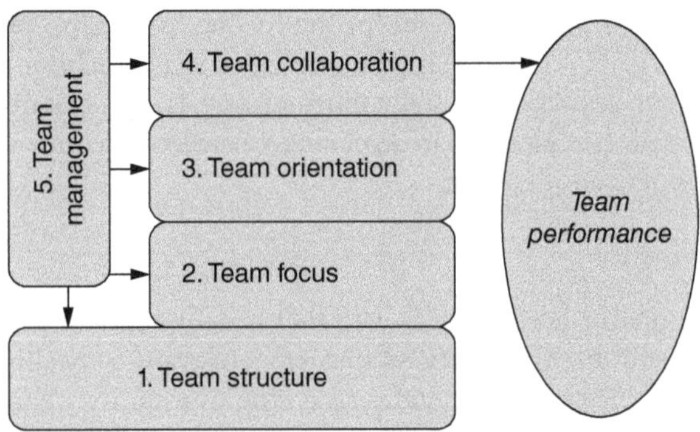

▲ Figure 6–2. Components of effective team performance.

Team Structure

David Ziegler, MD, was leading rounds in the surgical ICU on Wednesday morning. The ICU was part of a teaching hospital in Washington State. Dr. Ziegler was the head of the unit. With him were 2 surgical residents, a clinical pharmacist, a physician assistant, and 3 medical students doing their clerkships in surgical intensive care (6-week training periods). The head nurse sometimes joined the group on rounds, but she was attending an administrative meeting that morning. Sometimes the social worker attached to the unit also joined the group, but that morning she was meeting with the family of a critically ill patient. As the group moved from patient to patient, the critical care nurse caring for each patient joined the discussion. When the clinicians were seeing a patient who could participate in the discussion, they included the patient too—although most of the patients were either sedated or too ill to join in. Dr. Ziegler frequently asked questions of the other members of the group. One or the other of the 2 residents had primary medical responsibility for each of the patients, and for each patient Dr. Ziegler asked the responsible resident for the details of the patient's progress and for the test results obtained since the group had rounded the evening before. He asked the medical students more general questions about the patient's medical problem or the significance of various test results. Throughout these interactions it was clear that Dr. Ziegler was in charge. The residents answered his questions quickly and respectfully, avoiding any extraneous comments. They also offered their viewpoints freely and showed no signs of hesitation in stating their views. The medical students answered as well as they could, but sometimes they did not know the answers. All 3 of them looked nervous but not intimidated. When a medical student could not answer a question, Dr. Ziegler would either answer the question himself or redirect it to one of the residents. He never belittled the students for answering incorrectly or for not being able to answer his questions. The pharmacist was often asked for information and judgments about the drugs being administered, and she often volunteered comments unprompted. The critical care nurses usually offered comments on the patient's progress after the resident responsible for that patient had summarized the key events during the past 18 hours or so. The critical care nurses often commented on whether the patient was agitated and whether the family members had visited. Dr. Ziegler's manner was purposeful and earnest. However, he did offer light-hearted remarks from time to time, especially when talking with patients who were able to converse with him.

Dr. Ziegler's team was a well-structured clinical team. The structural characteristics of effective teams are shown in Table 6–2.

Table 6–2. Characteristics of effective teams: team structure

1. A shared goal, understood by all team members
2. Shared responsibility across team members for achieving the goal
3. Well-defined membership for the whole team or for the core team, with or without defined peripheral membership
4. A clear leader, acknowledged by all team members as the leader
5. Sufficient hierarchy to enable quick decision making if needed
6. Adequate authority for the team to take action to achieve its goal
7. Stability of membership; the more stable the better

First, like all other effective teams, the members not only had a shared goal but understood it very well and could have stated the goal clearly if asked (Thompson, 2011, p. 76). The first priority was to provide safe and effective care so that patients could quickly move through the ICU to a regular surgical unit in the hospital. In addition, they aimed to provide for the psychological and emotional needs of the patients and their families. For this second purpose the team relied especially on the nurses and the social worker.

Second, all of the team members understood that they shared responsibility for achieving their goal, that is, providing excellent health care for their patients.

Third, the membership of the team was well defined (Hackman, 2002, pp. 44-50), and the members' roles were well defined (Thompson, 2011, p. 79; Mitchell et al, 2012, pp. 9-13). The team consisted of Dr. Ziegler, the residents, the critical care nurses, the head nurse, the pharmacist, the physician assistant, the social worker, and the health unit coordinator (a clerical staff member). The coordinator never participated in rounds but did participate in other team functions. The medical students were not core team members. They might be regarded as peripheral or secondary members. They were present to learn, not to care for the patients; and everyone understood this distinction. Although each patient was a member of his or her care team, in this case the patients' participation was quite limited because of their medical conditions. In many cases, family members served as surrogates in making decisions about care. In total, the core team had 10-13 members, depending on the number of critical care nurses working at any given time. In other words, it was small enough for all of the members to interact directly with all of the other members and have complex, detailed conversations when such conversations were required for good patient care. We discuss the important question of team size, especially the advantages of small size, in Chapter 12 when discussing the design of teams.

Fourth, the team had a clear leader in Dr. Ziegler, and he was acknowledged by all other team members to be the leader. This feature of the team is implied by the clear roles for the members, but it merits special mention because of its importance, which is well recognized in health care (Firth-Cozens and Mowbray, 2001). The leadership need not be vested in one person. Some teams are genuinely co-led by 2 people. Co-leadership by 3 people usually reflects a political compromise, and is usually not functional for a long period of time—unless the arrangement is actually rotating leadership and not true co-leadership. This ICU care team in fact had rotating leadership since the attending surgeon changed every month. Dr. Ziegler would be replaced by another surgeon when his month as ICU head was completed.

This ICU team was led by a physician as is commonly the case for clinical teams. Must the leader of a clinical team always be a physician? Many physicians think so. For example, in the statement of principles for patient-centered medical homes, issued in 2007 jointly by 4 national physician associations, the second principle is that a medical home is a "physician-directed medical practice" (American Academy of Family Physicians et al, 2007). Many advanced practice nurses do not agree. In Chapter 8, we take up the contentious question of whether clinical team leaders must be physicians.

Fifth, the team had a steep enough hierarchy to provide for its needs. Hierarchies of authority enable decisions to be made quickly. Hierarchies also enable teams to maintain order and give people an understanding of what authority they have in the team (Leavitt, 2003). In this ICU team, Dr. Ziegler had final decision-making authority for treatment decisions requiring quick action, for example, decisions about whether rapidly deteriorating patients need to return to the operating room for the management of postoperative complications such as bleeding inside the chest. On the other hand, Dr. Ziegler did not demand frequent acknowledgements of his superior standing, and he welcomed information, opinions, and suggestions from the pharmacist, the nurses, and other team members—although probably not the medical students. All teams need some hierarchy of authority to maintain order; authority differences beyond the minimal level required to maintain order need to be justified because differences in status and authority within teams threaten communication as discussed in Chapter 2.

Sixth, the team had clear authority to do its work (Thompson, 2011, pp. 76-77). The team was expected to provide health care for the patients in the ICU without seeking input or approval from anyone except for the patients and their families, whom they regarded as team members in any case. Ultimately, the ICU, represented by Dr. Ziegler, the head nurse, and the unit's administrator, were accountable to the senior leadership of the hospital (the Chief Medical Officer, Chief Nursing Officer, and Chief Executive Officer), but this accountability did not imply the need for any action by the senior leaders in the care of individual patients.

Seventh, the team had some degree of membership stability. As in all teaching hospitals, there was turnover in the team according to a calendar known to everyone well ahead of any changes. Dr. Ziegler was the attending surgeon this month, but there were 5 other surgeons who also served as attending surgeons, rotating each month. The residents changed every other month. Meanwhile, the head nurse, the other critical care nurses, the pharmacist, the social worker, and the health unit coordinator changed only rarely. As discussed in Chapter 2, stability of team membership is conducive to good performance. Thus even greater stability would likely make the team more effective. However, the attending physicians also had other duties to fulfill, and the residents were in training and needed to gain experience in surgical areas besides the ICU. Changes every month or two are preferable to changes every week. The team was as stable as it could be, given the other responsibilities of the surgeons. It was not a true team like the primary care team in Chapter 1 or the colonoscopy team in Chapter 2, but neither was a rapidly changing template team like the emergency room teams described in Chapter 2. It was somewhere in between. One might call this team a *slow-turnover template team*.

The value of membership stability is particularly well recognized in primary care (Willard and Bodenheimer, 2012), but stability is valuable for any team, for reasons detailed in Chapter 2. This has important implications for the scheduling of physicians, nurses, and other clinicians in template teams. Specifically, scheduling of whole teams is preferable to scheduling individuals separately because separate scheduling of individuals to comprise template teams results in constantly changing membership (Hackman, 2002, pp. 54-59). There are many factors that stand in the way of scheduling of whole teams in health care, and these factors are not unique to health care: tradition, union contracts, desires of clinicians to set their own schedules, and concerns about costs—although experience in some other industries indicates that costs are often reduced by scheduling whole teams (Hackman, 2002, pp. 58-59). If institutions continue to prefer scheduling individuals, they should at least acknowledge that this practice is second-best, and they should keep template teams intact whenever possible.

As depicted in Figure 6–2, a sound structure is the platform or foundation that enables a team to function well in the 4 areas to be discussed next. If pieces of the platform are missing, the team will be hampered in its performance. For example, if the membership of the team is not well defined, then the team will have difficulty in making decisions that last over time. And if a team is not stable, then it will be difficult for the team to develop a sense of identity.

Team Focus

The Chief Executive Officer (CEO), Chief Nursing Officer (CNO), Chief Medical Officer (CMO), Director of Pharmacy, attorney for the hospital, and Theresa Fournier, MD, were meeting on a Wednesday morning in 1992 to discuss the care of Bobby Harrington, a 5-year-old boy with leukemia, specifically, acute lymphoblastic leukemia (ALL). Dr. Fournier was a pediatric oncologist at a children's hospital in North Carolina. She and her team had been treating Bobby.

Bobby had developed fatigue and severe nosebleeds about 6 weeks earlier. Investigation quickly revealed that he had ALL. His white blood count at the time was extremely high, placing him at higher risk of death than other children of similar age with ALL. Mr. and Ms. Harrington wanted to understand all they could about the disease and the treatment options available for Bobby. The initial treatment was evidence-based and well established. It consisted of chemotherapy aimed at achieving control (remission) of the disease in the short run, to be followed by other treatment aimed at achieving cure in the long run. Assuming that control would be achieved, the next step in Bobby's treatment might include eradication of Bobby's bone marrow, followed by bone marrow transplantation with disease-free bone marrow. This step, which carries considerable danger, warranted serious consideration because of Bobby's high white blood cell count at the time he was found to have ALL. In other words, Bobby's higher than usual risk of death from ALL warranted consideration of more aggressive treatment early in the disease to prevent the disease from recurring in a form that would be resistant to further treatment. Mr. and Ms. Harrington spent many hours reading and talking with one of the pediatric oncology nurses on the team, Dr. Fournier, a clinical pharmacist, and a radiation oncologist (who might be involved in the bone marrow transplant if that treatment pathway was chosen). Bobby's parents anticipated deliberating with Dr. Fournier and other team members about whether a bone marrow transplant should be done. The decision would be made after it was known how Bobby responded to the initial treatment. In the meantime, the pediatric oncology team was engaged in supporting both Bobby and his parents as they coped with the disease.

Bobby's initial treatment regimen included intravenous (IV) vincristine, a potent anticancer drug. Three weeks prior to the meeting of the CEO and others, Bobby had been given 10 times the intended dose of vincristine. The error had originated in the pharmacy, where 10 times the required amount of the drug was mixed with IV fluid in the plastic bag used in administering the drug. It was unclear how the error had occurred. The bag was transferred to the patient care area with the amount of the drug indicated on the bag's label. Despite the label showing the high dose of vincristine, the oncology nurse treating Bobby that day had administered the drug.

Over the next 3 weeks, Bobby had lost sensation in his feet and had developed some difficulty walking because of weakness in his lower legs and inability to lift his feet normally. The symptoms had advanced gradually and had been plainly evident for only 2 days prior to the Wednesday meeting. The loss of sensation was discovered only after the muscular weakness was noted by his parents. Bobby, being only 5 years old, had said nothing about his feet being numb.

The question addressed at the Wednesday meeting was what to tell Bobby's parents—and how and when. The attorney raised the possibility of saying nothing and waiting out the symptoms, which were likely to resolve completely with time. The CEO, who was an administrator without a clinical background, responded firmly that hiding the error was out of the question. He told a brief story about being counseled 15 years earlier by an attorney to disclose nothing to the parents of a child who had died because of a surgical error. After talking with the child's parents without acknowledging the error, he had pondered what had happened and vowed that he would never again mislead or lie to parents in dealing with a healthcare error causing harm. The question, said the CEO, was simply how and when to tell Mr. and Ms. Harrington what had caused their son's symptoms.

The meeting was short. Dr. Fournier offered to speak with Bobby's parents. She and the CEO met with Mr. and Ms. Harrington that morning and explained in detail what had happened. Dr. Fournier took the lead in the discussion. She told Bobby's parents what the future might hold for Bobby, acknowledging that no prediction could be made with certainty. She pledged that the hospital would do everything possible to see that the error did not occur again—in Bobby's care or in the care of any other patient. By his presence, the CEO conveyed to the parents that the hospital accepted responsibility for the error and stood with Dr. Fournier in dealing with the consequences. He apologized on behalf of the hospital. Bobby's parents expressed their anger about what had happened, but they strongly emphasized their gratitude for being told promptly and openly what caused the problem. They asked what was being done to assure that the error was not repeated, and they expressed their confidence in Dr. Fournier and the other members of the pediatric oncology team who were caring for Bobby.

This pediatric oncology team was squarely focused on the interests of Bobby Harrington and his parents. Actually, there were 2 teams at work here, a clinical team and a management team. Both teams were effective in interacting with Bobby and his parents. The characteristics of effective teams as they focus on patients and families are listed in Table 6–3.

Despite the serious medication error, Dr. Fournier and her clinical team were able to maintain an effective relationship with Bobby and his parents. The senior leadership team of the hospital, which was a management team, also had a good relationship with the parents. The CEO was directly involved. He did not leave the handling of the calamity to the CNO or CMO. What accounts for both teams being able to maintain good relationships in this highly regrettable situation?

Table 6–3. Characteristics of effective teams: team focus

1. Respect for the interests of patients and families, above all other interests
2. Generation of trust in patients and families
3. Support for patients as partners in their care or managers of their own care (if they want to be partners or to be in charge)

First, all of the healthcare people involved—including the attorney, who felt obliged to play devil's advocate briefly—respected Bobby's parents (and Bobby) as persons and set their interests ahead of those of the hospital and everyone who participated in Bobby's care. The clinicians and administrators sought to understand not only the parents' and Bobby's goals but also the parents' experience of Bobby's health care. They sought to provide for the parents' wants as defined by them. Before the medication error, they responded without reservation to the parents' wishes for information and for discussion of the available treatment options. After the error, their dedication to Bobby's and the parents' interests was even more obvious. As voiced by the CEO in the Wednesday morning meeting, the hospital's interest was less important than giving the parents what they wanted, namely, the truth about what had happened. In 2012, this approach to dealing with a medical injury is becoming common worldwide although there are still obstacles and nay-sayers (Iedema et al, 2011). In 1992, providing full and prompt disclosure was unusual, even courageous. At that time, fear of litigation and damage to reputation commonly led both administrators and clinicians to put their own interests and the interests of their organizations ahead of the interests of the patients and their families. In contrast, Dr. Fournier and her colleagues put the patient's and family's interests first.

Second, the oncology team succeeded in garnering the trust of Bobby and his parents. Clinical teams face this challenge with every new patient and family.

(Management teams are not often called on to gain the trust of specific patients and their families although they need to do so occasionally, as in this case.) If this trust in the team had not existed prior to the medication error, it is doubtful that good relations would have prevailed when the causes of the error were disclosed. During the process of diagnosis, treatment planning, and initiation of treatment, the team had engendered in Bobby's parents the belief that the team had both *competence* and *integrity*. These 2 components of trust are separate, and both are necessary. A healthcare team might bring a patient to believe that the team is competent but prone to hide shortcomings or even to lie to avoid blame. In that case, the team would not have succeeded in generating the full trust that is achieved by an effective team. On the other hand, a team might generate in the patient the belief that the team has high integrity but not generate the belief that the team can perform its technical tasks reliably. In that case, full trust would also not be present. If Bobby's parents had had doubts about the team's integrity, they most likely would not have accepted the explanation of the error as true or complete. If they had had doubts about the team's competence, they would have had difficulty accepting Dr. Fournier's pledge that the error would not be repeated. Either way, ongoing care for Bobby and his parents would have been compromised.

The trust at issue here is trust in the whole team. Of course, the behavior of individuals determines whether trust is achieved, but the flawless behavior of most team members will ordinarily not compensate for the flawed performance of 1 or 2 members. Some patients and families will differentiate among team members, but most will not and probably *should* not for 2 reasons. First, the team members operate interdependently so that the poor performance of 1 or 2 members affects the results achieved by the whole team. Second, as patients with knowledge of behavior in organizations will know, the performance of any and all members of the team is heavily influenced by the systems or context in which they work. So poor performance by 1 or 2 members may well indicate a flaw in the forces that affect the whole team. In Bobby's case, the initial error was made by a pharmacist or pharmacy technician. This may have been a matter of poor individual performance, or it may have resulted from a system defect within the pharmacy. Regardless, others also participated in Bobby's care and contributed to the injury. The error is best attributed to the whole team, including its system or processes for doing its work. The question on Mr. and Ms. Harrington's minds is whether they can trust the whole team.

Third, the oncology team demonstrated its commitment to serving the parents' interests by supporting the parents in their desire to be partners in Bobby's care. As soon as Bobby was found to have ALL, his parents expressed their desire to learn as much as they could about the disease and Bobby's treatment. They did not want to be in charge (like the lawyer with coccidioidal meningitis in Chapter 4), but they did want to be actively involved in making the decision about whether a bone marrow transplant should be done and in making any other decisions that lay ahead. The team showed that it understood the parents' viewpoint, respected it, and was willing and able to support Mr. and Ms. Harrington in their chosen role in Bobby's care.

In other situations, supporting patients as partners would also include providing them with assistance for self-management as discussed in Chapter 4. Patients with chronic diseases such as rheumatoid arthritis need more than information if they are to manage their own diseases day-to-day. They need skills in identifying and solving problems. When serving patients with these needs, additional activities are manifest in effective teams, for example, motivational interviewing and referrals to programs providing self-management education.

The ultimate purpose of any healthcare team—whether it is a clinical team or a management team—is to protect and restore the health of the people who are served, or, if prevention or cure is not possible, to minimize symptoms and decrease suffering. To say that effective teams are focused on the patient is simply to say that they are focused on the purpose of health care without distraction or compromise by secondary goals. As shown in Figure 6–2, team focus is the second element needed for a team to be effective. Focus provides the aim for the rest of the team's activities. We turn next to how effective teams function to achieve the object of their focus.

Team Orientation

Dr. Kimpell, Dr. Gomez, Penny Mills, RN, and their colleagues provide primary care to about 9000 people in a large clinic in North Dakota. They were introduced in Chapter 1 as the members of one of 4 primary care groups in their clinic. There are 11 members of the team, including physicians, a nurse practitioner (NP), a registered nurse, medical assistants, and receptionists. They are known throughout the medical group as Red Family Medicine or the Red Team.

Red Family Medicine meets once monthly. The main purposes of the meetings are to troubleshoot operational issues and to keep the team's process improvement projects moving forward. Dr. Kimpell always wants everyone on the team to attend the meetings. The only exception is that one of the 2 receptionists needs to be at the front desk to answer the telephone and help any patients or parents who arrive unexpectedly. The 2 receptionists alternate this duty every other month. Having everyone attend the monthly meetings is important to Dr. Kimpell and the other team members because it repeatedly reminds everyone that all team members are important for the team's success in providing patient care.

Over the years, largely through decisions made at the monthly meetings, the team has developed a standardized approach to doing its work. For example, telephone calls from patients seeking healthcare advice are normally directed to Ms. Mills. However, any patient who requests to speak with a physician is either connected with a physician or, more often, is told that a physician will call the patient back within 4 hours. Also, laboratory test results are reviewed first by the physician or NP who ordered the test. In the days before the electronic health record, the medical assistants reviewed all test results first and passed along to the ordering clinicians only those results that were abnormal. This routine delayed action on abnormal results but saved time for the clinicians in handling the paperwork for normal results. This same sequence was used briefly after the records were automated, but it became apparent quite soon that with the electronic record this routine saved very little time for the clinicians. The delays in acting on abnormal results could be eliminated without any significant inefficiency for the clinicians.

In conversation inside and outside of the team, the members of the team identify themselves as members of Red Family Medicine. They can easily say what is distinctive about their group and how they fit into the larger whole. Being members of the team largely defines their work lives and their places in the larger organization. Last year one of the medical assistants came to work one Tuesday wearing a red scarf. She suggested that every Tuesday should be Ruby Tuesday and that people should wear something red to celebrate the team. The other medical assistants, Ms. Mills (the registered nurse), and the receptionists quickly joined in as did Dr. Gomez. The other physicians and the NP were a bit embarrassed by this idea, but Dr. Kimpell did wear one or another red tie each Tuesday for a while. Eventually the idea died out except for the occasional red sweater or tie.

Dr. Kimpell is the leader of the team. He is very attentive to what he calls the morale of the team. Others call it the social climate. Every summer he invites all of the team members and their families to his home, which is located on a river west of town. He and his wife host a picnic; and toward the end of the afternoon, the team members give each other joke awards. One year, Dr. Gomez, who is well known in the team for becoming agitated when things do not go smoothly in the clinic, was given "an Ativan (antianxiety drug) the size of a hockey puck," in other words, a hockey puck painted white. She enjoyed the ribbing as much as everyone else. It was all in good fun. Members of the group rarely miss these picnics. They appreciate both the fun and the contribution that the social interaction makes to the functioning of the team.

Red Family Medicine also engages in behavior that often surprises other physicians and nurses who happen to visit the unit. The team members point out each other's omissions and mistakes. For example, one afternoon after the clinic session was finished, Carrie Tanaka, CMA, one of the medical assistants, saw Dr. Lewis walking away from her down the hallway with his overcoat on and briefcase in hand. "Just a minute," she said and then reminded him that earlier in the day he had said that he would telephone one of their patients himself to report that the patient's Pap smear was mildly abnormal and needed to be repeated. Both Ms. Tanaka and Dr. Lewis knew the patient well and knew that she would be upset by the news, even though the abnormality was very unlikely to be an indication of anything serious. They also knew that she would be put at ease more fully by hearing the explanation of the test result from Dr. Lewis rather than Ms. Tanaka or anyone else because she had a particularly strong relationship with Dr. Lewis. With a quick thank-you to Ms. Tanaka, Dr. Lewis went straight to the telephone. On another occasion, Dr. Pearson was preparing to inject an anti-inflammatory medication (methylprednisolone) into the knee joint of a patient with severe arthritis. April Simpkins, CMA, another medical assistant, was working with Dr. Pearson, and had just returned to the procedure room with a new vial of the medication. Ms. Simpkins noticed that Dr. Pearson had placed a packet of iodine (Betadine) swabs on the instrument stand. The swabs were to be used to clean the patient's skinned knee prior to inserting the needle into her knee. Flustered, Ms. Simpkins could think of nothing else to do except to ask Dr. Pearson to come with her to take an urgent telephone call. In the hallway, Ms. Simpkins explained that there was no telephone call. She recalled for Dr. Pearson that the patient had suffered a severe allergic reaction to iodine when she was in the hospital for surgery last year, as Dr. Pearson knew but had overlooked on this busy day in the clinic. Dr. Pearson thanked Ms. Simpkins for preventing a mistake that could have been quite serious. A different antiseptic solution was used in doing the knee injection.

The members of Red Family Medicine are oriented to being members of a team. They continually think about the performance of the whole team, and its capacity to perform well. They appreciate that simply carrying out their own individual tasks well will not be enough to meet the needs and wants of the patients, and they know that they need to spend time contributing to the team as well as time performing their own tasks. Table 6–4 lists the characteristics of teams whose members are effectively oriented to being a team.

Table 6–4. Characteristics of effective teams: team orientation

1. Agreement on common values
2. Agreement on a common set of processes to be used in doing the team's work
3. Team identity
4. Attention to the social climate of the team
5. Mutual accountability for achieving the team's goal
6. Spending time on activities that build and maintain the team

First, the team members agree on common values. The fact that all team members attend the monthly meetings symbolizes an important team value. All of the team members value the contributions of all other members, including the contributions of the receptionists, who are the most junior members of the team. Everyone is important to the team's success; no one is regarded as performing menial tasks that are taken for granted. Service to patients is also an important value. Dr. Lewis's delay in going home reflects the fact that the team regards service to patients as more important than convenience for physicians and others in the team. These values and many others are agreed on by all of the team members. In most effective teams, these values are rarely verbalized. They develop with time but require nurturing and protection by everyone, especially by the senior people in the team—in this case, the NP, the physicians, and the registered nurse. Dr. Kimpell's insistence that everyone attend the monthly meetings is an example of protecting the value that everyone has important contributions to make in serving the patients.

Second, the team has come to agreement on a common set of processes for doing their work. Some writers on teams regard this characteristic as sufficiently important to include it among the defining characteristics of a team (Katzenbach and Smith, 2006, pp. 56-59; Scholtes et al, 2003, pp. 1-2). In this primary care team, there is agreement that the different members have their own roles and that there will be monthly meetings plus additional ad hoc meetings to deal with issues that need rapid resolution. Some of these "rules of the road" have been established explicitly by the senior members of the team, and some have been established through group discussion at the monthly meetings (for example, the rule that patients should be addressed by their last names unless they request otherwise). Other behavior was acquired long ago in the course of the education and training of the team members in nursing school, medical school, and other educational institutions. Standardization of routines through professional training is typical of professional bureaucracies, discussed in Chapter 5 (Mintzberg, 1979, pp. 348-379).

Third, the team members identify with the team. This is evident in their calling themselves *Red Family Medicine* and the like. They take pleasure in celebrating their team as was apparent in the Ruby Tuesdays even though wearing red on Tuesdays was short-lived. Some writers on teams regard a work group as a work team only if its members identify with the team and its purpose (Reeves et al, 2010, pp. 40-41). In other words, they regard team identification a defining characteristic of work teams. Scholars of organizational behavior distinguish between what they call *group entiativity* and *group identity* (Thompson, 2011, p. 99). Group entiativity is the belief by the people in a group that they actually are a group or team. It is difficult to imagine how a team could function without entiativity. In order to work together interdependently, the members of a team must recognize that they constitute a group that has both a common purpose and some established methods for collaborating. In contrast to entiativity, group identity is the belief by people in a group that membership in the group is an important part of who they are. Teams can function without group identity, but those that have it benefit from it. When team members identify with the team, they are more likely to take to heart the team's goal and perform up to their full potential. To the extent they believe that their membership in the team defines who they are, their self-esteem is at stake. Few motivators are as powerful as the desire to preserve and strengthen self-esteem. Team identity also contributes to group cohesion, which is an emotional attraction among team members that helps to bind the team members together (Thompson, 2011, pp. 106-109). Cohesive teams are less prone to high turnover and more productive in performing various tasks than are teams that lack cohesion.

At the same time, as a practical matter, not all healthcare teams can aspire to having group identity—even though they have entiativity. Many healthcare template teams do not persist long enough for members to develop any sense of identification with the team. For example, a nurse who participates in a code blue team with other nurses, physicians, and pharmacists whom she does not know will not regard membership in this team as defining her identity in the workplace because the team is too short-lived. So too an administrator who works for 2 weeks on a team that drafts a budget will most likely not identify with the team even though she takes the assignment seriously and does her best. Still, when team members regard team membership as part of their personal identity, the team benefits and is likely to be more effective.

Fourth, the members of the Red Team are also attentive to their social or interpersonal dealings. Dr. Kimpell understands very well that the social climate of the team affects its ability to provide good health care to its patients, and he is not alone among Red Team members in having this understanding. The medical assistant who started Ruby Tuesdays may have worn red and promoted the idea because she thought it was fun and wanted to express her pride in being part of a first-rate healthcare team. On the other hand, she may have understood that Ruby Tuesdays would contribute in some measure to patient care by strengthening team identity and reinforcing interpersonal bonds within the team. Most of the team members regularly attended Dr. Kimpell's summer picnics in part because they understood that the picnics fostered social cohesion, which was carried back to the clinic. And everyone responded to Dr. Kimpell's occasional interventions to resolve relationship conflicts. Even if a team member remained annoyed with someone else, she or he knew that relationship conflicts interfere with serving the patients well and need to be resolved for the sake of the team's effectiveness.

Teams that ignore the social side of their activity, do so at their peril—and, for clinical teams, at the peril of their patients. Clinicians whose training emphasizes biological science, especially pharmacists and physicians, are often intensely focused on getting the patient-care job done and are often neglectful of interpersonal dealings with colleagues, expecting everyone "to just do their jobs." Fortunately, nurses and social workers are usually more attentive to interpersonal relations and can counterbalance the inclinations of the more task-oriented team members. Administrators vary more widely; some are well attuned to social interactions, but some are heavily task oriented.

Michael West, an organizational psychologist, has devised a helpful framework for understanding how a team's attention to task interacts with its attention to social climate in shaping the team's task effectiveness, its stability over time, and other aspects of its performance (West, 2012, pp. 6-10). A simplified interpretation of West's framework is depicted in Figure 6–3.

Most clinical teams that include physicians are at risk of having high task orientation without adequate orientation to social climate. These teams (upper, left quadrant of Figure 6–3) can be called *coldly efficient teams.*

Orientation to task \ Orientation to social climate	Low	High
High	*Coldly efficient team* High short-run task effectiveness Poor social climate Unstable over time	*Functional team* High task effectiveness Good social climate Stable over time
Low	*Dysfunctional team* Low task effectiveness Poor social climate Very unstable over time	*Comfortable team* Low task effectiveness Average social climate Unstable over time

▲ **Figure 6–3.** Task and social climate orientation in teams. (West MA. *Effective Teamwork: Practical Lessons from Organizational Research.* 3rd ed. Chichester, UK: John Wiley & Sons, Ltd.; 2012:6-10.)

They have high task effectiveness, at least in the short run, but their inattention to establishing a favorable social climate has adverse effects. For example, the poor social climate results in team members quitting or drifting away. These teams have "short-term viability," to use West's phrase. In other words, they are unstable over time. Also, these teams commonly have some members who are not fully engaged, especially the more junior members. The more senior members of the team often do not appreciate the junior members' contributions, or their appreciation is not expressed. As a consequence, the junior members become reluctant to offer new ideas because they fear being criticized. The junior members' contributions are therefore withheld, and so the task effectiveness of coldly efficient teams is usually lower than it could be.

Teams that are highly attentive to social climate but inattentive to task can be called *comfortable teams* (lower, right quadrant of Figure 6–3). Not surprisingly, these teams have poor task effectiveness. In addition, despite their attention to social and interpersonal dealings, comfortable teams achieve only a mediocre social climate because their members eventually become frustrated and dissatisfied due to the team's ineffectiveness. For this reason, comfortable teams, like coldly efficient teams, are unstable over time. Among clinical teams, comfortable teams are unusual; they are more frequent among management teams but still uncommon.

Dysfunctional teams (lower, left quadrant of Figure 6–3) are teams that do not attend adequately to task or to social climate. Obviously this combination is to be avoided. These teams have low task effectiveness. Working in them is unpleasant. And they are the most unstable of the 4 types represented in Figure 6–3.

Finally, *functional teams* (upper, right quadrant in Figure 6–3) attend well to both task and social climate. They enjoy sustained high task effectiveness. Their good social climates reinforce their effectiveness. And they are stable in the long term.

West posits 5 components of overall team effectiveness: task effectiveness, team member well-being (reflecting the social climate and opportunities for individual growth), team viability, team innovation, and inter-team cooperation (West, 2012, p. 7). By the word *viability*, West means the team's capacity to remain intact and effective over time. By the phrase *inter-team cooperation*, he means the team's capacity to work effectively with other teams to achieve its purpose. West sees each of these 5 components as an end in itself. All 5 components are included in West's full framework. We view member well-being, viability, innovation, and inter-team cooperation as important because they are key contributors to the team's being able to be effective in performing its task. In other words, we believe that they are very important means to the end of effectiveness but not ends in themselves.

The attitudes of team members toward the social climate of their teams are central to the team's ability to come together as a unit and perform well. The leader has a major role to play in shaping these attitudes, as Dr. Kimpell demonstrates in the preceding vignette. There are also organized methods for building teams, as discussed in Chapter 15.

Fifth, Red Family Medicine displays mutual accountability. Mutual accountability, discussed in Chapter 2, is shared responsibility taken to a higher plane. In a team with mutual accountability, the members actually take action, when appropriate, to hold each other accountable for doing what is needed for the team to be effective. In this vignette, Carrie Tanaka, a medical assistant, held Allen Lewis, a physician, accountable for making a telephone call to a patient. April Simpkins, another medical assistant, held Dr. Pearson accountable for neglecting the iodine allergy of a patient. In both cases, the physician thanked the medical assistant for her intervention. What is more remarkable is that both medical assistants did not hesitate to intervene. In Ms. Simpkins's case, she was briefly uncertain about what to do, but this was only because she sought a way to prevent Dr. Pearson from using iodine swabs without embarrassing Dr. Pearson or diminishing the patient's regard for Dr. Pearson. To avoid these potential undesirable effects of intervening, Ms. Simpkins invented the fictional telephone call so that Dr. Pearson would go into the hallway where they could talk confidentially. Both stories bespeak the excellent working relationships in Red Family Medicine.

Some writers on teams regard mutual accountability as a defining feature of work teams and would not regard a work group as a team if the team members did not hold each other accountable (Katzenbach and Smith, 2006, pp. 60-61). In health care, many teams lack mutual accountability. Some template teams are comprised of team members who have worked together so little that they never get comfortable about speaking up to hold each other accountable. In some teams, the difference in status between the senior and junior members is great enough to inhibit the junior members from saying anything that might be construed as impertinent—or might generate retaliation. Nonetheless, mutual accountability is desirable, and in many healthcare teams the degree of mutual accountability is lower than it can and should be. When it can be achieved, mutual accountability makes a team's effectiveness more secure because tasks are more likely to be done correctly and the risk of social loafing is decreased.

Finally, the members of Red Family Medicine devote a portion of their work time to activities that build and maintain the team. In the vignette, the 2 examples are their regular participation in the monthly meetings and their attendance at the summer picnics hosted by Dr. Kimpell. There are many other examples evident in healthcare teams: interviewing candidates to become members of the team when there is turnover, orientation of newly hired clinicians and staff, participation in performance improvement projects, and so on.

The members of an effective team are aware that they comprise a team, and they consciously contribute to the team's capacity to function effectively. They understand that individual patient-centered work by clinicians and managers is not enough to assure that the team will succeed. They know that they must also perform work that is team-centered. As depicted in Figure 6–2, team orientation is added to team structure and team focus to enable team members to collaborate effectively. We turn next to collaboration.

Team Collaboration

Jane Ryan, RN, placed a retractor (a surgical instrument) in the gloved hand of Leann Wang, MD. Dr. Wang was doing an open cholecystectomy (gall bladder removal) for a middle-aged woman who was healthy except for her gallstones. Throughout the procedure, Dr. Wang called for various instruments by saying the name of the instrument and putting her hand forward with the palm upward. Ms. Ryan, the scrub nurse in the team, would then place the instrument in Dr. Wang's hand and repeat its name. Little was said during the 40-minute procedure. Once Dr. Wang asked the nurse anesthetist for the patient's blood pressure reading. Once the circulating nurse briefed Dr. Wang on some details of her next case. Dr. Wang had a heavy schedule that day.

Ms. Ryan was concerned about how the case had started. During the "time-out" immediately before the procedure, Dr. Wang, as is customary, had recited the patient's name, stated that a cholecystectomy would be done, and asked whether anyone in the operating room (OR) had any questions or concerns. She made her statement and asked her question very quickly without looking up from the anesthetized patient. She did not ask the individuals one by one whether they had questions or concerns. After she spoke, she paused only about 3 seconds before making the incision to start the surgery. While Dr. Wang's actions might meet the letter of the required procedure—barely—they did not match the intended spirit. Someone in the OR could have had a question or concern that he or she did not voice fast enough. Moreover, by speaking rapidly without looking up, Dr. Wang signaled that she would not welcome a delay caused by anyone raising a concern about whether this was the right patient, whether a cholecystectomy was indeed the planned procedure, whether this patient's numerous allergies to medications were duly noted, or anything else.

After the surgery was completed, Ms. Ryan sought out Dr. Wang and told her that she was concerned about the way that the time-out was conducted. If this manner of doing the time-out was used regularly, Ms. Ryan said, a patient might some day be put in jeopardy because the surgical team might fail to prevent a wrong-site surgical procedure or some other mistake. The cholecystectomy done that morning was completely straightforward, and everyone in the OR knew that a careless time-out carried no risk. Nonetheless, Ms. Ryan was concerned about the precedent.

Some might think that Ms. Ryan's comments were brave or perhaps disrespectful to Dr. Wang, but both Ms. Ryan and Dr. Wang regarded them as normal and appropriate. Dr. Wang responded by saying, "Yeah, you're right. I should do it properly. It takes only a minute or two." She said that she should not have moved so quickly and that she had been concerned about her tight schedule that morning. She thanked Ms. Ryan for pointing out that what she had done might be dangerous in other situations. Ms. Ryan thanked Dr. Wang for "being so professional."

This OR template team exemplifies several characteristics of collaboration in effective teams. These characteristics are listed in Table 6–5.

First, the members of the surgical team respected one another. This feature of their interactions was not particularly striking during the surgery as there were no events that tested whether team members respected each other. However, following the surgery, mutual respect was apparent in the conversation between Ms. Ryan and Dr. Wang. Some surgeons would have reacted to being called to task by becoming annoyed or responding dismissively. Dr. Wang's response showed that she valued both Ms. Ryan and her viewpoint. Ms. Ryan showed respect for Dr. Wang by choosing to have the conversation when she and Dr. Wang were alone so that Dr. Wang did not feel attacked or ridiculed in front of the whole surgical team.

Second, the members of the surgical team trusted one another. As noted earlier in discussing the vignette about the medication error in Bobby Harrington's care, there are 2 components to trust: trust in competence and trust in integrity. In an effective team, all of the team members trust the other members in both respects. At a minimum, this trust is *swift trust*, mentioned in Chapter 2. Swift trust is characteristic of template teams even if they consist of members who have never met before (Meyerson et al, 1996). Teams that come together with clear purpose and well-defined roles can enjoy mutual trust very quickly as long as each member knows that all of the other members have become team members as a consequence of a reliable process that attends to the members' suitability to be on the team, for example, the process of scheduling surgical procedures. Swift trust will persist as long as team members perform in their assigned roles. If they depart from their assigned roles and perform additional tasks, then the other team's members may doubt that they have the competence to perform these additional tasks well. Moreover, swift trust can be lost if a team member behaves even briefly in a manner that puts his or her interests above the interest of the team in achieving its goal—because this behavior would suggest that the team member may lack integrity. In the surgical template team in the vignette, trust was based on more than confidence in the institutional processes that bring together team members to perform in well-defined roles. Ms. Ryan and Dr. Wang knew each other because they had worked together many times before, and their mutual knowledge contributed to their trust. Ms. Ryan's tactful challenge of Dr. Wang's behavior was not part of the customary role of a scrub nurse. Nonetheless Dr. Wang trusted that Ms. Ryan was behaving with competence. Dr. Wang also trusted that Ms. Ryan was not acting out of some ulterior motive, that is, that she was acting with integrity. Trust is commonly cited as a feature of team-based health care, and members of effective teams are often said to have earned each others' trust (Mitchell et al, 2012, pp. 14-16). This is true of true teams and of other teams whose members have worked together long enough to have the opportunity to earn each others' trust. Some template teams are formed of members who have no experience working together at all. Nonetheless, these teams commonly also have trust, namely, swift trust.

Third, the team members were actively interdependent. In other words, they requested each other to take action to achieve the team's goal. In the OR, this interdependence is quite unremarkable because the roles of the various team members call for them to take various actions on cue, for example, for the nurse anesthetist to

Table 6–5. Characteristics of effective teams: team collaboration

1. Respect by all team members for each other and for the patient
2. Trust
3. Active interdependence
4. Use of scientific evidence in making decisions about clinical matters and work processes
5. Effective communication
6. Prevention and management of relationship conflicts

track the patient's blood pressure and be prepared to report it immediately when asked. In other teams, reaching out to other team members for contributions to the team's effort is not so routine and requires calling on the other members in a timely manner, using knowledge of what those other team members can do. For example, in a primary care setting, a middle-aged male physician may sense that a 20-year-old female patient is being physically abused by her boyfriend. At the same time, he might also know that the social distance between him and the patient would make her reluctant to talk to him about physical abuse. The physician would be able to advance the patient's interest by relying on his 30-year-old NP colleague, finding a reason to ask the NP to come into the examination room and replace him in interviewing the patient. We say more about interdependence when discussing team member competencies in Chapter 7.

Fourth, effective teams use scientific evidence, when it is available, to establish their work processes and in general to inform their collaboration. In the vignette about Ms. Ryan and Dr. Wang, this characteristic of effective teams was not illustrated although it might have surfaced if there had been any disagreement between Mr. Ryan and Dr. Wang about whether the "time-out" checklist routine was effective. There is evidence that such checklists decrease surgical complications (de Vries et al, 2010); and, if Dr. Wang had doubts about the value of the "time-out," it would have been appropriate for Ms. Ryan to bring the evidence into the conversation. As it happened, Dr. Wang did not have doubts.

Fifth, the team exhibited excellent communication. For example, during the surgical procedure Ms. Ryan used a standard communication technique called *check-back* (Agency for Healthcare Research and Quality, 2006). When she placed an instrument in Dr. Wang's hand, she stated its name, repeating Dr. Wang's words. This repetition conveyed to Dr. Wang that her request for the instrument had been heard correctly and that Ms. Wang was giving her the instrument she needed. The team members also spoke to each other respectfully and showed no signs of ethnic stereotyping. We also discuss communication in Chapter 7 and in Chapter 14, where team training is covered.

Finally, collaboration in effective teams includes prevention and management of relationship conflicts by the team members themselves. Ms. Ryan took prompt action to prevent a conflict. Instead of observing Dr. Wang conduct a perfunctory time-out repeatedly until Ms. Ryan became truly annoyed and resentful, she dealt with the issue straightaway. Preventive action of this kind goes beyond the attentiveness to social climate described in the discussion of Red Family Medicine. In the story about that team, members were described as responding to Dr. Kimpell's requests for conflict resolution. Ms. Ryan took care of the problem before it reached that stage. Clearly Ms. Ryan and Dr. Wang had a good working relationship, making it easier for Ms. Ryan to do what she did. If team members do not prevent conflicts or take steps to resolve them (or otherwise manage them), then someone in authority needs to intervene, that is, the issue then becomes a management issue.

Team collaboration is the operational component of teamwork. As shown in Figure 6–2, it is the proximal or immediate source of benefit to the patients. It requires far more than coordination of members' actions, which would be achieved by members simply making sure that their activities did not conflict or interfere with one another. Collaboration requires the members to interact with each other productively, using each others' capabilities so that they can achieve together what none of them could achieve alone. In order for team members to collaborate effectively—and to maintain the necessary structure, focus, and team orientation—the team and its members need to be well managed. We turn next to team management.

Team Management

The Department of Pediatrics, part of Cypress Medical Group, was having its monthly meeting. The department Head was Sandy Malinin, MD, but the meeting was chaired by Joan Tschida, BSN, CPNP. Long ago, Dr. Malinin had realized that she was not effective in chairing meetings because she tended to neglect the clock and encourage people to speak at length about any topic that they felt strongly about. Ms. Tschida, in contrast, ran very effective meetings, and so Dr. Malinin had asked her to perform this role. There were 12 people in the department: 3 pediatricians, 2 pediatric NPs, 5 medical assistants, and 2 front desk clerks. With some exceptions, everyone attended the monthly meetings.

At this meeting, the main topic of discussion was how to improve the scheduling of patients to see either pediatricians or NPs. Some patients were being scheduled to see pediatricians for ear pain when this problem could be handled by NPs. Some patients with high fevers and lethargy were being scheduled with NPs when they should be seeing pediatricians. The front desk clerks and the medical assistants had difficulty determining on the telephone which patients should see pediatricians and which should see NPs.

Dr. Malinin suggested that the group generate ideas for solving the problem by having everyone write down 1 or 2 ideas and then report their suggestions out loud to the group as Ms. Tschida called on them, moving person by person around the room. This was not a new routine for the group; they had used it in the past from time to time. Everyone contributed ideas. Very quickly, they had a white board filled with 17 possibilities for how they might schedule more effectively. Next came a discussion of the pros and cons of the various solutions suggested. At this point nearly everyone joined in the discussion. However, one of the medical assistants and both front desk clerks said very little. Still, they did not appear to be intimidated or disengaged. Most of the suggested solutions included some training to enable the medical assistants and front desk clerks to use algorithms in determining which clinician a particular patient should see. Two of the medical assistants noted that they would need to have time for training and that this would be somewhat difficult to schedule, although it could be done if everyone was willing to do a bit more work to cover for those who were absent for training.

Ultimately the team decided by common agreement to appoint a sub-group of 3 people—1 front desk clerk, 1 medical assistant, and 1 NP—to review the ideas and bring back a proposal to the whole group next month.

This pediatric department was well managed. The characteristics of well-managed teams are listed in Table 6–6. Note that while all of the people described in the vignette are care givers, when they came together for their monthly meetings, they were a management team, specifically, an operational team—even though no administrator was present. (An administrator would have been helpful, but the medical group could not afford management expertise for meetings at the department level.) The sound management of the team is seen in several characteristics apparent in the vignette.

Table 6–6. Characteristics of effective teams: team management

1. Unity of purpose and structure (no sub-groups operating independently of the whole)
2. Favorable social climate
3. Enjoyment of work by team members
4. Effective building of the team
5. Effective team-level operations
6. Management of unresolved relationship conflicts
7. Timely and effective training
8. Systematic performance improvement
9. Effective sponsorship of the team
10. Support from the larger organization

First, the team had unity of purpose and unity of structure. Unity of purpose is one of the structural characteristics of an effective team (Table 6–2), but it comes up again in discussing management because preservation of this unity requires attention and maintenance. For example, in discussing the scheduling problem, the convenience of one or another sub-group of the team might have been asserted as a reason to adopt one of the proposed solutions. If convenience supersedes the interests of the patients in the eyes of a sub-group of team members, then unity of purpose has been lost. As the leader, Dr. Malinin would have needed to remind everyone of the team's purpose—unless someone else made the point first. The team also had unity of organizational structure. There were no separate sub-groups operating without accountability to the whole team. The scheduling problem was seen as a team problem, to be solved with input and participation by everyone. It was not seen as a problem to be solved by the pediatricians—or by the pediatricians and the NPs—acting without the medical assistants and front desk clerks.

Second, it is also apparent that the team had a favorable social climate—at least as far as can be determined from this meeting. All of the pediatricians were comfortable with an NP chairing the meeting. And everyone contributed suggestions in the brainstorming session. During the open discussion of the various suggestions, some of the junior members remained quiet, but this is to be expected in any group that has gradients of authority and prestige. It is not necessary or realistic that all the members of a healthcare team have equal influence and standing. A favorable social climate rarely arises without deliberate action as exemplified in a previous vignette by Dr. Kimpell's picnics for Red Family Medicine. The social climate requires management.

A particularly important component of the social climate is an atmosphere of psychological safety (West, 2012, pp. 131-133). In other words, it was important that the members of the pediatrics team believed that they could offer suggestions and ask questions without risking an angry response, humiliation, or punishment. A safe atmosphere is not the same as a comfortable atmosphere. A safe atmosphere is highly desirable, but a comfortable atmosphere may interfere with good performance if the team members respond by becoming complacent and feel that less than best effort is acceptable. Those at the Pediatrics Department meeting did not feel comfortable in the sense that they felt lackadaisical; they were aware that genuine effort was required. On the other hand, they felt safe in speaking up. They were not concerned that they would be penalized for making remarks that others might regard as foolish, ill informed, or incorrect.

Third, the members of an effective team enjoy their work. In other words, they find the work gratifying. In the vignette this feature of team effectiveness was not obvious, except perhaps in the high levels of participation apparent in the problem-solving discussion. Team members' enjoyment of their work is often not obvious, but their lack of enjoyment can be very obvious, as seen in a later vignette in this chapter. Whether one's work is gratifying is an individual matter, which may or may not be something that team members choose to discuss with each other. But the presence or absence of this sense of satisfaction is central to the team's success. Without ongoing pleasure in what they do, team members are likely to hold back from best effort or leave the team to find work that does afford them satisfaction. Healthcare teams do not exist to serve the psychological interests of their members, but their members must find that they gain satisfaction from the team's activities or the team will not be able to achieve its ends. For clinical teams, the end is serving the patients. For management teams, the end is achieving whatever purpose the team pursues in support of patient care. As with social climate, assuring that team members find their work enjoyable requires management—of the social climate, of the content of various team members' assignments of work, of training, and, when necessary, of relationship conflicts.

Fourth, a team's membership needs to be carefully built and maintained over time. This requires close attention to the team's mix of different professionals and clerical personnel, to hiring practices, and to orientation and integration of new people into the team. Generally, these activities are supervised closely by the team leader or directly carried out by the leader although, as a team grows in size, some activities are delegated. Building the team is central to the role of the leader as is discussed in Chapter 8. However, all of the team members should participate, for example, in interviewing candidates and in orienting them. This participation distributes the workload and assures that all team members have a sense of ownership of how the team is growing or turning over. Specific interventions can also be used to build the team, as presented in Chapter 15.

Fifth, all teams perform team-level operations that are distinct from direct service to patients. These operations need to be well managed. In the Department of Pediatrics, there are monthly operational meetings. These meetings need to be well run. By appointing Ms. Tschida to chair the meetings, Dr. Malinin provided for more effective meetings and showed her understanding that the leader does not have to be a superwoman and do everything herself. In the meeting described above, the team engaged in a structured exercise to generate creative solutions to the scheduling problem. We say more about team creativity in Chapter 10. Resolution of the scheduling problem will eventually require a decision about which solution to pursue. Team decision making also needs to be managed, as discussed in Chapter 9. All of these whole-team activities—problem solving, decision making, creative planning, and so on—require management.

Sixth, in the event that team members do not prevent or adequately manage relationship conflicts themselves, these conflicts need to be managed, as noted earlier. Occasionally, conflicts among team members will not be prevented so easily as happened with the scrub nurse and surgeon whose story was told earlier, nor will actual conflicts always be promptly resolved by the involved parties. If conflicts do occur and are not quickly resolved by the conflicted parties, someone on the team needs to step in to counsel or, as a last resort, to impose a solution. This intervention is commonly handled by the leader, but others can do it too. We address conflict management in Chapter 11.

Seventh, effective teams use training when it is appropriate. The type of training needed by different teams varies greatly, as noted in Chapter 2. Template teams, like the OR team described earlier, need training especially in role definition, communication routines, and the handling of predictable emergency situations. True teams, like the primary care teams in Red Family Medicine and Dr. Malinin's Department of Pediatrics, do not have the same need for well-understood, standardized roles or for standard communication routines. Members of those teams are more likely to benefit from training in the tasks that they routinely perform and cross-training in those tasks usually performed by other members of the team (Bodenheimer, 2007). For example, the Pediatrics Department was contemplating solving its scheduling problem by having the medical assistants and clerks use algorithms when talking with patients on the telephone to schedule visits. If this approach is chosen, then the medical assistants and clerks will need training to be able to perform this new task. We deal with team training at greater length in Chapter 14. For the present, the point is that the provision of training for a team needs to be managed. Needs for training should to be assessed from time to time. Some training needs to be provided directly by some members of the team for other members. Other training needs to be obtained from outside of the team. In very small organizations, most training obtained from outside of the team is purchased externally. In larger organizations, training is commonly provided from a centrally organized source although it may also be purchased.

Eighth, well-managed teams engage in systematic performance improvement. First, an effective team periodically identifies what portions of its performance either have defects or could be improved even though there are no frank defects. This identification of potential areas for improvement requires the team to evaluate its performance, as discussed in Chapter 13. In canvassing for potential improvement topics, the team should consider whether it is accomplishing its goals and is functioning well as a team. An effective clinical team also will examine whether its patient care processes meet established standards, and an effective management team also will examine whether its management methods are sound (for example, its techniques for project management). The team then prioritizes these topic areas, chooses what to focus on, sets goals, and pursues improvements using several different means. These means include training, team building, process improvement, and a wide variety of other management actions. Process improvement is improvement of the sequences of events that constitute the operations of a team. Follow-up on process improvement projects was mentioned in the vignette about Red Family Medicine as one of the purposes of their monthly meetings. The project to improve scheduling in Dr. Malinin's Pediatrics Department is another example of a process improvement project. There are several methods for carrying out process improvement, including Plan-Do-Study-Act (PDSA), Lean Production, and Six Sigma. Process improvement is discussed in Chapter 16.

Ninth, like other well-managed teams, the Pediatrics Department has effective sponsorship from the larger Cypress Medical Group. Dr. Malinin is accountable to the Medical Director, a surgeon. He established the Pediatrics Department years ago in the second year of his tenure as Medical Director. As noted in Chapter 1, we call the Medical Director the *sponsor* of the pediatric team, that is, the person to whom the team leader is accountable. (Sometimes the sponsor is not a person but a committee.) The Medical Director provides feedback to Dr. Malinin on the department's performance, coaches her, and is available to help her troubleshoot problems when she needs help. Team sponsors also have other functions, discussed in Chapter 12.

Finally, the Cypress Medical Group also supports the Pediatrics Department in several other ways—providing money for salaries, providing leadership training for Dr. Malinin plus other kinds of training for other department members, maintaining an organizational culture and reward system that foster teamwork, and so on. This broad supportive role, which is shaped and directed by the senior leaders of the organization, is explained in Chapter 18.

Team management, as shown in Figure 6–2, keeps the other components of effective performance (team structure, team focus, team orientation, and team collaboration) functioning well and functioning in harmony. Good team management requires action by the team leader but also by various other team members who are designated by the leader for particular management tasks. It also requires the team sponsor to perform various functions and requires the senior leaders of the organization to exercise their authority and skill in the support of teams.

HAZARDS FOR TEAMS

Tables 6–2 through 6–6 and Figure 6–2 summarize the structure and operating attributes of an effective team. The picture of an effective team can be made more vivid by contrasting it with some undesirable alternatives. These alternatives illustrate hazards that are especially common. Teams must avoid or manage these hazards in order to perform well. These commonly encountered hazards are listed in Table 6–7.

Failure to Have Meetings

Montgomery Digestive Care is a single-specialty medical group of 6 gastroenterologists and 2 NPs, located in a mid-sized city in the Indiana. The group is organized legally as a partnership in which 5 physicians in the group are the partners. The other physician will be eligible to become a partner after she has worked in the group for another year. The partners meet every other month over dinner. They review recent financial reports with their business manager and discuss any contract issues pending with insurance companies and health maintenance organizations. Occasionally leases for their practice space, personnel problems within the office staff, and other business matters are discussed.

Day to day, the physicians and NPs see their patients at 3 clinic locations and 2 hospitals. Questions of office procedure often come up, for example, how long to schedule various types of patient visits and how to handle telephone and e-mail messages. The physicians, NPs, and office staff address these questions as they arise, and generally the offices function smoothly. However, over the past few months, there have been several problems concerning waiting times for patients to get appointments and, in a few cases, delays in reporting important test results to patients. The physicians have tried to add these issues to their bi-monthly dinner meeting agendas, but the topics are always listed last on the agendas and rarely receive thorough consideration. As a consequence, the problems continue.

Table 6–7. Hazards for teams

Failure to hold meetings
Working as a completely virtual team
Marginalizing junior members of the team
Generating fear that suppresses dissent and the expression of novel ideas
Reaching consensus prematurely

Montgomery Digestive Care may well deliver first-rate gastroenterological care, but they manage their clinical work poorly. They regard themselves as very busy doing clinical work, and they actually are. They are very reluctant to have meetings concerning operations and management of the clinic. They never have meetings together with the NPs, nurses, technicians, and clerical staff who are employed by the group. They deal with—or try to deal with—the inevitable needs for solving problems and planning by using hallway conversations and the like. The result is that they have become disorganized, and have begun to accumulate resentments due to role conflicts, vagueness in procedures, and other unmet needs. When the practice consisted of 2 physicians and associated staff working in one office, all worked well, but the practice no longer functions smoothly.

The work of healthcare teams cannot be managed without having meetings of the people who do the work. There is no substitute. Most clinical professionals dislike meetings. Also, for the physicians and other clinicians reimbursed by insurers, the fee-for-service payment system used in most of the United States makes the visible, immediate cost of clinician meeting time very high—while the longer-term cost of *not* meeting is unknown and sometimes higher. One hour spent by a gastroenterologist in a meeting means 2-3 fewer colonoscopies performed, with the fees for those procedures foregone. Failure to have operational meetings is common. In one study of 6 general practices in England, only 1 practice set aside time for regular practice meetings (Field and West, 1995). The same is true of many medical groups in the United States, especially smaller medical groups. In a medical group, this failure to hold meetings results in teamwork that is disorganized if not chaotic; and, presuming that the operational decisions are made by physicians acting alone (as they commonly are), the nurses, medical assistants, and other staff become disengaged and sometimes alienated. To function well, teams must meet.

Working as a Completely Virtual Team

Moreover, at least some of the meetings need to be face-to-face. The advent of e-mail and videoconferencing (in addition to the older technology of telephone conferencing) has suggested to some people that face-to-face meetings are no longer needed. When work groups, including healthcare teams, are geographically dispersed, the temptation to eliminate face-to-face meetings and use fully virtual teams becomes very strong. But eliminating the face-to-face meetings is not prudent (Hackman, 2002, pp. 130-132; West, 2012, pp. 125, 235-238). Even when a team meets in person, the team members face a substantial challenge when they seek to achieve a common sense of purpose, a set of agreed values and work routines, and a favorable and reliable social climate. Without face-to-face interaction to help the team members to become engaged personally, these team tasks become even more challenging. There has been very little rigorous evaluation of the use of face-to-face meetings to supplement electronic communication (or of virtual meeting methods in general), but there is evidence that introductory face-to-face meetings improve the performance of business students formulating business strategy online (Hill et al, 2009). It seems plausible that this finding would generalize to teams in general, but more research is needed. Teams composed of members who are geographically dispersed need to meet at least when the team is forming and then periodically, perhaps once a year at a minimum. Within health care, to date most virtual teams have been management teams. However, with the advent of telemedicine, for example, for cardiac intensive care using cardiologists connected by videoconference to cardiac ICUs, virtual teams will soon become common in clinical care too. Investment in travel for these teams will be needed to assure that they function well.

Marginalizing Junior Members of the Team

Jeannine Revere, MD, was a cardiologist practicing with 16 other cardiologists in a single-specialty medical group, Riverside Heart Clinic. The group had 2 offices, one on the east side of the city and the other on the west side. The cardiologists hospitalized patients and performed cardiac procedures at 2 hospitals. At each of the offices, they employed medical assistants, 2-3 NPs, and several clerical staff, most of whom interacted directly with patients at the reception desks and in the scheduling cubicles. The medical assistants and clerks at each office were supervised by managers, one at each office. The managers both had long experience in health care but did not have clinical backgrounds.

At one of the offices, the physicians, NPs, and manager met on the third Wednesday of each month to deal with issues of clinic operations. Dr. Revere saw patients at this office, and routinely chaired these meetings. Most of the other physicians attended the meetings although 2 had never attended, and often one or more physicians were absent because they were busy in the hospital. (In a separate series of meetings, the 11 physician partners in the group met every other month with their contracted business manager to deal with business matters.)

The medical assistants and clerks never attended the operations meetings because they were not asked to attend. Decisions were often made about their roles, the procedures they were to follow in the office, and whether their numbers should be increased (or decreased through attrition, not lay-offs). Sometimes the manager spoke up when she anticipated that proposed changes would burden the staff, but for the most part—with 5-8 physicians and 2 NPs in the room—she said very little. Changes in the roles and procedures for the medical assistants and clerks were communicated to them by the manager.

Dr. Revere and others had long noticed that several of the medical assistants and clerks were taciturn and sullen most of the time although they always did their work. They left the office promptly at 5 p.m. every day. They rarely volunteered to do anything beyond their regular duties. If Dr. Revere had asked them about their dispirited demeanors, she might have learned the cause, but there was no way that she could have a candid conversation with them on this topic.

Dr. Revere and her colleagues had pushed the medical assistants and clerks to the periphery of activity in the office. These staff members were excluded from the operations meetings—unlike the staff in Red Family Medicine and Dr. Malinin's Pediatric Department in earlier vignettes. Their only line of communication with the physicians and NPs was through the manager, who was moderately intimidated by the clinicians. For the most part, no one asked the staff for their opinions or even paid much attention to them except as was required in the course of direct patient care in the office. The exclusion of the staff from a larger role in the office was not deliberate. They were simply taken for granted and generally ignored except when they were expected to perform their duties. No one benefitted from their insights and ideas, including the patients. They did their jobs in accordance with their job descriptions with little or no creativity or positive affect. They had come to believe that their roles were not important. Their work was not gratifying or enjoyable for them. And turnover among the medical assistants and clerks was high.

Some healthcare teams alienate their junior members by neglect. The ill effects of this alienation are mainly losses of contributions from the junior members—although occasionally there are angry outbursts caused either by frustration or by being undervalued. In fact, junior staff in this state of mind can be unintentionally dangerous if they sink so low that they come to believe that what they do makes no real difference to patient care. Patient experience and even patient safety can be put at risk. The absence of contributions from the staff is usually not obvious, and so the alienation can develop slowly over time without being noticed by those who are causing it. Teams need to be on the alert to this pitfall, which is an issue for management teams as well as clinical teams.

Generating Fear that Suppresses Dissent and the Expression of Novel Ideas

In some teams, a more serious variant of this problem occurs. Suppose that Dr. Revere were arrogant and harsh, from time to time sharply criticizing the manager, medical assistants, and clerks for their shortcomings in the presence of other people. The effect of this behavior would be to generate fear and suppress almost any disagreement with her. And if she or other physicians or NPs were to mock the manager or others for making novel improvement suggestions, then even the expression of new ideas would be suppressed. Teams with this atmosphere clearly do not have psychological safety. A similar but less oppressive situation can arise in hospitals and medical groups where the physicians have a distinctly higher status than anyone else. In these circumstances, other people will commonly acquiesce to whatever is desired by the physicians and will not voice novel ideas unless they can anticipate that the ideas will be welcomed by the physicians.

Unfortunately, these states of affairs are not rare. A demoralized atmosphere caused by fear or suppression of dissent is another pitfall for teams, both for clinical teams and for management teams. The avoidance or correction of this problem is in part the responsibility of the team leader, but most of the responsibility lies with the senior leaders in the organization. They are responsible for the organization's culture, including its values and norms of behavior. Establishing a supportive culture is a challenge, and changing a dysfunctional culture can be very difficult, but it can be done. We deal further with this topic in Chapter 18.

Reaching Consensus Prematurely

Mark Weldon, MD, was regarded by everyone at St. Margaret's Hospital as a reincarnation of Dr. Marcus Welby of television fame—and not just because of his name. Dr. Weldon was knowledgeable, kind, thoughtful, courageous, and interpersonally very skillful. His age was 58. He had graying hair and wore well-cut suits, usually blue or gray and never garish.

Dr. Weldon was often chosen by the Medical Staff Executive Committee and the hospital Chief Executive Officer to lead task forces and other committees. He enjoyed bringing fractious doctors and nurses to consensus. He chaired meetings masterfully—ordinarily. The meetings he chaired were frequently marked by sharp controversies. Dr. Weldon always made sure that every person who wished to speak had his or her say. Sometimes he would be mistaken about some consideration relevant to the committee's task at hand, and other committee members would correct him. When information was presented to show that he was in error, he characteristically accepted the correction with grace. Occasionally, when dealing with a self-righteous nurse or an arrogant physician, he would become angry, but his anger was visible only if one looked very carefully at his jaw muscles and face. He never let his anger get the better of him.

Two years ago, Dr. Weldon was the chair of the Credentials and Privileges Committee of the Medical Staff. Harrison Simms, MD, a surgeon, had recently moved into the community and applied to become a member of the hospital staff. In his application, he requested privileges to perform many common surgical procedures and a few advanced procedures, including thyroidectomy (removal of part or all of the thyroid gland). For surgeons requesting to be permitted to do thyroidectomies, the application form called for a statement of the applicant's training to do the procedure. Dr. Simms listed his general surgery residency, completed 22 years earlier. Dr. Weldon noted that this training alone was not regarded by the Committee as adequate for a surgeon to have privileges to do thyroidectomies. All of the other Committee members and the hospital staff to the Committee agreed that this was the policy. There was ample precedent for requiring that any surgeon doing thyroidectomies at St. Margaret's must have more than basic general surgical training for this procedure. Dr. Weldon said he would entertain a motion to approve the application but not to grant privileges to perform thyroidectomies. Someone said, "So moved," and someone seconded the motion. At this point, 2 of the Committee members were thinking that taking this action on Dr. Simms' application would be a mistake. They agreed that basic residency training was inadequate for privileging Dr. Simms to do thyroidectomies, but perhaps there was more to be learned that would be relevant to Dr. Simms' application. Perhaps he had been trained as a resident by an eminent thyroid surgeon and had performed the procedure for 22 years 3 or 4 times a year with a superb record. Despite their misgivings, the 2 Committee members said nothing and voted in favor of the motion. Their regard for Dr. Weldon was so high and Dr. Weldon's prestige in the eyes of all of the Committee members was so great that the 2 doubters did not want to disagree with his judgment, especially when he had explicitly proposed that the application be approved except for thyroidectomy privileges.

As it turned out, Dr. Simms was very experienced indeed in doing thyroidectomies and had an exemplary record of success. He was also very proud of his skill in performing the procedure, which is technically difficult and requires careful attention to detail. He was insulted by the action of the Committee and annoyed because they took action without seeking discussion with him beforehand. Six weeks later, the hospital was served with papers for a lawsuit claiming $4 million in damages. Dr. Simms alleged unlawful denial of privileges and damage to his professional reputation.

Premature consensus is another hazard for teams. The Credentials and Privileges Committee suffered from too much agreement—and, ironically, for a positive reason. Dr. Weldon was held in such high esteem by the committee that no one wanted to dispute what he suggested. The Committee members had disagreed with him on factual grounds many times in the past, and they might have disagreed with him in the handling of Dr. Simms' application if the issue had been a matter of black-and-white fact. But the issue this time was a matter of judgment and was less clear cut, and so they remained quiet. Consensus without due deliberation can also occur because all of the people on the team are similar with respect to education, prior experience, or even ethnic background. In the presence of these similarities, possibilities for action outside of what is customary often do not occur to anyone—and if they do, these possibilities may not be expressed because no one wants to risk being belittled for having made an unconventional or eccentric suggestion. Teams can also come to agreement too quickly when they choose a course of action that is consistent with long established habit that no one wants to set aside. Sometimes teams come to agreement too quickly because they are impatient and choose the first solution that appears to be minimally adequate. This hazard is called *satisficing* (West, 2012, p. 129). Finally, in almost all teams there is some degree of pressure to conform.

The list of hazards for teams in Table 6–7 covers 5 hazards that are especially common in healthcare teamwork. The list is far from complete; many more hazards could be added. We deal with other hazards in Chapter 8 in the discussion of team leadership, in Chapter 9 in the discussion of decision making, and in Chapter 12 in the discussion of sponsorship.

CONCLUSION

Effective teams are teams that achieve their goals. For clinical teams, these goals can be understood as the IOM 6 aims for improvement of health care. For management teams, the goals vary across teams and need to be specified team by team. On the path to achieving their goals, effective teams exhibit a number of characteristics that are similar for clinical and management teams. The characteristics of effective teams can be summarized in 5 categories: structure, focus on patients, orientation of the team members to the team, collaborative work, and management of the team (Figure 6–2). Five hazards are of particular importance for healthcare teams: failing to have meetings as part of doing their work, excessive reliance on remote communication such as videoconferencing, marginalizing junior members of the team, generating fear that suppresses dissent and innovative thinking, and premature consensus of various causes.

Having portrayed how effective teams are structured and function, we are now ready to begin dealing with how team members, leaders, sponsors, and senior leaders can contribute to team effectiveness. In the next chapter, we deal with the competencies needed by all team members.

REFERENCES

Agency for Healthcare Research and Quality. *TeamSTEPPS Fundamentals Source: Module 6.* Washington, DC: Agency for Healthcare Research and Quality; 2006. http://www.ahrq.gov/teamsteppstools/instructor/fundamentals/module6/slcommunication.htm. Accessed May 6, 2012.

American Academy of Family Physicians, American Academy of Pediatrics, American College of Physicians, American Osteopathic Association. *Joint Principles of the Patient-Centered Medical Home.* Leawood, KS: American Academy of Family Physicians; 2007. http://www.medicalhomeinfo.org/downloads/pdfs/jointstatement.pdf. Accessed June 9, 2012.

Begun JW. Realistic evidence-based management. *Health Care Manage Rev.* 2009;34:214-215.

Bodenheimer T. *Building Teams in Primary Care: Lessons Learned.* Oakland, CA: California HealthCare Foundation; 2007. http://www.chcf.org/~/media/MEDIA%20LIBRARY%20Files/PDF/B/PDF%20BuildingTeamsInPrimaryCareLessons.pdf. Accessed June 10, 2012.

de Vries EN, Prins HA, Crolla RMPH, et al. Effect of a comprehensive surgical safety system on patient outcomes. *N Engl J Med.* 2010;363:1928-1937.

Field R, West M. Perspectives on teamwork from general practices. *J Interprof Care.* 1995;9:123-150.

Firth-Cozens J, Mowbray D. Leadership and the quality of care. *Qual Health Care.* 2001;10(Suppl 2):3-7.

Hackman JR. *Leading Teams: Setting the Stage for Great Performances.* Boston, MA: Harvard Business School Press; 2002.

Hill NS, Bartol KM, Tesluk PE, et al. Organizational context and face-to-face interaction: influence on the development of trust and collaborative behaviors in computer-mediated groups. *Organ Behav Hum Decis Process.* 2009;108:187-201.

Iedema R, Allen S, Sorensen R, et al. What prevents incident disclosure, and what can be done to promote it? *Jt Comm J Qual Patient Saf.* 2011;37:409-417.

Institute of Medicine. *To Err Is Human: Building a Safer Health System.* Washington, DC: National Academy Press; 2000.

Institute of Medicine. *Crossing the Quality Chasm: A New Health System for the 21st Century.* Washington, DC: National Academy Press; 2001.

Katzenbach JR, Smith DK. *The Wisdom of Teams: Creating the High-Performance Organization.* Collins Business Essentials ed. New York, NY: HarperCollins Publishers; 2006.

Leavitt HJ. Why hierarchies thrive. *Harv Bus Rev.* 2003;81(3):96-102.

Meyerson D, Weick KE, Kramer RM. Swift trust and temporary groups. In: Kramer RM, Tyler TR, eds. *Trust in Organizations: Frontiers of Theory and Research.* Thousand Oaks, CA: Sage Publicatons, Inc.; 1996:166-195.

Mintzberg H. *The Structuring of Organizations: A Synthesis of the Research.* Englewood Cliffs, NJ: Prentice Hall; 1979.

Mitchell P, Wynia M, Golden R, et al. *Core Principles & Values of Effective Team-Based Health Care.* Discussion paper. Washington, DC: Institute of Medicine; 2012.

Porter ME. What is value in health care? *N Engl J Med.* 2010;363:2477-2481.

Reeves S, Simon L, Espin S, et al. *Interprofessional Teamwork for Health and Social Care.* Chichester, UK: John Wiley & Sons, Ltd.; 2010.

Scholtes PR, Joiner BL, Streibel BJ. *The Team Handbook.* 3rd ed. Madison, WI: Oriel Incorporated; 2003.

Thompson LL. *Making the Team: A Guide for Managers.* 4th ed. Upper Saddle River, NJ: Prentice Hall; 2011.

West MA. *Effective Teamwork: Practical Lessons from Organizational Research.* 3rd ed. Chichester, UK: John Wiley & Sons, Ltd.; 2012.

Willard R, Bodenheimer T. *The Building Blocks of High-Performing Primary Care.* Oakland, CA: California HealthCare Foundation; 2012. http://www.chcf.org/publications/2012/04/building-blocks-primary-care. Accessed May 3, 2012.

Competencies for Healthcare Team Members

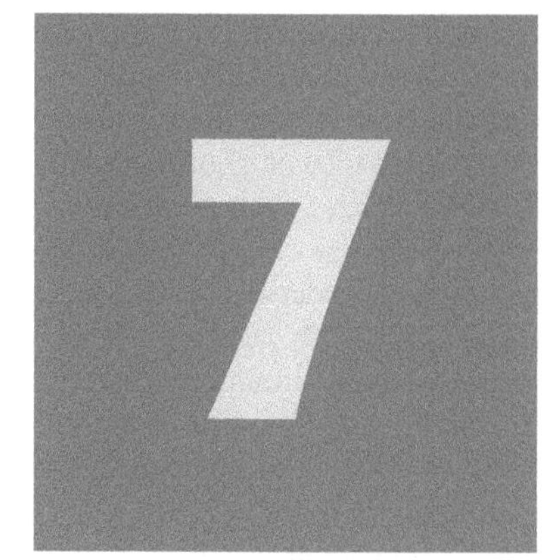

As indicated in Chapter 1, teamwork competencies are the combinations of values, knowledge, and skills that team members need in order to work effectively in teams. In the last few years, health professional groups in the United States and Canada have developed lists of competencies for interprofessional or collaborative healthcare practice. These competencies pertain equally to nurses, physicians, administrators, psychologists, social workers, and others working as members of a healthcare team. The previous chapter, Chapter 6, delineated characteristics of effective teams. In this chapter we discuss the competencies required of individual team members to achieve effective teamwork. In later chapters, we cover additional competencies specific to team leaders (Chapter 8), team sponsors (Chapter 12), and senior leaders of organizations in which teams function (Chapter 18).

TEAMWORK COMPETENCY FRAMEWORKS

A variety of groups and researchers have concentrated on the development of competencies for interprofessional healthcare practice in the past 2 decades, meaning that consensus-based competency frameworks for interprofessional practice are relatively current. In 2011, 6 professional associations in the United States—American Association of Colleges of Nursing, Association of American Medical Colleges, American Association of Colleges of Osteopathic Medicine, American Association of Colleges of Pharmacy, American Dental Education Association, and Association of Schools of Public Health—issued a joint statement of core competencies for interprofessional collaborative practice (Interprofessional Education Collaborative Expert Panel [IECEP], 2011). Interprofessional competencies are defined by that expert panel as "integrated enactment of knowledge, skills, and values/attitudes that define working together across the professions, with other health care workers, and with patients, along with families and communities, as appropriate to improve health outcomes in specific care contexts" (IECEP, 2011, p. 2). The panel's framework separates 38 competencies into 4 domains: values/ethics (10 competencies), roles/responsibilities (9 competencies), communication (8 competencies), and teamwork (11 competencies).

The study of interprofessional collaboration has a more extensive history in the United Kingdom, Europe, and Canada than in the United States. Those countries have a longer and deeper experience base with collaborative care, probably due to their stronger public systems and the lower levels of fragmentation in their systems of healthcare financing and delivery. A Canadian group, the Canadian Interprofessional Health Collaborative (CIHC), issued a National Interprofessional Competency Framework in 2010, after 2 years of work that included a review of literature and existing competency frameworks (CIHC, 2010). The Canadian Collaborative defined competency as "a complex 'know act' that encompasses the ongoing development of an integrated set of knowledge, skills, attitudes, and judgments enabling one to effectively perform the activities required in a given occupation or function to the standards expected in knowing how to be in various and complex environments and situations." The competencies are customized around interprofessional collaboration, which is defined as "a partnership between a team of health providers and a client in a participatory, collaborative, and coordinated approach to shared decision making around health and social issues" (CIHC, 2010, p. 24). Six competency domains or clusters are identified in the Canadian framework, with a total of 39 competencies: team functioning (7 competencies), role clarification (7 competencies), interprofessional conflict resolution (8 competencies), collaborative leadership (8 competencies), patient/client/family/community-centered care (4 competencies), and interprofessional communication (5 competencies).

The US and Canadian frameworks are quite alike. Both the US and Canadian groups define competencies in a highly abstract way, with the US group using the phrase "integrated enactment" and the Canadian group using the phrase "complex 'know act.'" This abstraction reflects both the breadth of the term "competency" and the fact that it is difficult to specify exactly what constitutes proficient workplace behavior.

The 2 definitions refer to integrated sets of knowledge, skills, and "values/attitudes" (US) or "attitudes and judgments" (Canadian). This is consistent with the delineation by teamwork scholars of competencies as consisting of knowledge, skills, and attitudes (Cannon-Bowers et al, 1995, pp. 336-337). Our definition of competencies as *integrated sets of knowledge, values, and skills* draws on this consensus and avoids the higher level abstraction of "enactment" or "know acts." We prefer the term "values" to "attitudes" because it is more foundational, in the sense that underlying values drive attitudes.

In terms of classifying types of interprofessional teamwork competencies, the most notable difference between the US and Canadian framework is that the Canadian framework separates leadership competencies (as do we, in a separate chapter, Chapter 8) and patient-centered competencies. In general, the 2 frameworks are remarkably similar in both scope and in specific competencies, which lends some support to the conclusion that there is general agreement about generic competencies. We draw on both the US and Canadian frameworks to ensure that our list is comprehensive.

We organize competencies into 4 categories: patient focus, team orientation, collaboration, and team management. The categories are the same as those employed in Chapter 6 to explain characteristics of effective teams, minus the category *team structure*. Team structure is beyond the purview of individual members (except the leader, whose competencies are addressed in Chapter 8). Our intent is to parallel the characteristics of effective teams with the specific expectations of individual members to produce those characteristics, so there is some overlap in the topics covered in this chapter and the previous chapter.

As noted above, competencies are combinations of 3 components—values, knowledge, and skills. Next, we define those 3 terms in more detail. Depending on the wording and content of specific competencies, different competencies emphasize each of the 3 components to different extents.

Some competencies clearly emphasize the values component, because values are fundamental to effective performance on teams. For example, "respect the other members of the team" is a competency worded so that it emphasizes understanding and acceptance of the value "respect." *Values* are broad preferences concerning useful, worthy, and important courses of action or outcomes. Values also may reflect preferences regarding what is considered "excellent" in important arenas of one's life, such as work and family relationships. As such, values reflect a person's sense of right and wrong, as well as what "ought" to be. Values are deeply held and difficult to change. They often are rooted in family, spiritual, and cultural socialization, established over several years, particularly the younger years. Socialization into a new arena of life, whether it be adopting a new religion, marrying into a new set of relatives, moving to a new part of the world, or entering a new profession, has the potential to alter previously held values and to create new ones. The period of socialization into a new health profession provides opportunities to develop new values around teamwork with other professions.

Several teamwork competencies require a strong knowledge base. *Knowledge* includes the key technical and contextual information, theories, and concepts needed to be competent. For example, we emphasize the need for professionals to have knowledge of the potential contributions of other professions to the team. Managing conflict, discussed below as a competency, benefits from knowledge of the options for constructively addressing conflict. Of the 3 components of competencies, knowledge is the easiest to obtain. Knowledge can be gained by reading, studying, and learning. Knowledge about teamwork can be conveyed to health professionals in their education and continuing education.

Many competencies are phrased such that they emphasize the third component of competencies, skills. *Skills* are the specific behavioral practices needed to be proficient in the workplace. For example, "communicate effectively" is phrased as a skill, although in the context of interprofessional teamwork, those who exhibit effective communication likely benefit from underlying knowledge and values, such as knowledge of effective communication practices and adherence to the value of respect for teammates. Skills are difficult to learn through reading and studying; developing skill requires practice in realistic settings. The applied learning of skills is a significant component of the training of all health professionals, including administrators. Teamwork skills can be learned by practicing them in "safe" settings such as classrooms and simulation laboratories and fieldwork projects, followed by practice in "real" settings under the guidance of mentors and preceptors. In practice, values, knowledge, and skills are all inputs that are synthesized or integrated into workplace behaviors.

TEAMWORK COMPETENCIES

Focus on the Patient

Three competencies in support of a patient focus are required of team members. Table 7–1 lists the 3 competencies, which begin with having respect for the interests of patients and family members. *Respect* is a value that has important behavioral implications that are detailed in the 2 other patient focus competencies. The importance of respect in all effective relationships has a deep foundation in human history (DeLellis, 2000). Respect is a way of regarding another person, specifically, attending to the person because one deems the person to be important, usually because of some special worth or excellence but also simply because the other person is a person. As argued in Chapter 4, patient interests are central to team-based clinical care, and they are central to the mission of healthcare delivery organizations and the management teams in those organizations. Unless team members are enrolled in respecting the role of patients and family members on the team, the members will vitiate or sabotage the underlying, shared purpose of healthcare teamwork.

Table 7–1. Competencies for team members: patient focus

1. Respect the interests of patients and families, as defined by them
2. Actively solicit and integrate the input of patients and families in the design, implementation, and evaluation of services
3. Perform professional roles in a way that respects the different cultures of patients and families

Respect is manifest in behavior and thoughts. Behavioral indicators of respect include listening to others, using appropriate language and forms of address, and seeking advice from others (DeLellis and Sauer, 2004). In demonstrating respect for patients, we particularly emphasize 2 individual member behaviors: soliciting and acting on patient and family input, and performing roles in a culturally sensitive manner.

Team members who respect patients listen to and incorporate patients' goals in receiving care (Competency 2 in Table 7–1). Patients are "experts in their own lived experiences and are critical in shaping realistic plans of care" (CIHC, 2010, p. 13). For clinical teams providing care for defined episodes, a full team meeting with the patient and family, early in the care planning process, is often useful when such a meeting is feasible (Mitchell et al, 2012, p. 7). Respectful listening to the patient and family, rather than conveying of information from the professionals to the patient, is the main purpose of the meeting. For patients with chronic disease, if they wish to manage their own care, support for self-management is implied by respect for the patents' goals. For management teams, inclusion of patients in teams is important as well. Team members who meet privately with the patient can share their learning with the team, if the patient is not an active member. To solicit input from patients and families, health professionals often must communicate technical information to them. It is important that team members do so in an understandable, jargon-free way. This behavior is discussed further below in the context of a competency for effective communication.

Effective involvement of patients in healthcare teams also requires sensitivity to cultural differences (Competency 3 in Table 7–1). The Canadian competency framework identifies a separate skill in cultural sensitivity (practitioners "perform their own roles in a culturally respectful way" [CIHC, 2010, p. II]), and the US competency framework urges team members to "Embrace the cultural diversity and individual differences that characterize patients, populations, and the health care team" (IECEP, 2011, p. 19). Cultural sensitivity is a key to effective communication when patients or clients are from different cultures than other care team members. In particular, cultural sensitivity includes collaborating to overcome linguistic and literacy challenges (Expert Panel on Cultural Competence Education for Students in

Medicine and Public Health, 2012, p. 8). Patients and families with limited English proficiency are a significant component of the population served by many clinical practices and healthcare delivery organizations.

We also note the need to involve patients and families in the *evaluation* of team outcomes as explicitly noted in the statement of Competency 3 in Table 7–1, and individual team members can assist in making that happen. This issue is discussed in Chapter 13 on evaluating teams and team members.

Cultural diversity is but one dimension of human diversity. Differences between the social status, economic position, sexual orientation, and other characteristics of patients and families all challenge healthcare professionals to treat patients and families with equity—to treat them the same regardless of their life condition other than their health concerns. As explained earlier in Chapter 6, equity in the delivery of services is a desired outcome of all clinical teams. Equity requires sensitivity to the wide range of potential differences between patients and team members.

"Generation of trust in patients and families" was noted as a characteristic of effective healthcare teams in Chapter 6. Patient and family trust will result from individual members demonstrating the 3 patient focus competencies of respect, involvement in service design, implementation and evaluation, and cultural sensitivity.

Team Orientation

In Chapter 6, the example of Red Family Medicine, an 11-member primary care team, was used to illustrate orientation to working in a team. Individual members contributed to team goals as well as their own. Five competencies, delineated in Table 7–2, are required for individuals to demonstrate a team orientation. First, individual team members should actively participate in setting the foundations for successful teamwork—agreement on basic values, goals, and processes. In particular, team members need to share feelings about ethical principles, such as patient confidentiality and transparency. The US Interprofessional Education Collaborative competency framework specifies the following competency: "Develop consensus on the ethical principles to guide all aspects of patient care and team work" (IECEP, 2011, p. 25).

Kerri Janus, MSW, LICSW, is a mental health social worker in a program that runs a suicide prevention hot line. Upon arriving at her team's Monday morning weekly meeting, she took one look into the meeting room and shook her head in resignation. The weekly meeting was already 5 minutes late starting, and Naomi Granville, RN, CNS, a psychiatric/mental health clinical nurse specialist, was nowhere to be seen. Already present were the other team members—another mental health social worker, a patient/family representative, a pharmacist, and a psychiatrist. Not only was Ms. Granville chronically late to these meetings, but she frequently skipped them, with no advance notice. She had attended the team's initial meeting, but had missed important discussions about the team's goal and members' underlying assumptions about the value of preventive care and the ethics of intervention. When Ms. Granville did attend, she was happy to voice her own opinion, but she never really got engaged in the team's discussions. She did not seem to care what other team members had to offer. The team would just have to "soldier on" without her.

In the suicide prevention team in the vignette, one member, Ms. Granville, was relatively uninvolved in the critical early stages of team formation, demonstrating an absence of a team orientation on her part. An important additional point, however, is that attending meetings (showing up) is not enough. Team members should demonstrate investment in the team by active participation. It is not enough to let others form the team, or to delegate one's participation to another team member. Participation ensures others that each member is committed to the final product.

Competency 2 in the team orientation cluster is the competency for team members to invest in building team identity and a positive social climate. This

Table 7–2. Competencies for team members: team orientation

1. Actively contribute to the formation of commonly agreed values, goals, and processes for doing the work of the team
2. Actively contribute to building team identity and a positive social climate
3. Acknowledge shared responsibility for the outcomes produced and hold other team members responsible for their contributions (in a respectful way)
4. Understand the characteristics of effective teams and common pitfalls for teams
5. Understand the competencies of effective team members and one's personal strengths and vulnerabilities relative to the competencies

competency is important to denote separately because it tends to be neglected by healthcare teams that are ready to "get down to business." As will be apparent in a later vignette in this chapter, healthcare team members sometimes are impatient with the investment of time in this important foundation-building step.

Next, recall that effective teams exhibit mutual accountability for achieving the team's goal (Chapter 6, Table 6–4). The statement of Competency 3 in Table 7–2 says that members should be able to "acknowledge shared responsibility for the outcomes produced." This acknowledgement is implicit, that is, implied by behavior, rather than overtly stated, though explicit discussion of the concept by the team may be useful. At the individual member level, members need to surrender any desire to assume sole responsibility for the outcome. This can be difficult for professionals who are accustomed to solo practice and autonomy, particularly those with high levels of power. It may be difficult for the chief executive officer of an organization, for instance, to participate as an equal team member on this dimension. Mutual accountability also includes the expectation that members will hold each other responsible for their contributions. For some, acknowledgement of shared responsibility ends with making a contribution to the team. Ideally, however, this competency includes holding other team members responsible for their contributions, in a respectful way. While the team leader is formally responsible for coaching, giving feedback and evaluating team members, individual members can contribute constructively by helping their teammates to perform better.

The competency of providing respectful feedback to others about their performance is not so easily attained or implemented because of the reluctance of many professionals to criticize each other and the natural defensiveness of individuals to criticism. Some tips for providing feedback to other team members are given in Chapter 13 on evaluation. In the vignette above, colleagues of "absentee" member Ms. Granville could ask her about her attendance with comments such as, "We really missed your input at the meeting." In this case, stronger intervention by the team leader is needed as well.

Finally, we note 2 competencies for demonstrating a team orientation that require a knowledge base about teamwork. Competencies 4 and 5 in Table 7–2 call for all team members to understand the characteristics of effective teams, pitfalls for teams, competencies of effective team members, and to have insight into their own level of team member competence. In other words, team members need to understand how teams work. The features of effective teams are discussed in Chapter 6, and here in Chapter 7 the corresponding competency for individual team members is that they understand these features and know their abilities to contribute (or not) to team effectiveness. Shared knowledge about what makes teams work empowers members to enact their own roles to maximum effectiveness and to enforce common expectations of fellow team members. Healthcare professionals need to add knowledge and understanding of teamwork competencies to the knowledge base of their own professions.

Dick Singletary, PharmD, was feeling great. He had just "schooled" his geriatric care team on the benefits and risks of various forms of antiplatelet therapy (mild blood thinning) for elderly patients with a history of stroke. While his explanation had taken longer than expected, he felt it was important to establish his credibility with other team members, none of whom really appreciated the depth of his knowledge. Sully Cowpen, RN, NP, was not so sure about Dr. Singletary's contribution to the team, however. He seemed to know his stuff, but never left time for others to question him, and rarely listened to others who offered input on their experience with a particular medication. Dr. Singletary's enthusiasm was great, but Ms. Cowpen wished that he would temper his contributions and become more of a "team player."

A team orientation is furthered when individual team members challenge themselves to improve. Improvement is only possible if team members understand their strengths and weaknesses in relation to the other competencies. Self-understanding requires personal reflection about ways to improve one's contribution to the team. Pharmacist Dick Singletary seems to lack self-understanding in the vignette above. If he had this understanding, he would be able to overcome his vulnerabilities and prevent unintended ill effects of his behavior. He would be more cognizant of the unenthusiastic reaction of his teammates. Self-reflection and realistic feedback from others are important in development of this competency. Some professionals devote very little time to developing an understanding of their teamwork skills. In particular, they do not take advantage of the feedback that they might obtain from other team members.

Collaboration

Another 8 individual competencies fall in the category of *collaboration*. They are listed in Table 7–3. The first competency for collaboration requires respect for fellow team members and those peripheral to the team (for example, front desk staff). For activities that are highly individualized, a person who is disrespectful may still be able to be productive. For example, a highly specialized technical specialist who is disrespectful in interpersonal interactions may be productive if left alone (away from direct patient care) to analyze materials (for example, images, blood samples, or tissue samples). For interdependent work to succeed, however, respect is a critical foundation of relationships with other team members. We already have discussed the importance of respect for patients and families. The phrase "other members of the team" in the statement of Competency 1 in Table 7–3 should be understood to include individuals who support the team, such as front desk staff, secretaries, and custodians. Respect for other team members and for team support workers encourages them to contribute fully to the team's goals.

A specific behavioral indication of respect for other members of the team is to engage other professionals and seek out their value to the team. Competency 2 in Table 7–3 calls for team members to "be constantly attentive to how people in other professions can contribute." It is unlikely that team members who do not believe that other professionals can make important contributions to patient care can function effectively on interprofessional teams. Ideally, the commitment to interprofessional practice is expressed proactively, such that input from other professionals is not only appreciated but is actively sought. Members who value interprofessional care will seek the counsel of other professionals, will build on the contributions of other professionals, and will express appreciation for the contributions of other professionals. Proactively seeking others' contributions, rather than relying on them to contribute as needed, is a sign of collaborative behavior.

Competency 3 in the Collaboration category states that team members should be able to explain their own roles, education, professional values, and responsibilities in the team. A sampling of such knowledge is given in Chapter 3. While this competency may seem simple or trivial to some professionals, team members who have not had to explain their backgrounds to others may have trouble doing so, especially in ways that communicate across professional boundaries. Note that individual members need to be clear about their roles on the team. The explanation of responsibilities reduces the risk that other team members will resort to unfounded or stereotyped assumptions about the individual's role. Explaining roles also opens up opportunities for team members to expand their use of other members' expertise.

Table7–3. Competencies for team members: collaboration

1. Respect the other members of the team and those peripheral to the team (for example, front desk staff)
2. Value the contributions of people in the various professions and be constantly attentive to how people in other professions can contribute to the care of the patient and other team goals
3. Be able to explain one's own education, professional values, role, and responsibilities in the team
4. Understand the education, professional values, roles, and responsibilities of all of the other team members
5. Work interdependently with other team members
6. Communicate (for operational purposes) effectively with other team members
7. Refrain from domineering or demeaning behavior that inhibits communication and the effective performance of others in the team
8. Apply the principles and methods of evidence-based practice

Early Monday morning, Joanna James, secretary to Regina Knotts, MD, a cardiac surgeon, placed a call to Gabriel Ibanez, MSW, a social worker. Dr. Knotts frequently worked with Mr. Ibanez to get placements for her patients after hospital stays. As a result, Dr. Knotts considered Mr. Ibanez part of the "patient care team" for several of her patients. Dr. Knotts asked Ms. James to call Mr. Ibanez about her patient Thor Springer, who was having some problems with family support in addition to his postsurgical recovery needs following cardiac surgery last week. Dr. Knotts simply wanted Mr. Ibanez to find Mr. Springer a nursing home bed. She asked Ms. James to forewarn Mr. Ibanez that Mr. Springer's family was divided on the question of whether Mr. Springer should go to a nursing home and so dealing with the situation might be difficult. Mr. Springer himself was rather passive about the issue, Ms. James told Mr. Ibanez.

Mr. Ibanez visited Mr. Springer in the hospital and asked Mr. Springer where he preferred to go after he was discharged. Mr. Springer said that he wanted to do "whatever the doctor and my family think is best." With Mr. Springer's permission, Mr. Ibanez met with several family members and helped them talk through the issues surrounding Mr. Springer's upcoming discharge. The family, once informed of Mr. Springer's needs, all agreed that he should go to a nursing home for a period of convalescence. Some of the family members had thought that his going to a nursing meant that he would never return home. Others thought that family members should care for Mr. Springer at home, but after the discussion they understood that he required skilled nursing care that no one in the family could provide.

Later that week Mr. Ibanez took the opportunity to let Dr. Knotts know about the family conference and its outcome. He added that helping to resolve family disagreements was part of his stock in trade as a social worker and that Dr. Knotts should feel free to ask him to manage family disagreements in the future.

Another Collaboration competency (Competency 4 in Table 7–3) is that team members should understand the roles, education, professional values, and responsibilities of all of the other team members. In the preceding vignette, Dr. Knotts did not foresee the contribution of the social worker, Mr. Ibanez. If asked to articulate the social worker's role, Dr. Knotts likely would have said, "Social workers arrange appropriate posthospital settings for patients." A more informed role description would add something to the effect that "Social workers work together with patients and families and community resources to strengthen the patients' networks of support." Attaining this competency requires taking the time and effort to understand, communicate, and clarify roles in interaction with other team members.

A fifth collaboration competency is working interdependently with other team members. This behavior flows from respect for and knowledge of the capabilities of other team members. Interdependent work requires adjusting one's own behavior or attitudes in light of another's. It means surrendering control of a process to a larger group, which is difficult for many autonomous professionals. It also means having the capacity to take action to prevent relationship conflicts and to resolve them if possible.

Benjamin Bodeen, MD, a family physician, leaned back and suppressed a groan. It was another meeting of the quality improvement team that had been assembled by clinic administration to address the lengthy wait times of many patients in the clinic's waiting rooms. One of his colleagues on the quality improvement team, Samantha Jones, MBA, an administrator, was at it again: "I was talking to the CFO yesterday, and our quarterly competitor benchmarks are way out of whack. We're at the 70th percentile on FTEs per adjusted annual patient visit, even though our ACGs are no different than anywhere else. And our ambulatory CAHPS scores are way down, too." Dr. Bodeen was tired of asking Ms. Jones to speak in plain English, or at least to translate all the administrative acronyms and buzzwords that peppered her presentation. Ms. Jones was a healthcare administrator and was proud of her Master of Business Administration (MBA) degree. It appeared to Dr. Bodeen that Ms. Jones was more interested in impressing the team with her esoteric knowledge than in really communicating information. He decided to just let it go over his head.

Sixth, team members should be able to communicate (for operational purposes) effectively with other team members, unlike Ms. Jones in the preceding vignette. Communication is dissected into several separate competencies in both the US and Canadian competency frameworks, reflecting the importance of the issue to healthcare teamwork. Research studies and commentaries have shown widespread acknowledgement of communication problems among professionals in healthcare delivery settings, for example, between nurses and physicians and between healthcare administrators and physicians (Mannahan, 2010; McCaffrey et al, 2011; Smith, 2003). Effective communication includes (1) using terminology that is understandable by the other parties and avoiding discipline-specific terminology when possible, and (2) using respectful language. Methods of standardized communications among healthcare professionals in certain types of teams are explored further in Chapter 14 on team training. Effective communication also requires (3) active listening, that is, concentrating on the speaker and being sure of what the speaker is trying to communicate (DeVany, 2010, pp. 38-45; Sapienza, 2004, pp. 117-121), and (4) sharing information. The sharing of information in health care is complicated by ethical and legal norms that protect the confidentiality of patient information. Ethical norms vary among professional groups; for example, mental health service professionals often are less willing to share patient information than are nurses and primary care physicians (Seaburn et al, 1996, pp. 60-61). These norms should be discussed early in the team development process. Finally, effective communication requires (5) facilitating interaction among team members. Energetic exchange among team members is a predictor of team performance, with face-to-face communication the most valuable form of communication and e-mail and texting the least valuable (Pentland, 2012). Equal participation among all members heightens effectiveness as well.

Both the US and Canadian frameworks also note the importance of using information systems and communication technologies to facilitate discussions and interactions that enhance team function, being sure to include patients in the communication loops. These information systems often are the responsibility of the organization in which the team functions, as discussed in Chapter 18, on senior leaders of organizations.

Next on the list of requisite competencies for collaboration (Competency 7 in Table 7–3) is the only competency among the 21 team member competencies that is stated in a negative form (something members should not do, as opposed to something they should do): members should "refrain from domineering or demeaning behavior that inhibits communication and the effective performance of others on the team." While this could be considered an aspect of effective communication (Competency 6), it is given separate attention because it is so important and so frequently violated, due to power differences inherent in many interprofessional teams. Avoidance of offensive behavior flows from the competencies of respecting other team members and understanding one's own strengths and weaknesses in behaving accordingly. Effective team members are effective self-monitors—they "think before they speak and act" in order to avoid words and behaviors that might demean others or discourage others from contributing. Often, the offending party does not intentionally or knowingly do offense to the party who feels demeaned. In such cases, respectful feedback to the offender from the team leader or the offended party is appropriate.

One of the features of effective team collaboration noted in Chapter 6 is trust. The swift trust of template clinical teams is based on role definitions and reliable processes for assembling teams and is not based on the exercise of any competency by individual team members. The more extensive trust that can be enjoyed by true clinical teams and by management teams flows the exercise of the first 7 competencies listed in Table 7–3.

A final collaboration competency (Competency 8 in Table 7–3) is knowledge and application of the principles and methods of evidence-based practice (the integration of available scientific research evidence into decisions). This competency gives healthcare teams a common language and a criterion for consensus decision making. Evidence-based clinical care has been a standard for several decades in much of the health services sector, and the approach has spread into the healthcare management arena as well (Kovner et al, 2009; Straus et al, 2011). Putting evidence-based decision making to work in team activities builds on members' shared knowledge base in scientific research methods. Assessment of evidence does not solve every problem, of course, as often evidence is lacking and team members may vary in their perspective on what constitutes evidence and whether the evidence is relevant to the particular case at hand (Begun, 2009). This difference in perspective is particularly likely between professions with a social science base (for example, healthcare administration) compared to a natural science base (for example, pharmacy). However, a shared assumption that research evidence is important in decision making provides an important foundation for individual participation in collaborative team processes.

Team Management

Another obligation of team membership is active participation in the management of the team, and team members need to be able to make contributions in this arena. Team members who leave the team's operational and social health up to others are shirking team member responsibilities. Participation in 5 management activities is emphasized in this final category of competencies. They are listed in Table 7–4.

First, members must be able to participate in the selection and orientation of new members of the team. Team members often have the best perspective,

Table 7–4. Competencies for team members: team management

1. Actively contribute to the selection and orientation of new members of the team
2. Actively contribute to both the operational effectiveness and social health of the team
3. Actively participate in the evaluation and improvement of the team's performance
4. Actively participate in training, team building, and process improvement activities
5. Actively contribute to the prevention and management of conflict in the team

and unique insights, into what it takes to be an effective member of their particular team. While leaders (or sponsors) of teams hold ultimate responsibility for team composition, team members usually can provide valuable input, or the team leader can delegate hiring authority to a team member or sub-group of members (with hiring of a particular candidate subject to the approval of the team leader). In addition to securing new team members who are a better match for team needs, involvement in the selection process by members increases the commitment of team members to making the new addition a successful one. If participation in selection is not possible because members are externally chosen (for example, appointed by a team sponsor) or predetermined (for example, all providers in a clinical group are on the team), then assisting with orientation of new members is even more critical for existing members. The new member likely will feel like an "outsider" when she or he joins the team. Existing team members should proactively make new members feel comfortable, particularly if they are joining a team with strong identity and trust among existing members.

Kerry Hilton, an expert on autism with a Doctor of Education (EdD) degree in Special Education, was anxious for the monthly meeting of the neurodevelopmental disabilities leadership education team to get going. Several team members were engaged in chit-chat, and the meeting should be starting. His blood pressure rose even more when team leader Margo Atler, MD, started the team meeting by announcing that they would go around the room and each person would say what they had done during the holidays that had fallen between this meeting and the previous one. Kerry wondered to himself, "Who has time for fun? And who cares anyway? Can't we just get on with business?"

A second team management competency of members, Competency 2 in Table 7–4, is that they contribute to both the operational effectiveness and the social health of the team. Effective teams require both, as argued in Chapter 6. Individual team members can help to make sure this characteristic of effective teams is realized. In the preceding vignette, the team leader, Dr. Atler, is attending to the social health of the team, but Dr. Hilton is not buying into it. Many busy health professionals need to suspend their "get-it-done-now" mentality in order to devote time to building the bonds necessary for effective teamwork. On the other hand, too much attention to the social climate inhibits task accomplishment. Hopefully, Dr. Atler in the scenario above is aware of the need to balance attention to social and task needs.

Contributing to the operational effectiveness of the team is a tall order, covering a wide range of behaviors. One deserves special note: members should be careful not to sabotage team management by forming subgroups that operate autonomously of the larger team. Sub-groups often are necessary in order to accomplish the work of the team, but unless they are sanctioned by the team leader and are part of the hierarchy (reporting to the team as a whole), they may subvert the operational effectiveness of the team.

The ensuing 3 competencies address 3 important aspects of contributing to operational effectiveness. No team works to perfection, and effective teams learn "on the job." Members should expect their teams to grow and learn. This requires that individual members participate in the evaluation and improvement of the team's performance (Competency 3 in Table 7–4). Chapter 13 discusses methods of team evaluation. Chapter 16 deals with performance improvement in general and with process improvement specifically. An additional competency expected of all team members is active participation in process improvement as well as training and team building (Competency 4 in Table 7–4). Methods of training and team building are explained in detail in Chapters 14 and 15.

Conflict among team members is not only to be expected but often is valuable in clarifying roles and responsibilities and producing team decisions. Conflict management is a broad and important fifth team management competency to which individual members should actively contribute. Effective team members resolve conflicts with other members of the team and cooperate in conflict resolution facilitated by the leader or other members. In the Canadian Collaborative competency framework, as mentioned earlier, interprofessional conflict resolution is highlighted as one of 6 clusters of competencies, with 8 competencies in the conflict resolution cluster: value the potential positive nature of conflict; take constructive steps to address conflict; know common sources of conflict; know strategies to deal with conflict; set guidelines for addressing conflict; work to resolve disagreements; establish a safe environment for diverse opinions; and allow all members to feel their viewpoints have been heard (CIHC, 2010, pp. III to IV). Many of the competencies apply to individual members as well as team leaders. In Chapter 11, more detailed aspects of managing conflict are presented.

CONCLUSION

To produce the effective team characteristics delineated in the previous chapter, individual team members should be competent in 21 areas. Competencies for individual team members fall into the categories of patient focus (3 competencies), team orientation (5 competencies), collaboration (8 competencies), and contribution to team management (5 competencies).

Effective patient focus is created on the team by individual members respecting patients and families, actively soliciting and integrating patient input, and performing their roles in culturally sensitive ways. A team orientation is created by individual members contributing to the development of shared values, goals, processes and team identity, and acknowledging shared responsibility for team outcomes. A team orientation requires an understanding of teamwork by team members, including the characteristics of effective teams and competencies of effective members, as well as self-understanding of one's competency strengths and weaknesses. Collaboration on the team requires that individual members respect each other, value the contributions of the various professions, and understand their own roles and the background and role of others on the team. A commitment to working interdependently is another competency of collaborative team members, as is effective communication with other team members. To communicate effectively, team members must refrain from demeaning or dominating others on the team. The use of evidence-based practice provides a foundation for effective communication and decision making. Finally, team members are responsible for actively contributing to management of the team, in the form of new member selection and building the social and operational health of the team. Participation in team building, training, process improvement, evaluation, and conflict management are all expected of effective team members.

REFERENCES

Begun JW. Commentary: realistic evidence-based management. *Health Care Manage Rev.* 2009;34:214-215.

Canadian Interprofessional Health Collaborative (CIHC). *A National Interprofessional Competency Framework.* Vancouver, BC, Canada: Canadian Interprofessional Health Collaborative; 2010. http://www.cihc.ca/files/CIHC_IPCompetencies_Feb1210.pdf. Accessed September 20, 2012.

Cannon-Bowers JA, Tannenbaum SI, Salas E, et al. Defining competencies and establishing team training requirements. In: Guzzo RA, Salas E, eds. *Team Effectiveness and Decision Making in Organizations.* San Francisco, CA: Jossey-Bass; 1995:333-380.

DeLellis AJ. Clarifying the concept of respect: implications for leadership. *Journal of Leadership Studies.* 2000;7(2):35-49.

DeLellis AJ, Sauer RL. Respect as ethical foundation for communication in employee relations. *Lab Med.* 2004;35: 262-266.

DeVany C. *90 Days to a High-Performance Team: A Complete Problem-Solving Strategy to Help Your Team Thrive in Any Environment.* New York, NY: McGraw-Hill; 2010.

Expert Panel on Cultural Competence Education for Students in Medicine and Public Health. *Cultural Competence Education for Students in Medicine and Public Health: Report of an Expert Panel.* Washington, DC: Association of American Medical Colleges and Association of Schools of Public Health; 2012. http://www.asph.org/competency. Accessed February 9, 2013.

Interprofessional Education Collaborative Expert Panel (IECEP). *Core Competencies for Interprofessional Collaborative Practice: Report of an Expert Panel.* Washington, DC: Interprofessional Education Collaborative; 2011. http://www.aacn.nche.edu/education-resources/IPECReport.pdf. Accessed January 29, 2012.

Kovner AR, Fine DJ, D'Aquila R. *Evidence-Based Management in Health Care.* Chicago, IL: Health Administration Press; 2009.

Mannahan CA. Different worlds: a cultural perspective on nurse-physician communication. *Nur Clin North Am.* 2010;45:71-79.

McCaffrey R, Hayes RM, Cassell A, et al. The effect of an educational programme on attitudes of nurses and medical residents towards the benefits of positive communication and collaboration. *J Adv Nurs*. 2011;68:293-301.

Mitchell P, Wynia M, Golden R, et al. *Core Principles & Values of Effective Team-Based Health Care*. Discussion paper. Washington, DC: Institute of Medicine; 2012.

Pentland AS. The new science of building great teams. *Harv Bus Rev*. 2012;90(4):60-70.

Sapienza AM. *Managing Scientists: Leadership Strategies in Scientific Research*. 2nd ed. Hoboken, NJ: Wiley-Liss; 2004.

Seaburn DB, Lorenz AD, Gunn WB Jr, et al. *Models of Collaboration: A Guide for Mental Health Professionals Working with Health Care Practitioners*. New York, NY: Basic Books; 1996.

Smith R. What doctors and managers can learn from each other: a lot. *BMJ*. 2003;326:610-611.

Straus SE, Richardson WS, Glasziou P, et al. *Evidence-Based Medicine: How to Practice and Teach It*. 4th ed. Edinburgh, UK: Churchill Livingstone; 2011.

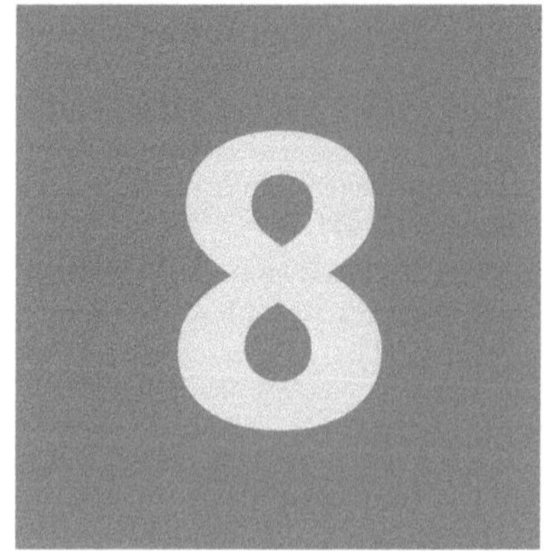

Leading Healthcare Teams

In Chapters 6 and 7, we cover the characteristics of effective teams and the competencies that team members need in order to contribute to making their teams effective. In this chapter we explain the leadership of teams, including the methods used to choose team leaders, the leader's role, and the competencies needed by a team leader. The subsequent 3 chapters provide more detail on team functions that are important for all team members but have special importance for team leaders because they oversee these functions or handle them directly. Chapter 9 describes decision making in teams; Chapter 10 deals with fostering creativity; and Chapter 11 explains managing conflict.

HOW ARE TEAM LEADERS CHOSEN?

Team leaders come to be leaders by various pathways. The most common paths are illustrated by the following 3 vignettes.

Vignette 1

Petronela Jarak, RN, MSN, started her nursing career at Central Valley Hospital immediately after completing her Bachelor of Science in Nursing (BSN) degree. She worked first on a medical-surgical floor and later on an oncology floor. After she had worked in oncology for 6 years, she became charge nurse on the evening shift. In other words, she was in charge of the oncology unit during one-third of the day. Within 2 more years she became head nurse for Central Valley's oncology services, including services provided on all shifts and in some outreach programs. During her years at Central Valley, Ms. Jarak often was asked to serve on task forces and committees. She gained experience in small group problem solving and eventually in chairing committees. She also continued her nursing education by earning a Master of Science in Nursing (MSN) degree in nursing administration at a university in a nearby city. She took some of her courses online and some on nights and weekends over 4 years.

Last year the Chief Nursing Officer (CNO) of the hospital retired. A search for her replacement was conducted. The Chief Executive Officer (CEO) made the hiring decision, with input from the Chief Medical Officer (CMO) and several others. She appointed Ms. Jarak as the new CNO, and her appointment was confirmed by the board.

Vignette 2

Frances Painter Medical Center is an integrated health system in Oregon. It was founded in 1920 by several physicians in various clinical fields—internal medicine, pediatrics, general surgery, orthopedics, and so on. It had functioned as a multispecialty group practice for 35 years before the group practice purchased the hospital that the physicians had been using since the group was founded, thus creating an integrated health system. By 2010, the Medical Center had grown to include 425 physicians, 52 nurse practitioners (NPs), about 500 registered nurses, and many other professionals. All of those who worked at Frances Painter were employed by the organization. Despite the expansion of the organization over the years, many of the original operating policies and procedures persisted.

Among the time-honored procedures was the election of department chairs. Archana Gupta, MD, was Chair of Primary Care Internal Medicine at the main center in Beaverton. Two years ago, she had been elected to her position for a 5-year term. The voters in the election were the 23 general internists who practiced at the main center. The NPs, registered nurses, and others who worked in this primary care unit did not vote.

For the present, election by physicians remains the method of choosing department chairs. However, there is talk of changing to a new method. A recurrent problem with using elections has been that some department chairs come into conflict with the organization's Medical Director, who is appointed by the CEO of the whole organization. Some think that the Medical Director should appoint the department chairs; with that method, most likely there would be fewer conflicts between the Medical Director and the department chairs. Also, the exclusion of the NPs from voting for department chairs is becoming a point of contention between the NPs and physicians.

Vignette 3

Mountain Lake Medical Group was formed in 1997 by 2 family physicians, Rodney Schreiber, MD, and David Hunt, DO. Over the next 15 years it grew steadily. By 2012 it had 9 physicians and 3 NPs. Eight of the physicians are family physicians, and 1 is a surgeon. The group is organized as a professional corporation, owned by the physicians who have been admitted into "partnership." Technically, these physicians are directors of the corporation, not partners, but everyone refers to them as the partners. Each year the 7 partners elect a president of the corporation. The partners take turns serving as president, 1 year at a time.

The leader of the group, however, is not the president. The leader is Dr. Schreiber. He recruited Dr. Hunt to join him in forming the group. Dr. Schreiber's interests go beyond practicing medicine; he is interested in the organization and its development. He is skillful interpersonally and knowledgeable about the business of medicine. He is trusted by everyone who works at Mountain Lake as competent and honest. Some find him to be domineering, and there are some in the group who routinely challenge his proposals. Nevertheless, everyone believes that he is and should be the leader.

Some people, for example, Ms. Jarak, become team leaders by appointment. Some people, for example, Dr. Gupta, are elected. And sometimes a leader emerges from the history of the team without ever having been formally designated as the leader, for example, Dr. Schreiber. All of these methods for choosing a leader can be successful. What is important for the effectiveness of the team is that the method results in a clear choice of leader and that the method is perceived by the team members as legitimate.

As described above, Ms. Jarak became head of the nursing leadership team at Central Valley Hospital by appointment. There is no question that she is the leader of the team, and all of the unit head nurses and others on the team regard her appointment as legitimate even though some of them wished they had been appointed and some others find her management style outdated. Ms. Jarak is accountable to the CEO, who appointed her. The CEO is also the sponsor of the team and owes certain forms of assistance to the team, as discussed in Chapter 12.

Dr. Gupta's position as Chair of her department at Frances Painter is also clear. She reports to the Medical Director of Frances Painter Medical Center, but whether she is, strictly speaking, accountable to the Medical Director is not clear. Because she was elected, she is seen by most members of her team as accountable first to them. It is also not clear whether the Medical Director is the sponsor of the team or whether the team even has a sponsor. For the moment, elections for department chairs are seen as legitimate means for determining who is a department chair at Frances Painter, but cracks are beginning to appear in the unanimous support for elections. A shift from electing leaders to appointing them is common as organizations become larger. One reason arises from the way that natural sub-groups develop and come into conflict as an organization grows. These sub-groups—family medicine, surgery, site-based teams, and so on—are the organization's genuine work teams, integrated by a senior leadership structure. A leader who is elected by a team tends to become a representative of that team, expected to protect the team's interests in interactions with the larger organization. This often leads to conflicts between team leaders and those responsible for integrating the multiple teams. Eventually the dysfunction results in a shift to top-down appointment of the team leaders. If the misgivings about elections at Frances Painter deepen over the next few years,

Dr. Gupta's elected successor may be acknowledged as the new leader but seen as doubtfully legitimate by many team members, especially the NPs, who are not permitted to vote. In that case, the successor will have difficulty functioning as the leader.

Dr. Schreiber at Mountain Lake Medical Group was not appointed or elected. He is the leader because he has worked at Mountain Lake from its beginning and has always been the leader. This basis for leadership can also be successful—as long as everyone accepts the result. At some point in the future of the group, a political disagreement is likely to arise, and maybe a crisis. At that point the group is likely to adopt a new means for determining the leader. Perhaps the president's role will come to consist of more than signing leases and contracts as the personal symbol of the group. Perhaps the person chosen by the board to be the president will be the true leader instead of Dr. Schreiber.

THE TEAM LEADER'S ROLE

What Do Effective Team Leaders Do?

One simple but incorrect answer to this question is that effective team leaders make decisions and tell the other team members what to do. This is the notion of leader-as-commander. The error of this answer can be seen from the nature of teamwork in health care. Most healthcare teams are interprofessional. A person with one profession will not have sufficient knowledge to direct people in other professions properly. For example, physicians, with rare exceptions, know very little about social work and cannot instruct social workers on social work interventions. However, they can call on social workers to use their knowledge and skills to contribute to patient care, and ordinarily that is what physicians do when they are leading healthcare teams. Nurses and other team members interact with social workers in the same way. The notion that leaders tell other people what to do arises from a certain picture of team organization in which there is a clear hierarchy and orders are issued top-down by a highly knowledgeable leader. This view of the leader's role is not tenable. First, it is based on an over-simplified military model of teamwork. In fact, it is doubtful that the military ever used this model. The military understands very well that a rigid top-down approach to team leadership is not effective (Marine Corps, 1996). Second, all effective healthcare teams have interdependent members who call on each other to take action, each member using his or her specialized skills. Those who prompt action from others adjust their own activities in response to that action. If team members were acting solely on the basis of orders from the leader, they would not be interdependent because each member would be dependent only on the leader. A team that functions in this way is in fact a dysfunctional team, as discussed later in this chapter.

If issuing orders is not what effective team leaders do, what do they actually do? The role of the leader can be summarized in 3 tasks (Hackman, 2002; West, 2012, pp. 61-63). Team leaders (1) create and maintain the conditions that enable the team to function effectively, (2) build and maintain the capacity of the team to do its work, and (3) coach the team to optimize its performance, or arrange for others to provide coaching. These tasks are listed in Table 8–1.

To create the necessary conditions for effectiveness means to enable the team to function at least at a minimal level of proficiency. The leader does not create the team or establish its goal. Those actions are taken by the team's sponsor as discussed in Chapter 12. The only exceptions are teams that constitute the whole organization, for example, Mountain Lake Medical Group, described in one of the vignettes at the beginning of this chapter. In those cases, the team leader and the team sponsor are the same person. In all other teams, the leader's role does not include creating the team or setting the goal. Assuming that the team has been created and its goal set, the leader's first task is to establish and maintain the conditions necessary for the team to exist and to function. The team needs all members to understand the goal, it needs its membership to be well defined, and so on, as detailed below. The leader must see that all of these conditions are in place. In other words, the leader must assure that the team has all of the defining features of a work team as discussed in Chapter 1 and listed in Table 1–1.

Building the team means adding new members to augment the knowledge and skills available in the team.

Table 8–1. Tasks for team leaders

1. Create the conditions that enable the team to function
2. Build the team's capacity to do its work
3. Coach the team to optimize its performance

It also means fostering development of the team's shared values, assuring that the team has the teamwork capabilities it needs to function well, and so on, as explained below. The leader does not exercise these capabilities himself or herself—at least not more than occasionally—but does make sure that the team has the capabilities that it needs.

Coaching the team means attending closely to how the team is performing, evaluating the performance, and providing advice and support for team members and for the team as a whole. Many team leaders provide coaching directly, but some leaders arrange for others to do it.

COMPETENCIES FOR TEAM LEADERS

The 3 tasks that define the team leader's role serve well to categorize the competencies needed by leaders. Team leaders need to be able to perform the 3 tasks, and performance of each task requires certain competencies.

Enabling the Team

Breslo Medical Center is an integrated health system that employs 325 physicians, 825 registered nurses, and 52 nurse practitioners. It operates 12 clinics and 2 hospitals. The Breslo clinics are scattered throughout a metropolitan area of 2 million people. The clinicians are divided into a Primary Care Division and a Specialty Care Division. Both divisions are headed by a physician-administrator pair or dyad.

The Specialty Care Leadership Team meets monthly to deal with both strategic and operational issues in the division. The members of the team are Thomas Steward, MD, and Cari Rebold, MHA (the dyad that leads the whole division) plus the physician-administrator dyads for surgical specialties, for medical specialties, and for the large sub-specialty services such as general surgery and cardiology. However, the physician members of these various dyads rarely attend except for Dr. Steward and the physician heads for surgery and medical specialties.

On one Thursday afternoon, the meeting was chaired as usual by Ms. Rebold. The topic of discussion was how to increase the proportion of primary care referrals going to specialists employed by Breslo Medical Center. For several years, 30% or so of referrals had been going to outside specialists—because of the long distances between some of Breslo's primary care sites and the 2 specialty centers and because of the referral patterns that had been established for certain specialty services before Breslo hired specialists in those fields. Breslo was trying to keep more of this referral business inside its own walls. Linda Lawson, the administrator for medical specialties, proposed that primary care physicians and nurse practitioners simply not be allowed to refer patients outside of the group, that is, that procedures be established to assure that all referrals remained inside the group, permitting exceptions only when Breslo could not provide the specialized service needed. Ms. Rebold asked whether other exceptions might be permitted, for example, for patients for whom travel to a Breslo specialist would be a hardship or for patients who had long-established relationships with specialists outside of Breslo. Ms. Lawson responded by saying that Breslo was having financial difficulties and that, while the conveniences Ms. Rebold suggested would be fine reasons for exceptions in better times, Breslo could not afford them at present. Ms. Rebold responded by saying that the considerations she had mentioned were not merely matters of convenience for patients. She said that insisting that patients travel long distances or give up trusting relationships with specialists would worsen the patients' experience of their health care. Dr. Steward added that the specialists at Breslo needed to find ways to appeal to the primary care clinicians and the patients so that more referrals would come their way. Dr. Steward then led a discussion of how Specialty Care might attract more referrals from Primary Care. He concluded the meeting by saying that he and Ms. Rebold would raise the issue with their superiors, the Clinical Services Administrator and Medical Director for Breslo, and explore with them how to achieve the goal.

In this team, Ms. Rebold and Dr. Steward provided genuine co-leadership. Although functional co-leadership can be difficult to achieve, using physician-administrator leadership dyads is increasingly common in larger medical groups and integrated health systems (Baldwin et al, 2011; Zismer and Brueggemann, 2010). At Breslo, the dyad of Ms. Rebold and Dr. Steward

Table 8–2. Competencies for team leaders: enabling the team

1. Establish and maintain a clear, common understanding of the team's goal
2. Establish shared responsibility for achieving the goal, or, better yet, mutual accountability for achieving the goal
3. Assure that the team has sufficient authority to do its work
4. Establish interdependency of members
5. Assure defined membership for the team
6. Keep the team unified, that is, assure that there are no subgroups operating independently of the whole
7. Relate effectively to the team's sponsor and to the larger organization

created and maintained the conditions that enabled their team to accomplish its goals. The competencies that leaders need to enable their teams' effectiveness are listed in Table 8–2.

At the meeting described in the vignette, Ms. Rebold, supported by Dr. Steward, assisted the team by helping it to maintain its common sense of purpose. The team had a vision for its future, that is, a picture of what care provided by the Specialty Division would be when the Division was performing as well as it possibly could. In the meeting, Ms. Rebold responded to Ms. Lawson's suggestion that patient-centeredness be compromised to serve the financial interests of the medical center. Her response reminded everyone that the goal of the team was to serve the patients' interests as defined by the patients. As Dr. Steward stated, having made the patients' interests the first priority, the team needed to seek a means to increase in-house referrals without coercing the patients. (The primary care physicians might have been coerced if the organization's financial condition required that referrals be made in-house and if the patients were not adversely affected. That is a different matter. The interests of the clinical providers have lower priority than those of the patients. Coercion of the primary care providers would not have been an attractive option, but it would not have been inconsistent with Breslo's goal of patient service.) Team leaders need to be able to remind team members of the team's goal, clarify it when necessary, and fend off challenges to the goal when they arise. At best, all of this needs to be done without offensive preaching. And, if possible, it should be done in a way that inspires.

Although not illustrated in the vignette, the team leader must also be able to foster a sense of shared responsibility so that various team members help each other in pursuit of the goal. For example, within the Specialty Care Leadership Team a sense of shared responsibility might lead one administrator to help another in estimating costs for a budget. Or a physician leader for one of the specialty services might help another physician leader to think through how to resolve a conflict between a nurse and a physician whose dysfunctional behavior is disrupting smooth operations. Ideally, the team leader creates a sense of mutual accountability in the team, as discussed in Chapter 6. The Specialty Care Leadership Team is stable over long periods of time, and mutual accountability might be achievable. It would be worthwhile for Ms. Rebold and Dr. Steward to pursue it.

The leader also needs to be able to assure that the team has sufficient authority to do its work without needing to seek continual approval or direction from outside the team. The team needs to have authority to determine how to reach its goal and to be confident that it will retain that authority. At Breslo, threats to this condition for effectiveness might take the form of rigid instructions from the Clinical Services Administrator and Medical Director (to whom Ms. Rebold and Dr. Steward report) about such matters as times when department meetings can be held or methods for making appointments for patients. The co-leaders of Specialty Care need to be able to protect the team from such intrusions while remaining sensitive to the needs of the whole organization and continuing to work with others outside Specialty Care to meet the needs of Breslo overall. They need to be able to balance their responsibility to their team with their responsibility to the whole organization.

Interdependency of members is a defining feature of work teams. Without it, there is no gain in having people work together and surrender the flexibility of working independently. If there is to be a team, the leader must be able to create and sustain interdependency. This is done chiefly by designing the work so that individual members will draw on the knowledge and skills of other members and by encouraging members to make best use of what other members have to contribute. In the case of the Specialty Care Leadership Team, Ms. Rebold and Dr. Steward could, for example, partner pairs of department administrators so that cardiology and cardiac surgery scheduling routines are designed jointly or so that procedures for handling surgical specimens are designed jointly by the Pathology Department and the Surgery Department.

A team also needs clarity about who is a team member and who is not. On this point, the Specialty Care Leadership Team may have a problem. Most of the physician heads of the specialty departments do not attend the meetings regularly. Are they team members or not? They probably think that they are team members and that they may attend any meeting and participate in decision making. However, the other team members may resent and resist infrequent participation because the infrequent attenders are not well informed about the team's methods of operation or its history of decisions made, that is, the precedents that shape the team's on-going decision making. Ms. Rebold and especially Dr. Steward need to make it clear whether the rarely seen physician heads are team members or not, and, if they are not, to make it clear to these physicians that they may not attend the meetings. One solution might be to make attendance at meetings a condition of membership.

The leader also needs to keep the team unified, that is, to keep everyone accountable to the whole team for actions that affect the work of other people on the team. For example, the physician-administrator dyad in charge of gastroenterological services at Breslo should not make decisions that affect the operations of the general surgery department without the participation and agreement of those in charge of general surgery. The leader needs to be able to recognize when sub-groups are functioning with inappropriate independence and bring them back into collaboration with the whole team.

Finally, Dr. Steward and Ms. Rebold need to be able to relate effectively to the larger organization. The discussion at the meeting touched on this issue. The challenge at hand was how to increase in-house referrals. Dr. Steward spoke of seeking help to meet this challenge by consulting with the senior leaders of the whole clinical enterprise. Also implied was a desire to avoid provoking conflict with Breslo's Primary Care Division. Another important aspect of relating to the larger organization did not come up at the meeting, namely, securing resources for the Specialty Care Division, for example, annual budget allocations and capital for major equipment purchases. Team leaders need to be able to secure funds and other forms of help from outside the team. They also need to assure that the team works smoothly with other parts of the organization and to obtain constructive evaluation of the team's performance from outside the team, especially from the team's sponsor, as discussed in Chapter 12.

Exercise of these 7 leadership competencies clustered under the heading of *enabling the team* establishes the possibility of effective team performance. However, for the team to move from possible to actual effectiveness, the team must also be developed and coached. We turn next to development of the team.

Developing the Team

George Mather, MD, was Medical Director of Cypress Medical Group. In 2002, he and the other leaders decided to establish a Mental Health Department. Prior to this time, the 63 clinicians in the group had referred patients outside of the group for treatment of depression, schizophrenia, and other mental and behavioral disorders. Dr. Mather hired William Chin, MSW, to chair the department. Mr. Chin was a mental health therapist with many years of experience as a therapist and as a leader of mental health teams.

Mr. Chin spent his first month at Cypress talking with family physicians, pediatric nurse practitioners, and other clinicians in the group about their perceptions of the needs for mental health services and of means that could be used to coordinate mental health services with general medical services. Then he began hiring. He first hired 2 psychiatrists, 1 PhD clinical psychologist, 1 RN, and 2 more therapists with Master of Social Work (MSW) degrees. He also hired 2 front desk clerks. More clinical staff members were added over the next 2 years. From the outset, the team had the help of a senior operations administrator at Cypress Medical Group. She was expert in handling appointment scheduling, use of the telephone system, and other routine aspects of the department's day-to-day activities. But she was not considered a member of the team, at least not a member of the core team.

As the new people joined the department, Mr. Chin brought them together as a team. At first the team had extended discussions of their values and operating philosophy. Then came efforts to establish operating procedures and behavioral norms. These efforts were accompanied by some jockeying for position and power within the team. At one point the psychologist attempted to use her credentials to assert authority over all matters of psychotherapy. The psychiatrists did not immediately object, being interested primarily in diagnosis and the use of medications. But the social workers rejected the psychologist's foray. Fortunately the episode was brief, and there were no damaging effects. Within 8-9 months the team had settled down into a highly functional and collaborative team, using regular case conferences and frequent informal consultations within the team.

Mr. Chin held a monthly operations meeting, attended by everyone in the department, including the clerks. Initially Mr. Chin chaired the meeting, but he turned this duty over to Dr. Green, one of the psychiatrists, an able chairperson, after a few months.

In the first 2 years, the mental health services clinical staff went off-site for an entire day twice annually to review what was going well and what problems the team was having in delivering service. The product of each of these off-sites was an action plan for the next year, to be revised in 6 months. As part of the planning, the team used 2 or 3 methods for brainstorming when they needed to solve particularly difficult problems. Conflicts were also addressed. Once the RN and social workers had a disagreement about the role of the RN in medication follow-up. The disagreement was worked through in a well-planned group discussion involving all of the clinicians.

During the first year, Mr. Chin met monthly with Dr. Mather, the team's sponsor. They discussed the team's rising capacity to receive new patients. Some new patients sought care directly, and others were referred from other departments at Cypress. Dr. Mather was frustrated that the capacity of the Mental Health Department was not increasing faster. Mr. Chin did his best to hasten development of the team's patient care operations, relying for some issues on the senior administrator provided to the department. Dr. Mather and Mr. Chin also discussed the pace of new additions to the clinical staff and began planning to remodel the department's consultation rooms to make them more suitable for psychotherapy. The rooms previously had been used as examination rooms for general medical care.

Table 8–3. Competencies for team leaders: developing the team

1. Oversee recruitment, orientation, and team formation
2. Establish the team's values and behavior norms
3. Assure a common understanding of the team's approach to doing its work
4. Maintain sufficient hierarchy for the team to achieve its goal—and no more
5. Foster team identity
6. Assure a favorable social climate, including psychological safety
7. Assure that the team can carry out team-level operations effectively

At the 2-year mark, all things considered, both Dr. Mather and Mr. Chin judged the venture to be a success. Mr. Chin had assembled and shaped an excellent team, all of whom made their own contributions to the team's development. Dr. Mather had provided excellent sponsorship.

Team leaders need to be able to develop their teams. The individual competencies required by a leader to develop a team are listed in Table 8–3. Mr. Chin's adept development of the Mental Health Department illustrates most of these competencies.

Establishing how many people will be on a team is a task usually performed by the team sponsor and team leader working together, as discussed in Chapter 12. Sometimes the sponsor also has a role in determining the mix of professions on the team. From that point onward, the leader needs to be able to recruit team members, assure their orientation to the team, and oversee the melding of the team members into a unified team. Mr. Chin showed his competence in these functions as he determined which professionals should comprise the team, hired them directly, and orchestrated a series of events to form them into a team. Adding new members to a team remains a central responsibility of the team leader throughout the history of the team. In teams of 12 or fewer people, the leader ordinarily should do the hiring directly to assure that each new member embraces the team's goal, shares the core values of the team, and fits well with the people already on the team. In larger teams—which are both unusual and riskier, as discussed in Chapter 12—some portion of the hiring process may be delegated to others, but even then hiring needs to be closely supervised by the leader. In either case, other team members should participate in the interviews that are part of the hiring process, especially members who have the same profession as the person to be hired. As the team grows, clarity needs to be maintained about who is a core team member and who is associated with the team but is a peripheral member or a resource for the team. As he built the Mental Health Department, Mr. Chin was clear about the senior operations administrator from Cypress Medical Group being a resource rather than a team member. She did not attend off-site meetings, and at the monthly operations meeting she was regarded as a respected advisor rather than a direct participant in decision making.

The process of team formation is something that the team leader must know well and be able to guide. While it is useful for the team members also to understand the process, commonly in clinical teams the members do not know the process, and this rarely makes a difference. Teams progress through a sequence of stages as they become competent as integrated units. This sequence has been characterized in different models proposed by various researchers in organizational behavior. The most commonly used model is the one devised by Bruce Tuckman. Its stages are memorably named *forming, storming, norming, and performing* (Tuckman, 1965; Tuckman and Jensen, 1977; West, 2012, pp. 89-91). This model is shown in Figure 8–1.

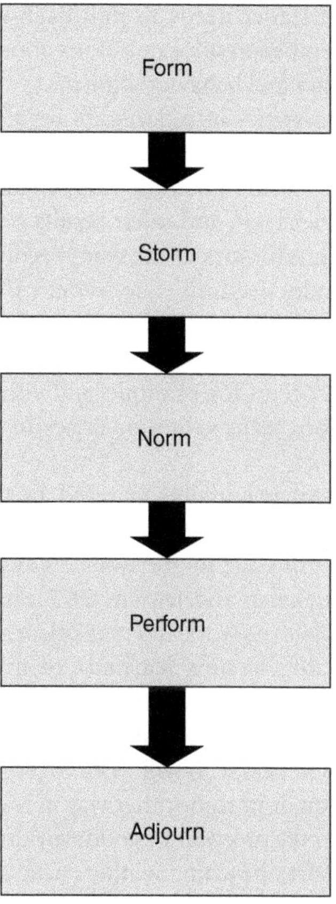

▲ **Figure 8–1.** Tuckman model of team development. (Tuckman BW. Developmental sequence in small groups. *Psychol Bull.* 1965;63:384-399. Tuckman BW, Jensen MAC. Stages of small-group development revisited. *Group and Organizational Studies*. 1977;2:410-427.)

During the stage of forming, the members learn the team's goal and what will be expected of them as individuals. They also become acquainted with the leader and the other team members. Mr. Chin used an off-site, 2-3 operations meetings, and 2-3 case conferences to take the team through this stage. Of course, there were also numerous one-on-one conversations involving many different pairs of team members. During the stage of forming, members determine for themselves whether they will commit wholeheartedly to the team. Commonly new members have not reached a firm decision on this issue before joining the team because they lack adequate information. If a member decides that the team is not a good fit, he or she may depart or may hold back psychologically, perhaps for a long period of time. Part of the leader's task during the forming stage is to convince the team members that the team's goal is worthy and that it can be achieved.

During the stage of storming, team members engage in testing assumptions about the team, and they may engage in outright conflict. The leader's conception of the goal and her or his competence are tested. Various members challenge the roles assigned to them and to others. Members elbow one another (hopefully not literally) to determine who has what knowledge and skills and who will have what authority as the team moves forward. In the preceding vignette, the psychologist's attempt to assert her authority in the new mental health team was characteristic of this stage. The social workers might have accepted some form of this authority, but they rebuffed her and insisted on their own independence as practitioners.

In the norming stage, team members establish the functional basis for doing the team's work. Norms of behavior are established, usually through group discussion, and people begin functioning in their roles. At this point, the leader needs to pull back and let the other team members resolve questions about communication routines and behavioral norms.

As the team settles into doing its regular work, it enters the stage of performing. The common understanding of the team's goal, the refinements of roles, the norms of behavior, and other results of the previous stages are put to work as the team becomes a functional and productive unit. The leader's direction of particular members usually decreases to a very low level from this time onward, rising again only when certain events occur, for example, individual actions that depart from team values or crises in staffing or financial support.

Although not originally included in the model, Tuckman, in response to work by other researchers, later added a fifth stage to the model, which he called *adjourning* (Tuckman and Jensen, 1977). In this stage the team completes its work and may celebrate achievements or catalog lessons learned. Team members acknowledge each other's contributions and say their good-byes. This stage is especially important for teams that include members who will work together again in some other team or in some other way in the organization. To sustain the prospect of good working relationships in the future, the team members need to close out their work and depart on good terms, sometimes expressing their sense of loss if the team has been particularly important to them. The Mental Health Department, of course, did not go through this stage since it was an on-going team. However, management project teams and time-limited consultative teams routinely do go through this stage and need to manage it well. (These and other types of teams are discussed in Chapter 2.) Clinical template teams usually do not attend to adjourning, but some probably would benefit from doing so, for example, surgical teams that carry out extended and complex procedures such as the multi-hour procedures done to remove certain cancers. Many clinical knotworks would also benefit from deliberate adjourning, but the opportunity to adjourn a knotwork is distinctly unusual.

The progression through Tuckman's stages is not a predictable march, invariable from team to team. In fact, Drinka and Clark (2000, pp. 18-27) hold that team development in health care usually has a different sequence of stages. The stages in the Drinka-Clark model are *forming*, *norming*, *confronting*, *performing*, and *leaving* (Figure 8–2). Forming and performing are

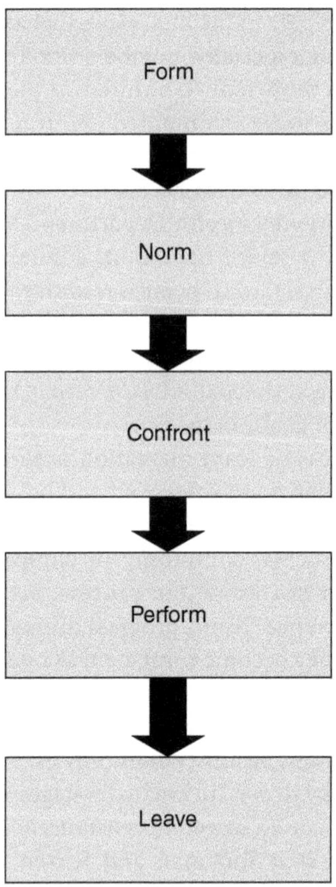

▲ Figure 8–2. Drinka-Clark model of team development. (Drinka TJK, Clark PG. *Health Care Teamwork: Interdisciplinary Practice and Teaching*. Westport, CT: Auburn House; 2000:18-27.)

the same in this model as they are in the Tuckman model, and the stage of leaving is equivalent to Tuckman's adjourning. The difference between this model and the Tuckman model lies in the second and third stages. In both the Tuckman model and the Drinka-Clark model, norming is a stage of clarifying roles, team procedures, and behavioral norms; but the discussions are pursued in the Drinka-Clark model without the benefit of a storming stage. In the Drinka-Clark model, the storming stage is passed over in the hope of avoiding all conflict. The reason offered for this behavior is that "health care practitioners do not like conflict and use many excuses for ignoring it" (Drinka and Clark, 2000, p. 26). But, of course, personal rivalries, doubts about the leader's vision for the team, and other sources of disagreement or conflict do not disappear. In time, the team members challenge one another and come into disagreement over goals, roles, and individual authority in daily operations. The term for this stage in the Drinka-Clark model is *confronting* instead of *storming*. The word *confronting* is apt because it suggests that disagreement is often more personal when it is openly expressed after having been suppressed for a time. In both models, a stage of conflict and negotiation occurs. Such a stage must occur for a team to develop into a unit that functions well. This stage can occur before norms are set, as in the Tuckman model, but if the team avoids this stage and proceeds directly to norming, team will need to go through a confronting stage later on. None of the stages can be omitted.

In the process of team formation, the leader needs to be able to recognize when the team is forming, storming (or confronting), norming, and performing and then to encourage the inevitable discussion and negotiation rather than suppressing it. The Mental Health Department's team formation generally followed the Tuckman model, but there was some blurring of the storming and norming stages—with no ill effect. Occasionally the leader will need to steer the team's development so that interpersonal conflicts do not become damaging; and occasionally damage will occur despite best efforts and will need to be repaired.

The Mental Health Department presents a simple illustration of team formation because it was a new team, and all of the team's members were becoming integrated into the team at the same time. Longer-standing teams need to cope with team members departing and new team members joining the team after the existing team has gone through its developmental stages. When new members join a team, there is almost always some repetition of one or more stages of team formation, including storming. The team leader needs to be able to recognize what stages are being repeated and manage those stages.

Mr. Chin also showed his competence in establishing the team values and behavior norms. In the first place, he held meetings at which the main topics of discussion were the team's values and operating philosophy. What degree of importance should team members attach to timeliness? When a patient has been seeing one therapist and then switches to another therapist without letting the first one know, should the second therapist notify the first one? These questions and many others were answered by common agreement as the team developed, and many of the questions would be revisited in the future.

The team leader also needs to assure that the team achieves agreement on an approach to doing its work, as discussed in Chapter 6 in connection with Red Family Medicine, a primary care team. In the case of the Cypress Mental Health Department, Mr. Chin made sure that the team fully discussed the different professional roles, the intake of new patients, the use of group visits, and numerous other aspects of its routine operations. It was not necessary or even desirable for all aspects of patient care to be standardized. For example, some therapists were likely to prefer cognitive behavioral approaches to therapy while others were likely to prefer psychodynamic approaches. However, it was necessary for all team members to agree on the conceptual frameworks in use and to agree on procedures for evaluating patients' needs, matching patients with clinicians, and providing therapy, drug treatment, or both. And the common understanding of routine operations needed to emphasize the interdependency of team members, a defining characteristic of the Department as a team.

A particularly challenging competency for team leaders is maintaining sufficient hierarchy within the team to enable the team to do its work while at the same time not establishing or condoning a hierarchy that stifles dissent and innovative thinking. In the case of the Mental Health Department, it was especially important for Mr. Chin to maintain his authority as the department was built. At the same time, he needed the team members to be candid and creative in the many meetings required to launch the department. Striking the right balance between these 2 needs requires substantial and unusual interpersonal skill, and Mr. Chin had this skill. It was primarily for this reason that Dr. Mather hired him.

An effective team leader also must be able to foster team identity. Mr. Chin did not use shirt logos, badges, and other visual devices to foster team identity as was done in Red Family Medicine in Chapter 6. He judged that his team members would regard this approach as juvenile and or sentimental. Instead, he relied chiefly on the use of off-site meetings. "Off-sites" are held away from the normal work setting and usually last for most or all of a day or even longer. Extended meetings without the interruptions of a normal workday enable team members to come to know one another personally. The vehicle for becoming better acquainted is discussion of work issues without any pressure to reveal personal information that members wish to keep private. The second off-site during the first year lasted a day and half and was held at a retreat center. It began on a Thursday afternoon, included an overnight stay, and continued through the whole of Friday. For this off-site, Mr. Chin hired a consultant in organizational development to help him plan the meeting and then to facilitate it so that Mr. Chin could participate without needing to chair the discussions. An overnight off-site is a particularly potent means for generating interpersonal connections and team identity.

Maintaining a favorable social climate is also a competency needed by team leaders. In a mental health department—for obvious reasons—it is not difficult to persuade the team members to lift their eyes from their immediate tasks and pay attention to the social climate. Nonetheless, maintaining a favorable social climate in a mental health department can be challenging. Mental health professionals bring to their work more interpersonal skill than most clinicians and managers possess. In other words, if rivalries and relationship conflicts develop, they can quickly become very serious because most mental health professionals have the ability to use their interpersonal skills effectively in pursuing their personal goals. For this reason, Mr. Chin was wise to move ahead quickly to foster interpersonal bonds within the group and to establish explicitly acknowledged and agreed norms of collaboration and openness, using group discussions and the off-sites. He did not need to intervene to mediate any disputes, but he was alert to the possibility that he might need to intervene and was attuned to the tenor of all of the interpersonal interactions in the team. For example, in all discussions, he was attentive to the presence or absence of psychological safety, a particularly important component of a team's social climate, discussed in Chapter 6.

Finally, a team leader must be able to develop the team's abilities to accomplish team-level operations effectively. Teams need to be able to perform various tasks as a group, and they need nurturing in order to develop these abilities. For example, they need to be able to conduct effective meetings in which decisions are made. This requires an effective chairperson. Mr. Chin regarded himself as an adequate chairperson but not a superb one. He also preferred to participate in discussions without having to maintain the neutrality required of a chairperson. He chaired the first operations meetings; but from the first meeting onward, he was watching for someone who could take over this function. He found such a person in Dr. Green. A team also needs the abilities to make durable decisions, plan creatively, manage conflicts, find resources elsewhere in the organization, train new members, and so on. The leader must be able to make sure that the team has all of these operational abilities. The leader does not need to be the central actor for any of these operations. Many team leaders in health care make the mistake of assuming that it is their responsibility (or burden) to chair meetings, locate sources of help elsewhere in their organizations, mediate disputes, and perform a host of other tasks. They think that these functions are all parts of the job description for the leader. Fortunately for many leaders, these functions can be performed by other members of the team although any leader may want to perform some of them.

In establishing the operational capability of a team, leaders can be helped by attending to Meredith Belbin's team roles (Belbin, 2010, pp. 19-31; West, 2012, pp. 45-48). Belbin distinguishes among 9 roles that need to be filled in nearly all teams. For example, a *coordinator* clarifies goals and promotes decision making in the team. A *shaper* is a dynamic, hard-driving person who challenges others and delights in removing barriers encountered by the team. A *completer finisher* is someone who seeks error-free performance for the team and attends closely to deadlines. There are 6 more roles in Belbin's list (Table 8–4). Not all teams need to have all 9 roles covered, but most of them are relevant to most teams. The leader can use the list as a checklist for team development, deciding for each role whether it is needed for the team and, if so, whether it is covered. Sometimes 2 or 3 roles can be covered by the same person.

Belbin's list of roles also provides help for leaders by showing them how much of their responsibilities can actually be delegated. All of the roles except for *specialist* are seen by some leaders as a portion of their responsibilities. However, all 8 of these roles can be delegated, leaving the leader free to enable, develop, and coach. Most team leaders do take on the coordinator role, shaper role, or both—at least sometimes. However, even those roles can be delegated. For example, in a postoperative cardiac surgery ward in one tertiary-care hospital, the person who runs the rounds each morning is a clinical nurse specialist, serving in a coordinator role. She moves the group along from patient to patient, making sure that all necessary topics are covered and all necessary decisions are made. A cardiologist participates, and sometimes the cardiac surgeons

Table 8–4. Belbin's team roles

Role Name	Function in the Team
Plant (or innovator)	Serves as a source of new ideas, innovation, unorthodox approaches; problem solver; sometimes provocative
Resource investigator	Searches for people and materials that can be useful to the team; makes contacts; connects the team with outside sources of help
Coordinator	Clarifies the team's goals; seeks to coordinate different components of the team's work; often chairs meetings
Shaper	Drives the team to higher levels of achievement; brings courage and determination to the team's work; sometimes pushes people too hard
Monitor evaluator	Serves as a critic of the team's performance; provides insight and good judgment; maintains broad perspective; sometimes overly negative
Teamworker	Brings a collegial, cooperative approach to the work of the team; listens well; diplomatic; has a manner that discourages relationship conflicts
Implementer	Practical doer; brings discipline, reliability, and efficiency; oriented to concrete action; usually brings a traditional approach to the team's work
Completer finisher	Provides thorough assessment of the team's services or work products; seeks to assure that the work is done well; insists on meeting timelines
Specialist	Brings special knowledge or skill to the team; focused on a narrow component of the team's work; dedicated; takes initiative

Source: Role names and definitions based on Belbin RM. *Team Roles at Work.* 2nd ed. Burlington, MA: Butterworth-Heinemann; 2010:19-31.

participate. However, they do not manage the rounds. One might be tempted to say that the clinical nurse specialist is the team leader, but in fact she is only coordinating the discussion on rounds. The leader of the team is the cardiologist, who has delegated coordination of rounds to the nurse.

In the vignette, Mr. Chin's developmental activities were focused on a new team. Eventually a new team becomes an established team, but the need for continuing development persists. The leader must continue to exercise the competencies listed in Table 8–3. In order for individual members and the whole team to function well over time, the leader also needs to coach the team or arrange for coaching, to which we now turn.

Coaching the Team

Diana Laguardia, RN, was the Director of Surgery at Rothesay Memorial Hospital, a voluntary hospital in a large city in the Northeast. She was in charge of the 10 operating rooms (ORs) and the staff who worked in and around the ORs. She was the leader of the OR nurses, surgical technicians, schedulers, and other staff who worked in surgical suite. The surgeons and anesthesiologists were members of the medical staff, that is, they had privileges to treat patients at Rothesay, but they were not employed by the hospital. Most of the surgeons also operated at other hospitals. The anesthesiologists worked at only one other hospital, which was closely associated with Rothesay.

Ms. Laguardia tried to spend about one-third of her time in the surgical suite talking with other nurses and staff and watching the work being performed, including activities in the operating rooms. Often surgeons would see her and make suggestions about the suite's operations or ask her to deal with problems. Spending time in the surgical suite, she frequently observed excellent teamwork. She also observed shortfalls in communication, behavior that suggested role confusion, signs of relationship conflict, and other difficulties.

Every weekday, Ms. Laguardia held a brief start-of-day meeting for all of the OR nurses and other staff. At these meetings she often would tell the group about innovative examples of teamwork she had observed recently in the surgical suite. Making these comments reinforced the good work she had seen and spread the word about the innovations to others. When she had noticed something suggesting lack of clarity about who should perform various tasks, she would question the group to confirm her impression and then usually ask 2-3 of the involved people to consider the issue outside of the meeting and bring back a proposal to her for solving the problem. Sometimes she would join these groups of 2 or 3 to make suggestions. Usually this step was followed by presentation of the proposed solution at the morning meeting for informal confirmation by the whole group or for surfacing difficulties which were then referred back to those who had devised the proposal so that they might revise it. Sometimes Ms. Laguardia drew people aside at convenient times during the day and made suggestions about how they could handle problems she knew they were dealing with, for example, conflicts among nurses or conflicts with surgeons.

Ms. Laguardia was an able leader of a group of people who were members of a series of template teams, namely, the operating room teams that functioned for varying lengths of time many times every day with ever-shifting membership. Fortunately all of the people in this group knew each other and worked together directly at least occasionally. Ms. Laguardia regarded the whole group as her team, but, using the concepts explained in Chapters 1 and 2, the individuals were actually too numerous to be a work team and were instead the people who constituted (with the addition of surgeons and anesthesiologists) the pool of people from which individuals were drawn to form the many template OR teams that performed surgery at Rothesay.

Ms. Laguardia liked to coach and did it often. Her competencies are noted in Table 8–5. Most of her coaching was focused on issues of teamwork such as role definition, but she also coached individuals about interpersonal relations at work (Thompson, 2011, pp. 276-278; West, 2012, pp. 72-76). Coaching requires careful gathering of information about the performance of individuals and teams, including genuine listening and mindful observation of team activity, often including not only what team members say but also the tone of voice they use, their facial expressions, and their body posture or body language. Using this information, a coach then evaluates the observed performance against expectations for good performance of individuals and the team. The expectations for individuals are the exercise of the team member competencies discussed in Chapter 7. For teams, the expectations are the characteristics of effective teams discussed in Chapter 6. Based on her or his evaluations, a coach then provides feedback and advice or guidance.

Table 8–5. Competencies for team leaders: coaching the team

1. Gather information on the performance of the team and individual team members
2. Evaluate performance
3. Provide feedback and advice

Sometimes a coach helps individuals to acknowledge feelings so that those feelings do not interfere with solving problems. For example, Ms. Laguardia once coached a scrub nurse about dealing with a circulating nurse who was so formal and abrupt in her manner that surgeons interpreted her to be antagonistic and refused to work with her, often refusing on very short notice so that delays occurred while alternative nurses were found. The scrub nurse was so infuriated by the circulating nurse's behavior that she could not think clearly about the situation and devise a way to deal with the problem. The nurse was in fact barely aware of her anger and so did not see it as a roadblock. By asking a series of questions, Ms. Laguardia was able to get the scrub nurse to express her anger and move past it to address the problem. At the same time, Ms. Laguardia was careful not to let the individual coaching stray into the arena of psychotherapy; she steered clear of any personal problems or internal conflicts the scrub nurse might have.

Team leaders functioning as coaches also provide advice to whole teams. For example, Ms. Rebold, the administrator in the Specialty Care Leadership Team described earlier, was coaching her whole team when, in a team meeting, she cautioned one of the team members not to let financial performance considerations cloud their understanding of the goal of the team, namely, to serve the interests of the patients.

Effective coaching is difficult and often time consuming. It is commonly informal so that checklists and step-by-step methods are usually not useful. Timing is critical. Choice of words and tone of voice are also critical. Some team leaders, because they recognize that their coaching skills are limited or that they have too little time to coach effectively, arrange for other people to do the coaching instead of doing it themselves. One option is to make use of team members who are good coaches. A leader can ask team members to work together on an issue, saying straightforwardly that one of the members is in a good position to help the other. Another option is to obtain coaching from outside of the team. The Human Resources Departments of many large healthcare organizations have coaches available to help with teamwork. Coaching may also be purchased from external sources. The level of expertise is often very high, but this approach is limited by its inflexibility. Since external coaches are not available on short notice for opportunistic coaching, they are ordinarily used for specific, well-defined projects such as planning and facilitating off-sites—in the way that Mr. Chin used a consultant in the mental health department described in the previous section.

The Team Leader as Enabler, Developer, and Guide

The portrait that emerges from this review of team leader competencies is not the picture of a martinet, task-master, or a dictatorial parent. In fact, effective leaders stand back from their teams and let them do their work. They provide the foundation (enabling factors), develop the team's capacity to function well, and coach when coaching is appropriate. Hopefully this portrait will put to rest the concept of team leader-as-commander, that is, the idea that effective team leaders make decisions on their own and issue orders to the other team members.

Leaders of Template Teams

As may be obvious already, the role of the leader of a clinical template team is not well characterized by the account of leadership in this chapter. Template team leaders might be regarded as exceptions among team leaders. However, it is more accurate to say that they have a different role. Template teams are typically short lived, for example, OR teams, emergency rescue teams, and emergency cesarean delivery teams. Time does not permit the leader to enable the team, develop it, or coach it. A clinical template team leader does have responsibility for maintaining a sense of common purpose in the team and keeping the team members focused on achieving the team's goal, but he or she cannot exercise the other competencies listed in Tables 8–2, 8–3, and 8–5 because time does not permit these activities. A template team depends heavily on the institutional arrangements that are in place before the team is formed and begins to function. These arrangements are the work of the team sponsor, which is often a committee. The role of the sponsor is discussed in Chapter 12.

The leader of a template team is an operational manager rather than a true leader. The distinction between leaders and managers is a common topic in the literature on leadership and is particularly well characterized by John Kotter (1996, pp. 25-30). Leadership is concerned with envisioning the future, establishing goals, maintaining alignment across the people working toward the goals, and motivating or inspiring. Management is concerned with getting the day-to-day work done, that is, execution, control, and problem solving. Template teams require managers, not leaders of the kind needed to head clinical departments or whole organizations. A surgeon leading an OR team, for example, is concerned much more with management than leadership. Some clinical template teams need to have a physician leader in order to direct operations. Other clinical template teams need to have a nurse leader or a dentist leader or a pharmacist leader and so on, depending on the nature of the work done by the team.

MUST THE LEADER OF A CLINICAL TEAM BE A PHYSICIAN?

In the second and third vignettes at the beginning of this chapter, the teams described are clinical true teams. Both are led by physicians, Dr. Gupta and Dr. Schreiber. (The team in the first vignette is a management team, led by Ms. Jarak, a nurse.) Must the leader of a clinical true team always be a physician? The short answer to this question is "No." This answer may surprise some physicians and perhaps other clinicians and managers. The answer warrants an explanation.

First, it should be noted that there is no widespread belief in health care that the leader of a *management* team needs to be a physician—or a nurse, pharmacist, or any other clinician. The CEOs of hospitals and integrated health systems are regularly people who are trained in management and have no clinical training or experience. There are, of course, nurse CEOs and physician CEOs, but they are uncommon. Administrators perform well as CEOs because they engage in administrative activities and rely on nurses to provide nursing, physicians to practice medicine, and so on. The CNO and CMO of a hospital are accountable to the CEO, but this does not mean that the CEO directs the nursing activity of the CNO or the medical activity of the CMO.

The CEO's role is limited to monitoring the work of the CNO and CMO to assure that they are performing well in their roles. In general, to do this monitoring properly, a CEO relies on the assessments that he or she solicits from nurses about the CNO and from physicians about the CMO. In the same way, the CEO of a large corporation with highly complex, technical operations does not need to be someone who has training in those technical matters. For example, the CEO of Shell Oil Company, does not need to be a geologist or petroleum engineer. And the CEO of Shell does not instruct the head geologist or head petroleum engineer in making decisions about geology or engineering.

Second, there are many interprofessional true teams headed by nurses, pharmacists, social workers, psychologists, or others who are not physicians. Nurse-managed practices consist of advanced practice nurses and other professionals and are led by nurses. Medication management programs are headed by pharmacists and sometimes include nurses. Mental health practices that provide counseling and psychotherapy may be headed by social workers in some cases and by psychologists in other cases. These are all examples of teams in which there is no physician, and therefore the leader is not a physician.

Third, for many years, interprofessional teams with physician members have functioned with leaders whose professions are not medicine. The case of the Cypress Mental Health Department, described above, is a real (but disguised) case. That department included physicians, and yet the leader was a social worker. In some medical groups, optometrists and ophthalmologists practice together with an optometrist as the department head. Some rehabilitation facilities employ primary care physicians or physiatrists who work in units led by nurses.

The idea that the leader of any clinical team must be a physician arises from a common but oversimplified concept of the leader's role, namely, the concept of leader-as-commander, discussed above in the explanation of what leaders do. Imbedded in this concept is the idea that the team leader rightly has the last say on any question that might arise in the team and that he or she exercises this authority from time to time. As applied to clinical teams—so the argument goes—the team leader must be a physician (1) because only physicians have sufficient knowledge to make decisions about any question that might arise, (2) because any other healthcare professional in the role of leader could and will overrule patient-care decisions made by other professionals (including physicians), sometimes causing harm to patients, and (3) because only physicians have the knowledge and breadth of vision to be able to define the future and lead the team to it.

This concept of the leader is a fiction. Even tyrannical CEOs and military officers do not have sufficient knowledge to exercise power effectively on this scale. The same is true of any thoughtful physician. First, physicians do not have sufficient knowledge to be able to decide any question that might arise in clinical practice. They rely on nurses, pharmacists, physical therapists, and many other professionals to use their knowledge in the care of patients; and physicians are routinely in no position to second-guess the other professionals—as they typically acknowledge. For example, in most states in the United States, the law requires physicians to order services that they do not understand. Any primary care physician can tell stories about asking a physical therapist what modalities of therapy a patient needs so that the physician's order can be written. Second, even if it were true that the team leader could overrule any patient-care decision made by another professional—by issuing an order countermanding the decision or by removing the other professional from the team—the likelihood that a team leader would do this is negligible or nil. Very unusual circumstances might cause a team leader to remove a team member—for example, because the individual is grossly incompetent or has diminished mental capacity—but in a case of this kind the reason for removing the team member is the disability or defect in the individual and not a disagreement over any particular decision that the individual has made. Oil company CEOs do not overrule the judgments of geologists about where oil is to be found, and hospital CEOs do not tell cardiologists (whether employed by the hospital or not) how to perform catheterizations. Of course, it is conceivable that a clinical team leader might begin issuing edicts beyond his or her professional competence because he or she has become delusional, morally corrupt, or mentally incapacitated. In that event, the person ordered to take action contrary to his or her professional judgment would have every reason to resist the team leader and to take action to have the team leader removed. Third, although physicians typically have more years of education and training than other healthcare professionals, their knowledge has limits. They also have their own distinctive values and perspective on health care as do nurses, pharmacists, and professionals in any other healthcare field. (See Chapter 3.) They are not uniquely well positioned to envision the future in health care. In fact, some of those who have had the most innovative and enduring visions for the future of health care were not clinicians at all, for example, William Beveridge in the United Kingdom (architect of the National Health Service) and Henry J. Kaiser of Kaiser Permanente in the United States.

Some writers on healthcare teams have noted the long-standing dominance of medicine in health care and have argued that this dominance is no longer justified in the current era of highly specialized professionals, many of whom use knowledge and skills that are not within the scope of medicine. The solution sometimes proposed is to shift the leadership within a healthcare team from one professional to another as the needs of the patient change so that there no longer is a single team leader (Reeves et al, 2010). This proposal is an attempt to side-step the issue, and it is also based on a misunderstanding of what effective leaders do. Every team needs a leader (or 2 co-leaders) as discussed in Chapter 6. Without a leader, the organizational needs of the team cannot be met. Switching leaders because the patient's needs have changed is unnecessary and only invites ambiguity and frustration. Of course, the patient's needs should be met by the professionals who can best meet them. A patient who has appendicitis needs a surgeon. If the patient later needs counseling about where he or she should reside during a period of convalescence, this need should be met by a social worker. But it is quite beside the point to shift organizational leaders from surgeon to social worker and later to a third professional who can meet some other need of the patient. Moreover, a healthcare team often serves several patients simultaneously. Which patient's needs should determine who the leader is? This approach to establishing leadership of the team has no defensible rationale because the leader does not provide health care in her or his capacity as leader. The leader is the person who maintains the conditions for team effectiveness, develops the team, and coaches; this person should remain constant during changes in the patients' needs. The determination of team leadership does not depend on the services needed by any of the team's patients at any given moment.

In the United States, challenges to medicine's traditional leadership in health care frequently come from the nursing profession. The tension between medicine and nursing has a long history (Stein, 1967; Stein et al, 1990). Although, as noted above, there are already some interprofessional clinical teams that include physicians and are led by someone in another profession, these arrangements are uncommon and usually exist in relatively small areas of health care, not in the core arenas of primary care, medical specialty care, and surgical care. Many nurses now seek equal status with physicians in these arenas. However, at present if a clinical team in one of these core arenas includes a physician, then the team leader is a physician. Exceptions to this pattern are rare. In the United States, there are a few nurse-managed practices that employ physicians, but they are rare (Hansen-Turton et al, 2010). We (the authors) have been unable to identify any practice that includes both advanced practice nurses and physicians practicing in a team that is led sometimes by a physician and sometimes by a nurse, a person in either profession being eligible to become the leader each time there is a change in leadership. In fact, there are substantial barriers to establishing a healthcare practice that handles its leadership in this way. State laws and insurance company payment practices generally reinforce the convention that healthcare practices must be led by physicians.

The nursing profession is increasing the educational requirements for nurses, expanding the scope of nursing, and seeking more leadership roles for nurses in health care. It is seeking to improve nursing care and to improve the standing of nurses relative to physicians. In 2011, the Institute of Medicine published *The Future of Nursing* (Institute of Medicine, 2011). The report recommended that Congress and state governments remove scope-of-practice barriers so that advanced practice nurses be permitted "to practice to the full extent of their education and training" and that nurses become "full partners, with physicians and other health professionals, in redesigning health care in the United States" (Institute of Medicine, 2011, pp. 7, 9). The response of the American Medical Association (AMA) was prompt and negative. The AMA spokesperson said that the United States needs a "physician-led team approach to care," and she continued:

> *Nurses are critical to the healthcare team, but there is no substitute for education and training. Physicians have seven or more years of postgraduate education and more than 10,000 hours of clinical experience. Most nurse practitioners have*

just two-to-three years of postgraduate education and less clinical experience than is obtained in the first year of a 3-year medical residency. These additional years of physician education and training are vital to optimal patient care, especially in the event of a complication or medical emergency (O'Reilly, 2010).

This statement reflects the misunderstanding explained above, that is, the mistaken belief that the leader's role in a clinical team is to supervise the clinicians on the team and issue instructions as she or he thinks best. The role of the leader is not clinical; it is organizational. The leader enables, develops, and coaches the team. This role can be performed by a physician, a nurse, a social worker, or any other healthcare professional. What matters is the person's competence in carrying out the functions of the leader, not the person's healthcare profession.

As explained earlier, the leader of a clinical template team has a limited role and is an operational manager rather than a true team leader. Template team leaders do not enable, develop, or coach their teams. Instead they manage minute-to-minute events. Some template teams need to be managed by physicians in the sense that they need minute-to-minute medical oversight by a physician. Perhaps the AMA spokesperson quoted earlier was thinking of certain template teams, but the needs of certain template teams—for example, OR teams—do not justify the generalization that all clinical teams must be led by physicians.

Clinical true team leaders do not need to be physicians. However, whether the leaders are physicians, nurses, pharmacists, or other clinicians, they do need to be effective leaders if their teams are to serve their patients well.

HAZARDS FOR TEAM LEADERS

To solidify the account of team leader competencies, it is useful to consider hazards that team leaders must be able to recognize and avoid (West, 2012, pp. 77-79). There are many hazards, of course. We deal here with only 4, chosen because they often are not recognized in practice.

The first error to avoid is managing the individuals on the team instead of the whole team. This is probably the most frequently encountered error among clinical team leaders, although it is not so frequent among management team leaders. Even in a leader who understands that he or she should focus on team function, the temptation to manage individuals can persist because the leader retains vestiges of the concept of leader-as-commander. The error is manifest in frequent one-on-one meetings by the leader with individual team members and by team meetings in which the leader directs almost all of his or her comments to individuals instead of the group. In order to develop an effective team, a leader should limit the number of team members with whom she or he meets individually as well as the frequency of meetings with any one team member. The leader also should encourage pairs and trios of team members to address and resolve procedural issues rather than resolving these issues by direct intervention. For example, in developing the patient intake process and other patient flow procedures for the new Mental Health Department described earlier, Mr. Chin could have met with the MSW therapists one at a time and asked each one to handle some portion of the planning. This would have been less effective for the long run than the choice he actually made, that is, to lead discussions in the monthly operations meetings in which he asked pairs or trios of team members to develop proposals to be returned to the group for consideration. This approach met the needs for establishing procedures and gave the team members practice working together. The practice in working together carried benefits for the future of the team. Mr. Chin also had the team engage in various group processes at monthly meetings and off-sites, for example, brainstorming, explicit role negotiation, and constructive controversy (discussed in Chapter 9), a method for assuring that several positions on a controversial issue are explored by a group (Tjosvold, 1998). Again, these assignments to the whole team nurtured the capabilities of the team.

Second, the leader must not assume that the team members are competent as members of a team. Leaders can appreciate fully that they need to give direction to individuals only sparingly but still overlook the fact that the team's ability to succeed is limited because the individuals do not know how to function as a team. In the eyes of many able team leaders, teamwork competencies appear to be matters of common sense; but many clinicians and some managers do not have intuitive teamwork competencies and need to be taught. Fortunately these competencies can be taught, as explained in Chapter 14. In the preceding vignette, Ms. Laguardia, Director of Surgery at Rothesay Memorial, spent much of her time teaching teamwork skills to the

OR nurses and technicians. Over time, the team members acquired the abilities to deal with the social climate, to communicate crucial information reliably, and to exercise the various other team member competencies discussed in Chapter 7.

Third, the leader needs to refrain from providing the team—or individuals—with detailed instructions on how to accomplish the team's goal. The leader's foremost responsibility to the team is to clarify and reinforce its goal, but the means to achieving the goal should be left to the team as much as possible (Hackman, 2002, pp. 73-83). If the members of the team devise the means for achieving the goal, they likely will be able to use each other's knowledge and skills more fully since they usually know each other better than the leader knows them. They will also be more fully engaged in the task and more likely to embrace the methods chosen since they will have psychological ownership of them. Consider the Breslo Specialty Care vignette, in which the Leadership Team was trying to increase the proportion of specialty referrals that were directed to in-house specialists. Ms. Rebold and Dr. Steward would be well advised to try to establish a task force comprised of people from Specialty Care and people from Primary Care. The task force would be charged with devising a proposal to achieve the objective. At the end of the vignette, Dr. Steward said that he and Ms. Rebold would take the issue to the leadership team for the whole medical group, suggesting that they expected to work out a solution in the more senior leadership team and bring the solution back to the Specialty Care Leadership Team for implementation. This approach would be less promising than asking for a proposed solution from those who will in the end have to make the solution work.

Fourth, a leader can stumble by failing to seek organizational support for the team. Teams cannot succeed unless they have the resources they need to do their jobs. Sometimes leaders clarify and reinforce the goal very well but then simply accept the resource constraints in place—often because they wish to avoid conflict with more senior people in the organization. Establishing a budget is to some extent a competitive sport, and team leaders must be prepared to represent their teams in this process. The leader must also protect the team from outside interference, either from more senior people in the organization or from other teams that seek to advance their interests by controlling other teams in some way. Sometimes institutional policies adversely affect the team, for example, compensation policies; and exceptions need to be sought by the leader when exceptions are needed for the team to function effectively. The leader is the team's agent in dealing with the larger organization. He or she must manage up the hierarchy as part of leading the team.

SELF-MANAGING TEAMS

Sometimes healthcare teams are described as self-managing. The term *self-managing team* suggests that the team has no leader at all, but this is not the case. The difference between self-managing teams and the teams described in this chapter is that the leader of a self-managing team stands far back from the team and does not function as a regular team member (Wageman, 2001). He or she sets the goal, establishes the size and composition of the team, and authorizes the team to evaluate its own work and make changes based on the team's own systematic consideration of its progress. The leader ordinarily does not attend team meetings but does receive progress reports regularly and may intervene. The team chooses someone other than the leader to coordinate its activities, monitor its progress, locate resources that team can use, and so on. In other words, it usually seeks to have all of Belbin's roles covered. Sometimes the person chosen to coordinate the team's activities is labeled as the leader, but this secondary leader is actually functioning as a manager and does not exercise all of the competencies listed in Tables 8–2, 8–3, and 8–5. Those competencies are exercised either by the hands-off true leader or are distributed throughout the team. For example, the whole team may be expected to foster team identity and assure that the team has a common understanding of its approach to doing its work.

Well-led healthcare teams are similar to self-managing teams in that the leader takes pains to foster the team's ability to design work processes, make decisions, solve problems, and so on. Fully self-managing teams and teams with strong top-down leadership can be seen as 2 ends of a spectrum. Well-led healthcare teams are somewhere in the middle.

Clinical teams are rarely truly self-managing. The leader almost always participates in the team even if she or he avoids directing individuals and avoids usurping the functions that should be exercised by team members working interdependently. Self-managing teams are more common but still unusual among healthcare management teams. In particular, project teams with clear objectives and a clear timeline are sometimes self-managing.

CONCLUSION

Team leaders can be appointed or elected; or they can become leaders as part of the historical development of a group or organization. Effective leaders are not top-down autocrats. Instead, they enable the team by attending to its basic needs, develop the team by adding members judiciously and nurturing the team's capabilities, and coach the team. Each of these 3 tasks requires certain competencies in the leader. The choice of the leader should not depend on the leader's profession because effectively leading a team calls for using organizational skill, not for exercising clinical skill or using clinical knowledge. Common hazards for team leaders are managing individuals instead of the team, assuming that team members have teamwork competencies when they do not, providing too much direction to the team, and failing to seek organizational support. In self-managing teams, the leader maintains distance from the team and encourages the whole team to manage most of its activities.

Having established the role and competencies of team leaders, we next deal in more detail with 3 areas that the team needs to develop under the leader's guidance—decision making, creativity, and managing conflict.

REFERENCES

Baldwin KS, Dimunation N, Alexander J. Health care leadership and the dyad model. *Physician Exec.* 2011;37(4):66-70.

Belbin RM. *Team Roles at Work.* 2nd ed. Burlington, MA: Butterworth-Heinemann; 2010.

Drinka TJK, Clark PG. *Health Care Teamwork: Interdisciplinary Practice and Teaching.* Westport, CT: Auburn House; 2000.

Hackman JR. *Leading Teams: Setting the Stage for Great Performances.* Boston, MA: Harvard Business School Press; 2002.

Hansen-Turton T, Bailey DN, Torres N, et al. Nurse-managed health centers. *Am J Nurs.* 2010;110:23-26.

Institute of Medicine. *The Future of Nursing: Leading Change, Advancing Health.* Washington, DC: National Academies Press; 2011.

Kotter JP. *Leading Change.* Boston, MA: Harvard Business School Press; 1996.

Marine Corps. *Command and Control.* Washington, DC: Department of the Navy; 1996. http://navsci.berkeley.edu/ma20/MCDP%20Books/MCDP%206,Command%20and%20Control.pdf. Accessed March 4, 2013.

O'Reilly KB. IOM urges greater role for advanced-practice nurses. *Am Med News.* October 20, 2010. http://www.ama-assn.org/amednews/2010/10/18/prsd1020.htm. Accessed June 30, 2012.

Reeves S, Macmillan K, Van Soeren M. Leadership of interprofessional health and social care teams: a socio-historical analysis. *J Nurs Manag.* 2010;18:258-264.

Stein LI. The doctor-nurse game. *Arch Gen Psychiatry.* 1967;16:699-703.

Stein LI, Watts DT, Howell T. The doctor-nurse game revisited. *N Engl J Med.* 1990;322:546-549.

Thompson LL. *Making the Team: A Guide for Managers.* 4th ed. Upper Saddle River, NJ: Prentice Hall; 2011.

Tjosvold D. Cooperative and competitive goal approach to conflict: accomplishments and challenges. *Appl Psychol.* 1998;47:285-342.

Tuckman BW. Developmental sequence in small groups. *Psychol Bull.* 1965;63:384-399.

Tuckman BW, Jensen MAC. Stages of small-group development revisited. *Group and Organizational Studies.* 1977;2:410-427.

Wageman R. How leaders foster self-managing team effectiveness: design choices versus hands-on-coaching. *Organization Science.* 2001;12:559-577.

West MA. *Effective Teamwork: Practical Lessons from Organizational Research.* 3rd ed. Chichester, UK: John Wiley & Sons, Ltd.; 2012.

Zismer DK, Brueggemann J. Examining the "dyad" as a management model in integrated health systems. *Physician Exec.* 2010;36(1):14-19.

Making Decisions in Healthcare Teams

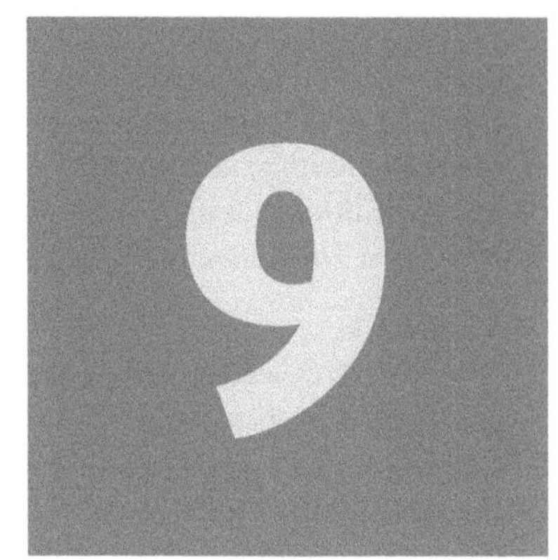

In Chapters 8-11, we explain the leadership of teams. Chapter 8 describes the choice, role, and competencies of team leaders. Chapters 9-11 deal more fully with topics that have special importance for team leaders although they are also important for other team members. This chapter examines decision making in teams. Chapter 10 deals with fostering creativity. And Chapter 11 covers managing conflict.

WHAT DECISIONS DO TEAMS AND TEAM MEMBERS MAKE?

The next 3 vignettes illustrate various decisions that are made within healthcare teams.

Vignette 1

Robert Jarna, MD, was an internist in a suburban practice of 8 physicians and 3 nurse practitioners (NPs). He had seen Michael Penine for general medical care for 11 years. Over the past 18 months, Mr. Penine's blood pressure had become consistently elevated, with 3 high readings in the past 4 months. Prior to starting treatment, Dr. Jarna took a history and carried out a physical examination. Mr. Penine reported that he occasionally had episodes of rapid heart beating without any apparent cause. There were no other symptoms accompanying the rapid heart beating. Dr. Jarna ordered various tests to detect kidney dysfunction and other possible underlying causes of high blood pressure (hypertension). Because of the episodes of rapid heart beating, he decided to include a 24-hour urine collection to check for the presence of a pheochromocytoma, a rare hormone-secreting tumor that causes high blood pressure in 0.1% of people with high blood pressure.

Vignette 2

Mary Thiessen, age 74, was a patient in the transitional care unit of a healthcare center that provided a wide range of services to elderly people and to some younger, disabled people. The services included long-term residential care, day care, and many others. Mrs. Thiessen had been admitted to the transitional unit after a hospitalization for a stroke. The purpose of her stay in the transitional unit was to determine her needs for nursing and other care for the longer term. The professional staff of the transitional unit consisted of several registered nurses, 2 social workers, 1 clinical pharmacist, and 1 internist-geriatrician. Over the 10 days Mrs. Thiessen was in the unit, her needs were evaluated by a nurse, a social worker, the pharmacist, and the physician. Options for her longer-term care were discussed extensively with Mrs. Thiessen and her family. Her stay culminated in a care conference attended by all of the professionals who had assessed her needs. Mrs. Thiessen was invited to join the discussion but deferred to her daughter. The meeting was chaired by the head nurse of the unit. All of the professionals had input to the discussion as did Mrs. Thiessen's daughter and the physical therapist who was asked to participate in the planning. In the end, the team reached a consensus that Mrs. Thiessen would be served best by moving into her daughter's home, where she and her daughter would be visited twice weekly by a home care aide. Mrs. Thiessen would be driven by her daughter once weekly to the healthcare center for a physical therapy session and would do strengthening and stretching exercises at home daily with the help of her daughter. In the short term, Mrs. Thiessen would see her primary care internist monthly; her internist, who did not work at the healthcare center, was agreeable with the plan. Mrs. Thiessen thought the plan sounded fine.

Vignette 3

Peter Lee, MD, worked with 4 other family physicians and 5 medical assistants in San Bernadino, California. A few years ago, Ann Morrison, one of the medical assistants, noted that patients were often unnecessarily delayed after preventive care visits because the physician had ordered an immunization, usually a tetanus-diphtheria (Td) booster or a flu shot. Patients would need to wait until a medical assistant was available to administer the immunization. Usually the wait was only a few minutes, but sometimes patients waited as long as 30 or 40 minutes. Ms. Morrison and Dr. Lee proposed to the whole team that a standing order be established so that a medical assistant could determine a patient's need for immunizations and administer them before the physician saw the patient. At one of the monthly team meetings, this proposal was discussed and agreed upon. A formal standing order was written and added to the practice's manual of policies and procedures.

These 3 stories illustrate 3 different kinds of decisions made in healthcare teams. In the first story, about Dr. Jarna and Mr. Penine, the highlighted decision is whether or not to test Mr. Penine's urine for biochemical compounds produced by a certain type of tumor. This decision was an *individual clinical decision*. Although Dr. Jarna worked in a team, the decision to do this urine test was not a team decision. It was appropriate for this decision to be made by Dr. Jarna alone, based on his medical knowledge and his assessment of Mr. Penine's symptoms. Dr. Jarna may have engaged Mr. Penine in making the decision, at least by asking him whether he would be willing to collect his urine for 24 hours. There is an immense literature on the topic of individual decision making in health care, including methods of reasoning and psychological pitfalls (Alfaro-LeFevre, 2013; Groopman, 2007; Kassirer et al, 2010). Decisions of this kind, however, are not team decisions and are not covered in this chapter, which deals with how decisions are made in teams and what hazards arise in team decision making.

In the second story, the team caring for Mrs. Thiessen made a *team clinical decision*. The decision about the plan recommended to Mrs. Thiessen required the input of people in several different professions as well as Mrs. Thiessen's daughter. It was also necessary—or at least highly desirable—for the different professionals and Mrs. Thiessen's daughter to agree on the decision because presenting a split decision to Mrs. Thiessen most likely would have distressed both Mrs. Thiessen and her daughter and would have left them without useful guidance. No one was in a position to "order" Mrs. Thiessen or her daughter to take a particular course of action, but Mrs. Thiessen and her daughter did expect guidance from the team. Team clinical decision making is covered in this chapter.

The other decisions covered in this chapter are *team management decisions*. The third vignette, about Ms. Morrison, Dr. Lee, and their team, illustrates this type of decision. The decision about standing orders for routine immunizations needed the input of both the physicians and the medical assistants to assure that the new process would function smoothly and to assure that everyone was comfortable with the change in the role of the medical assistants. For example, the team would have needed to address any legal concerns among the team members. However, the decision did not pertain to any particular patient, and for this reason it is not labeled a *clinical decision*. Instead it was a decision about how the team would manage its work. In this case, the management decision was made by a group of clinicians functioning as a management team. Of course, management teams comprised solely of managers often make similar decisions about processes that they use in their work. Team management decisions can be decisions about process issues such as the immunization process in this case, or they may be decisions about other management issues, including capital expenditures or competitive strategy for a whole healthcare organization.

METHODS FOR MAKING TEAM DECISIONS

The 4 basic choices available for team decision making are listed in Table 9–1. The method used by a team in making team decisions is a crucial element in the design of a team, as explained in Chapter 12. The issue is central to specifying the role and authority of the

Table 9–1. Models for decision making in teams

Strong central authority
Voting
Unanimous agreement
Consensus

team leader. The 4 options are illustrated in the next vignettes.

Strong Central Authority

John Smith was transported by emergency ambulance to the Emergency Department of County General Hospital, a Level I Trauma Center. He had suffered multiple gunshots to his chest. He was rapidly wheeled into Trauma Room #1, where he was assessed by Roy Chapman, MD, a trauma surgeon and head of the trauma team that evening. A nurse measured Mr. Smith's blood pressure and pulse. A technician applied electrocardiographic electrodes to Mr. Smith's chest. Mr. Smith's blood pressure was low, and his pulse was rapid. A quick physical examination revealed that he was unconscious and bleeding from 2 gunshot wounds, one in the center of his chest and one on the left side. Within 3 minutes, Dr. Chapman ordered administration of intravenous fluid at a rapid rate as well as transfusions of red blood cells, fresh frozen plasma, and platelets to control bleeding. Dr. Chapman suspected that Mr. Smith's aorta had been perforated by a bullet. Within a few more minutes, Mr. Smith was taken to the operating room.

This vignette illustrates team decision making by *strong central authority*. Although input from various professionals was relevant to the decision, time did not permit a decision based on deliberation by the team. The structure of the trauma team provided for strong authority vested in the leader, who on the evening in question was Dr. Chapman. If the leader is well informed and has good judgment, action proceeds rapidly and effectively. This approach to team decision making is often described as *autocratic* or *military*, and it is appropriate in situations of high risk in which rapid action is required to achieve desirable results or to avoid serious adverse outcomes. In health care, use of this model is not common. The number of acute emergency team decisions is a tiny portion of the team decisions made daily in clinical settings. Although vignettes about decision making by strong central authority are easily understood and often cited as examples of admirable team leadership, they are actually unusual. Decision making by strong central authority does not serve well as a general paradigm in health care even though it is entirely appropriate in some situations.

Some effective teams use strong central authority for making decisions even though time would allow for discussion and joint decision making by team members. Decisions that are regarded as trivial by team members can be handled efficiently by central authority without consultation. For example, deciding on the color of a replacement carpet is seldom a matter calling for input from all the team members. In other cases, the leader may seek consultation with one or several team members before making a decision using his or her own authority. Many healthcare administrative leadership teams function in this way.

Voting

Riverside Heart Clinic was introduced in Chapter 6. Twelve cardiologists and 5 NPs practiced at Riverside Heart. About 4 years ago, nearly all of them came to acknowledge that they had a problem with scheduling vacations. Although the cardiologists and nurse practitioners (NPs) were ready and willing to cover for their absent colleagues in the clinic and at the 2 hospitals they used, sometimes there were too few cardiologists and NPs in town to see all the patients who needed care. On these occasions, in the clinic the cardiologists and NPs would triple-book appointments (schedule 3 patients at the same time). Patients often waited 2-3 hours to see the clinicians with whom they had appointments. Cardiologists also would dash from one hospital to the other to perform catheterizations that were tightly scheduled even though they were scheduled at different hospitals.

The group called a special meeting of all 22 practitioners, chaired by Sam Lawrence, MD, the senior cardiologist in the group. Nineteen attended. No explanation of the problem was needed because everyone understood the issue.

Dr. Lawrence explained that he and 2 others had met and devised 3 possible solutions for their consideration: (1) separately limit the number of cardiologists and NPs who could be gone at any one time and have everyone sign up on a master calendar on a first-come-first-serve basis, (2) set a date for vacation requests to be submitted for the coming year and then draw lots for those weeks requested by more people than the number of people permitted to be gone, (3) use option 1 but set aside the Christmas-New Year period and possibly other particularly popular times to be handled with a rotation in 3-year cycles instead of using the first-come-first-serve method. Dr. Lawrence was not manipulating the situation. He genuinely wanted a solution to a problem that had become a point of distress for many people in the practice, and he did not have a favorite solution.

Dr. Lawrence invited everyone at the meeting to propose additional options for solving the problem. However, none were proposed, and this was not surprising since no one except Dr. Lawrence knew in advance what would happen at the meeting because Dr. Lawrence had not thought to tell anyone. Dr. Lawrence told the group that they would have ample time to discuss the options and would then vote unless they had reached general agreement through discussion. There followed a 90-minute, heated discussion of the 3 alternatives, including many suggestions for modifications of all 3. Eventually, it became clear to Dr. Lawrence—and everyone else—that agreement would not be reached. He then called for a vote. There were 9 votes for option 1, 6 votes for option 2, and 4 votes for option 3. Wanting a majority decision, Dr. Lawrence then deleted option 3 and asked the group to vote again. Thirteen people voted for option 1 and 6 people for option 2. Dr. Lawrence announced the result and said that vacations would be scheduled in accordance with option 1 as soon as further details had been settled by him and Riverside Heart's 2 office managers.

The 6 members of the group who had voted for option 2 left the room angry. In addition, 5 of the 13 who had voted for option 1 left annoyed because they preferred one or another variant of option 1.

Voting is an alternative to decision making by strong central authority. Sometimes it works well, but often it does not. In the case of the team management decision made at Riverside Heart, a majority of the team left the room dissatisfied; this did not auger well for the implementation of the scheduling process that had been chosen.

There are many different rules that can be used to come to a decision by voting (Thompson, 2011, pp. 157-158). For example, each voter can be asked to rate each option on a scale, say, of 1 to 10. The ratings can then be averaged across all voters, and the option with the highest average rating is declared the winner. Or, the option with the highest median rating can be declared the winner. More commonly, voters are asked to vote for the option they prefer without weighting the options, and the option that wins a plurality of votes is regarded as the winner. The plurality of votes is the highest vote total, regardless of whether that number is a majority of the votes cast, that is, regardless of whether that number is more than half of the votes. Plurality rule is used in almost all US elections and is often used by teams. In the meeting at Riverside Heart, Dr. Lawrence stipulated that the group would use majority rule rather than plurality rule, and so he deleted the option with the fewest votes on the first ballot and had the group vote again, thereby assuring that one of the options would receive a majority of the votes. This rule is also often used when teams vote. Majority rule and plurality rule generally perform quite well in reaching decisions that later can be assessed against some objective standard, for example, when groups choose among proposed solutions to problems and those solutions are later tested to determine whether they were successful (Hastie and Kameda, 2005). Of course, not all group decisions can be evaluated in this way since some decisions concern matters of personal preference—for which there is no standard available to use in testing the soundness or accuracy of the group's decision. Nonetheless, there is no need to use decision rules for voting that are more complicated than plurality rule and majority rule, except in very unusual situations.

Despite their strengths, majority rule and plurality rule have several disadvantages in team decision making. For example, neither procedure takes account of the strength of conviction among those who are voting. A vote backed with passion counts the same as a vote from someone who is almost indifferent. Thus the majority may consist mainly of people who care little about the choice at hand while a minority cares deeply. A result of this kind is likely to cause resentment and difficulties later on. Voting tends to polarize the team and interfere with negotiation to reach a compromise that might yield a solution acceptable to a larger number of people than a simple plurality or a majority. At the meeting at Riverside Heart, the team might have been able to work through variations on options 1-3 and arrive at a more broadly supported solution if they had not thought they were headed toward a vote at the end of the discussion. Also, since voting does not encourage collaborative interaction to construct new options, it does not foster support for the decision that is ultimately made. Voting can provide a quick route to a decision, but it often has significant longer-term ill effects.

On the other hand, voting does have a very useful role in team decision making. It is a rapid, simple method for deciding issues in which no one in the team is heavily invested. For example, the choice of the restaurant for a holiday gathering is sometimes a matter in which team members want to have a say although commonly no one is heavily invested in any particular outcome. In this kind of situation, 3 choices can be put forward and a quick vote taken.

Incidentally, voting does have a central and valuable role in groups that are not teams, specifically, in groups that consist of competitors, for example, hospital Chief Executive Officers (CEOs) gathered at a hospital association meeting. In this type of setting, making decisions by common agreement is often much slower than making decisions by voting, and the effort to reach agreement risks generating interpersonal conflict and frustration rather than support for the decision made (Tjosvold and Field, 1983). In situations in which the participants do not share a common goal but do share some interests, voting is ordinarily superior to other methods for group decision making.

Unanimous Agreement

Instead of guiding Riverside Heart's cardiologists and NPs to a majority vote, Dr. Lawrence could have stated at the outset that the group would make its decision by agreement across the whole group present, that is, by *unanimous agreement*. This is a third model for team decision making.

Using unanimous agreement as the basis for the team's choice forces the team members to listen to each other and work through various alternatives to a proposal that everyone endorses. This process tends to produce a decision that is widely approved while it simultaneously builds support for the implementation of that decision.

The disadvantage of requiring unanimous agreement for decisions, of course, is that the team may not be able to make a decision. Suppose, for example, that Dr. Lawrence had required the group to achieve unanimous agreement on its decision about vacation schedules. Under this scenario, one or more members of the group who did not celebrate Christmas might have objected to treating Christmas week differently from other portions of the year. And similarly, members who celebrated Christmas might have felt strongly that Christmas week should be handled in a manner that assured anyone interested in vacationing during that week that she or he would be able to do so at least every 3-4 years. Under these circumstances, unanimous agreement would have been impossible. Requiring every member of the team positively to affirm the final decision is a very demanding rule for decision making, and it can easily result in time-consuming negotiations or in stalemate. Nonetheless, when strong support for a decision is needed to assure durable commitment for its implementation, requiring unanimous agreement can be entirely appropriate.

Consensus

The pitfalls of voting and of decision by unanimous agreement can be avoided by relaxing the standard of unanimous agreement just a bit. Instead of requiring that all team members positively affirm the choice made, one can require only that every member be willing to accept the choice made or "live with it." We use the term *consensus* for agreement by general acceptance rather than by positive affirmation, and we distinguish between decision by consensus and decision by unanimous agreement.

For example, suppose Dr. Lawrence had proposed that Riverside Heart's clinicians decide how to handle scheduling vacations by basing the decision on consensus as defined here. As the 90 minutes of discussion progressed, someone wanting to be assured of a Christmas-week vacation at least every 3-4 years might have proposed rotating the people who can take vacation during this week only to find that she or he was opposed by someone who had no special interest in this week but did wish to be absent for Rosh Hashanah as often as possible (or someone who wished to be absent as often as possible for the end of Ramadan or for some other favored week during the year). At that point, someone in the group might propose that each person could designate one and only one of these especially popular times as his or her "prime vacation time." All of those choosing Christmas week as their prime vacation time would participate in a rotation, those choosing Rosh Hashanah would participate in a separate rotation, and so on—regardless of their religion or lack of religion or any other basis for choosing a particular period as their prime vacation times. This arrangement would imply that those choosing Christmas week could never be absent on Rosh Hashanah, those choosing Rosh Hashanah could never be absent during Christmas week, and so on. Everyone would gain something by this arrangement, but everyone would also lose flexibility. Some members might be quite annoyed by the loss of flexibility although willing to accept it because they would be assured of a vacation during their prime vacation time at least every 3-4 years. Under these circumstances, there might well be some people who would not positively affirm the proposal even though they could accept it. So, if Dr. Lawrence were to test for consensus by asking whether everyone could "live with this," it might happen that agreement was present throughout the room even though the enthusiasm associated with unanimous agreement was not present. Decision by consensus can permit the team to make a decision and move ahead when requiring unanimous agreement would result in an impasse.

An important reason that consensus is easier to achieve than unanimous agreement is that consensus permits team members to say that they oppose the choice made even though they also say that they will accept it. There may be several reasons for a team member to acquiesce in this way, for example, a desire to support the group in coming to a decision instead of getting stuck, an expectation of future consideration when some other difficult choice is faced, or a desire to return the team's favor of considerate treatment sometime in the past.

Using consensus decision making often requires some preparation prior to having the team make a decision. In the case of Riverside Heart, it would have been useful for a small group of, say, 4-5 people to talk through options and discover what conflicts and compromises might be anticipated and then present 2-4 thoughtful options to the group instead of expecting that a workable compromise might be constructed in the heat of discussion in the large group.

Choosing a Method for Making Decisions

Different situations call for different methods of team decision making. For example, situations of extreme urgency and high risk call for decision by strong central authority as in the case of the emergency room team treating a gunshot victim. Voting is suitable for a choice among alternatives that are all more or less acceptable to all team members.

However, most healthcare teams repeatedly use the same method for most of their decisions. Emergency room teams and other clinical template teams usually use decision making by strong central authority because they generally function under circumstances of moderate to high urgency. In the operating room, surgeons exercise central authority in making decisions—although this authority passes to the anesthesiologist for certain decisions. In rare situations of high urgency in matters of public relations, the CEO of a hospital may exercise similar authority. In contrast, most true teams prefer to make decisions by consensus, routinely avoiding voting. This choice is based on a desire to avoid conflicts and to generate broad support for decisions even though this desire is usually not stated explicitly and is often not even fully conscious among the team members and leaders.

Decisions in clinical knotworks (see Chapter 2) are sometimes problematic for 2 reasons. First, it is often unclear whether the members of a knotwork are functioning as a team or not. The referring physician, oncologist, and radiation oncologist treating a patient with pancreatic cancer may see themselves as a team, or they may see themselves as individual physicians practicing in their separate specialties. If they see themselves as individual physicians, they will construe all decisions to be made as individual clinical decisions and give no thought to how team clinical decisions should be made. If some members of the knotwork conceive of the knotwork as a team, they will see other members who operate autonomously as usurping the authority of the whole team, and conflict will result. Second, even if the knotwork members do think of themselves as a team, the question of how decisions will be made is often not raised. Sometimes one of the team members, for example, the oncologist, assumes that he or she has decision-making authority for all decisions except those requiring expertise outside of his or her field, for example, decisions about the dose and timing of radiation therapy. At the same time, the referring family physician may have the same (unstated) assumption, resulting in conflicts and inadequate communication from the point of view of both the oncologist and the family physician. The best approach to avoiding these difficulties is to address at the outset the questions of whether there is a team at work and, if so, how communication and decision making will be handled. Unfortunately, it is common for physicians and other clinicians not to be conversant with teamwork concepts, and so addressing these questions is often difficult.

At times, a team will change from using its customary decision-making method to using a different method. A team that ordinarily uses consensus will sometimes need to switch to requiring unanimous agreement. This change is appropriate when ill effects or high risk for some team members will result from one or more of the choices being considered. In the vignette about Riverside Heart, Dr. Lawrence was attempting to guide the team in its method for decision making although he did not succeed very well. The team often used voting with plurality rule for making decisions. As the voting progressed, he changed the basis for decision making from plurality rule to majority rule. Most likely the team would have fared better using consensus.

An interesting historical example of a shift from the extreme of decision by central authority to the opposite extreme of decision by unanimous agreement occurred when Hernán Cortés and his captains considered whether to burn their ships on the east coast of Mexico when beginning the conquest of the Aztec Empire in 1519. Burning the ships eliminated retreat as an option for Cortés' army, thus spurring on the soldiers. On the other hand, the risk for everyone in the group rose dramatically. Cortés was accustomed to making decisions on the strength of his own authority, with or without conferring with trusted captains. In addressing the question of burning the ships, however, he used his authority to pass the decision entirely to his captains (Díaz, 1963, p. 130). This action was suitable under the circumstances and provided a brilliant means for securing the support of his captains for burning the ships. Of course, he took the risk that they might have decided not to burn the ships.

The method used for making decisions in a healthcare team often is based either on expectations generated through professional acculturation during training or on long-established precedent in a given team. Physicians usually make decisions in groups of their peers by consensus or by voting because the culture of physicians is individualistic and egalitarian. Nurses working in hospitals or other institutions commonly make decisions by central authority but only after consultation within the team. The culture of nursing is both hierarchical and collegial. Healthcare administrative teams usually seek consensus but are prepared to use central authority if consensus cannot be achieved swiftly. The culture of healthcare administration is hierarchical. Regardless of the effects of professional culture, the method used in any particular team almost always varies in response to the nature of the issue to be decided and the context.

One of the responsibilities of the leader is to attend to how decisions are being made and to assess whether the method used for a particular decision meets the team's needs for reaching its goal and for development and maintenance of the team's capacity to function well over time. If leaders have strong authority, they can alter the method of decision making as they see fit as in the case of Cortés and his captains. Similarly, Dr. Lawrence at Riverside Heart Clinic, while not an autocrat, also had sufficient standing in the group to be able to specify how the decision about vacation scheduling would be made. However, if a team is long accustomed to decision making by consensus, ordinarily a switch to the use of strong central authority or to voting cannot simply be stipulated by the leader. In effect, the leader will need to seek broad approval from the group for the change. In these cases, the leader will usually propose the switch and then watch to see whether there are objections, rarely explicitly seeking formal action to confirm the switch that is proposed. Changing from consensus decision making to the use of unanimous agreement is more easily achieved because the methods are similar.

DECISION-MAKING PITFALLS AND THEIR SOLUTIONS

Some pitfalls in group decision making are discussed in Chapter 6 under the more general heading *Hazards for Teams*. In that chapter, suppression of dissent and novel

Table 9–2. Pitfalls in team decision making

Allowing personality factors, status, or hierarchy to interfere with deliberation
Production blocking
Hidden profile
Group polarization
Defensive routines
Groupthink

ideas is discussed as well as reaching consensus prematurely, for example, because of the overwhelming influence of one person in the group. In this chapter, we consider additional pitfalls for teams making decisions. A list of pitfalls is shown in Table 9–2.

Allowing Personality Factors, Status, or Hierarchy to Interfere with Deliberation

The Adult Medicine Department at Marina Medical Clinic was having its monthly lunchtime meeting. The department consisted of 10 internists and 5 NPs. The meetings always began with discussion of an interesting clinical case and then proceeded to consideration of operational issues. By 12:20 p.m. the clinical discussion had ended. At that point, Bernadette Morin, DO, the department chair, turned to the list of 3 operational issues that had been circulated by e-mail the day before. She asked whether anyone had any additional issues to consider. Mary Snyder, NP, who had been with the group for 2 years, said that she would like the group to consider whether it should stop using pharmaceutical samples provided by drug company representatives for distribution to patients. Dr. Morin responded by saying that she thought this issue was more important than the ones already on the agenda and should be considered first. Several physicians and NPs spoke up in favor of Ms. Snyder's proposal that the department stop distributing medications from the "drug sample cabinet." They cited the risks of providing the wrong drug, hurried and incomplete patient education about the drugs, and other potential problems. Three internists raised doubts about the proposal, saying that distributing samples was very convenient for some patients. Daryl Teasdale, MD, an internist who had been with the group for 18 years, spoke up in opposition to the proposal. He was highly regarded in the department as an excellent clinician. He said that providing drug samples for seniors was convenient for them and saved them money. He spoke loudly and derisively about the comments that had been made by Ms. Snyder and a young internist who had supported the proposal. Dr. Teasdale continued by saying that Ms. Snyder and the internist were typical of younger practitioners who favored using bureaucratic rules instead of relying on physicians and nurses to use their professional judgment. It was clear that he was angry. By the time Dr. Teasdale spoke, the hour allotted for the meeting was almost over. Dr. Morin brought the discussion to a close by saying that the group would need to return to the issue at some later time. They did not return to the issue for 9 months.

The decision being addressed by Marina Adult Medicine was whether to stop distributing drug samples provided by pharmaceutical company sales people. The deliberation was derailed by one person, Dr. Teasdale. His ability to end the discussion was based on his personality and his status in the group. He was most likely someone whom Dr. Morin would call a "difficult person" if she were candid. Dr. Teasdale's primary tactic was a personal attack on younger practitioners who wanted to change a policy that he wanted to preserve. His position was probably also strengthened by his gender, and perhaps by his age. Strictly speaking he did not have any positional authority, that is, no senior place in any organizational structure. However, his longevity with the Clinic and his prestige as an excellent clinician gave him authority similar to or greater than the department chair, Dr. Morin.

Team decision making is sometimes distorted by factors of personality, status, hierarchy, and customary obedience to authority. These distortions present substantial challenges to team leaders and other team members. Sometimes they cannot be overcome. In this case, Dr. Morin could have counterbalanced Dr. Teasdale's manner and insult by eliciting responses from other members of the team to the reasons that Dr. Teasdale stated for opposing the proposal—not responses to his irrelevant personal remarks and tone. But time ran out. She could have approached him privately sometime after the meeting to confront him about being derogatory and demeaning, thereby preparing the way for rediscussion of the topic at next month's meeting. She did not confront him; she withdrew. She could have enlisted another internist of similar standing in the group to talk with Dr. Teasdale. She could have asked the medical director of the medical group to join her in serving notice to Dr. Teasdale that his manner needed to change. The approach to managing the behavior of people like Dr. Teasdale is necessarily personal. It is difficult, and there are no recipes. It requires courage and some ingenuity. Early action is preferable to waiting. Once a pattern of abusive behavior has been tacitly approved by being accepted, the pattern commonly becomes extremely difficult to change. The handling of difficult team members is further discussed in Chapter 17.

Production Blocking

Team decision making can also be inhibited by a phenomenon known as *production blocking*, which is considered briefly in Chapter 1 (Diehl and Stroebe, 1987). As team members discuss the decision to be made, they are both generating new ideas and listening to the other team members. Nascent ideas need some time to be developed to point that they can be expressed coherently. The silent development often takes no more than a few seconds, but it is not instantaneous. During the give-and-take of group discussion, some of the nascent ideas are voiced to the group but others never reach this point because team members cannot formulate their new ideas well enough to be able to state them. In other words, listening interferes with the generation of new thoughts. In addition, some embryonic thoughts are simply forgotten as team members await their turns to speak. This problem can be overcome by certain formal procedures that are presented in Chapter 10. The purpose of these procedures is to provide time for individuals to formulate new ideas.

Hidden Profile

The quality of decision making in teams is sometimes degraded by what is called the *hidden profile* phenomenon (Thompson, 2011, pp. 130-131). In face-to-face group decision making, more attention is paid to information that is already widely shared in the group prior to the group beginning its discussion. Suppose that one or two people know of the superior characteristics of one possible solution to the problem at hand but the rest of the group does not have this knowledge before the group starts its discussion. For example, suppose that an interprofessional team is considering treatment options for an elderly patient with Parkinson's disease and mild cognitive impairment. The speech pathologist and occupational therapist know that one well-done study has shown that certain cognitive exercises improve cognitive performance in patients with Parkinson's disease (París et al, 2011). The nurse, physician, and other members of the team do not know about this option until they are told by the speech pathologist. In other words, the "profile" of this possible treatment—that is, the description of the treatment and its effects—is hidden from most of the group until the speech pathologist reveals it. Under these circumstances, the option with the hidden profile is likely to be neglected or regarded as not meriting serious consideration. The hidden profile phenomenon has been shown to interfere with making correct diagnoses in an experimental setting involving medical students, interns, and residents working in teams of 3 members. Diagnostic information possessed by only one of the team members and reported to the other 2 tended to be ignored by the other 2, leading to incorrect diagnoses in many of the teams (Christensen et al, 2000).

The solution to the hidden profile problem is, ideally, to share the hidden information with everyone prior to the group's discussion. If this is not possible, then the chair of the meeting has the burden of directing the group's attention to information newly shared by someone in the group. The chair must also depersonalize the discussion so that it is not perceived as a competition among team members to outshine one another with new information but instead is regarded as an opportunity to solve a problem.

Group Polarization

Group polarization is another pitfall for teams making decisions. Groups tend to make decisions that are more extreme than those that would be made by the group's members if they were making the decisions alone (Main and Walker, 1973). Group discussion often intensifies the viewpoints of individuals, causing a shift either toward taking more risk or toward exercising more caution. These effects can be very difficult to combat, and sometimes the group is not even aware of the effect of discussion on the views of individual team members. In healthcare settings, the effects can be quite dangerous. For example, pharmacists individually inclined to use a moderately high dose of an antibiotic in a patient at risk for the drug's side effects may find that their inclinations to downplay risk are reinforced in a group discussion and that they finish the discussion deciding to use an even higher dose. There is no reliable means to prevent group polarization except for the team members (especially the leader) to be aware of the phenomenon and to revisit any decision that seems extreme to anyone on the team, that is, to review systematically the considerations for and against the decision.

Defensive Routines

Many teams also have *defensive routines* that interfere with making decisions to solve problems and innovate (Argyris, 1990). Defensive routines are habits of thought and discussion that serve to protect the self-esteem of team members and the status quo in a team or organization. For example, surgeons and nurses confronted with the continuing occurrence of postoperative infections may respond by saying that the rate of postoperative infections can never be reduced to zero. This response protects the team's sense that it is providing good surgical care and provides a rationale for not having to do the hard work of reducing the infection rate. A particularly common defensive routine is one that assigns blame for a problem to some other team or to unalterable circumstances. For example, primary care practitioners may blame specialists for long waiting times experienced by patients who need to see the specialists. At the same time, the specialists may blame the primary care providers for the long waiting times, saying that the primary providers refer patients who do not need specialty care and send inadequate information so that care of the patients takes more time. Defensive routines are difficult to overcome, sometimes even difficult to recognize, because the arguments offered seem so well founded and are so familiar. Teams can avoid this pitfall by continually asking *what* is going wrong rather than *who* is wrong and by seeking to learn more about the causes of difficulties even if the difficulties appear unsolvable at first. Also, repeated uses of the same reason for not taking action should alert leaders and other team members to the possibility that a defensive routine is blocking improvement.

Groupthink

A particularly interesting roadblock to good decision making is called *groupthink*. Sometimes this word is used loosely to refer to any instance of similar thinking in a team, regardless of the cause. Homogeneous thinking in a team can occur for any number of reasons, including dominance of the team by one dictatorial person, lack of educational or other diversity among the team members, and so on. In a narrower and more useful sense, *groupthink* refers to agreement that occurs because the team values consensus more highly than it values coming to a good decision (West, 2012, pp. 128, 136-138). The original case study of groupthink by Irving Janis focused on President John Kennedy and a set of senior White House officials as they dealt with American support for the 1961 Bay of Pigs Invasion in Cuba (Janis, 1972). President Kennedy's team made a series of disastrous decisions that flew in the face of strong evidence that the anti-Castro invasion would fail and would harm American foreign relations. The invasion failed, and many lives were lost. Janis attributed the team's poor decisions to a barely recognized desire on the part of President Kennedy's inner circle to maintain a mindset of tight-knit unanimity, regardless of what decisions they made. Since Janis's study, many other studies have investigated groupthink occurring in other settings (Thompson, 2011, pp. 157-165). Several factors can contribute to the phenomenon. The risk factors that seem to be most relevant to its occurrence in healthcare settings are time pressure, exaggerated loyalty to a decisive leader, intentional rejection of information and viewpoints coming from outside of the team, fear that conflicts will develop within the team, and a sense of vulnerability to criticism by people outside of the team. Both management teams and clinical teams are at risk for groupthink.

The key to avoiding groupthink is recognizing that the team is at high risk because of the presence of one or more of the risk factors. Once the problem is recognized, the team leader and other team members need to adopt strategies that have been identified to combat groupthink, for example, keeping the team small, inviting presentation of disparate viewpoints, and appointing a devil's advocate to challenge the team's emerging decisions (Thompson, 2011, pp. 161-165).

ADDITIONAL METHODS FOR IMPROVING TEAM DECISION MAKING

Each of the pitfalls discussed in the previous section has its corresponding solutions, permitting the pitfalls to be overcome so that good decisions can be made—although some of the pitfalls are stubbornly persistent. In addition to these solutions, there are several other

Table 9–3. Additional methods for improving team decision making

Using evidence
Constructive controversy
Devil's advocacy
Encouragement of minority viewpoints
Negative brainstorming

techniques available to increase the likelihood that decisions will serve the team well in achieving its goals and will stand the test of time. These additional techniques are listed in Table 9–3.

Using Evidence

As discussed in Chapters 6 and 7, effective teams and team members use scientific evidence in decision making when evidence is available. In clinical decision making, interest in the use of evidence dates from at least 1972, when A. L. Cochrane published *Effectiveness and Efficiency* (1972), explaining and advocating the use of randomized, controlled trials to determine the value of treatments and other clinical interventions. This interest evolved into an approach to medical practice called *evidence-based medicine* (Straus et al, 2011), which has been generalized to evidence-based nursing (Dicenso et al, 2005), evidence-based health care (Gray, 2001), and evidence-based clinical practice in general. More recently the methods of evidence-based practice have been advocated for management (Kovner et al, 2009) although at this time the amount of evidence available for making leadership or management decisions is small.

Discussion of the development and methods of evidence-based practice is beyond the scope of this book. The subject is intertwined with the development of chronic disease epidemiology and statistical methods over the past 60 years, and it is highly technical.

In any case, evidence from systematic observations in scientific studies should be used whenever it is available for making decisions in any clinical field. Evidence provides a guide to clinical practice as well as common ground for clinicians in different professions. In addition to randomized, controlled trials, studies with several other research designs are used to gather evidence, and the strength of evidence provided by various designs differs. Clinicians sometimes disagree about whether adequate evidence exists to support the use of a given drug treatment, nursing procedure, diagnostic test, or other healthcare intervention. And sometimes there is disagreement about whether certain kinds of information count as evidence at all, for example, case reports about new treatments. Of course, sometimes there are no research findings available to answer a particular question. In those situations (which are common), clinicians must use the best evidence available. This evidence may be as weak as the experience of practitioners who have often dealt with the clinical issue at hand. As the years pass, research findings accumulate, and expert testimony is superseded by solid scientific observation.

When evidence is available on management questions (and it frequently is not), it should also be used. In the management arena, there is even more disagreement about the kind of information that counts as evidence and whether the available evidence is sufficient to answer questions such as what action would be best to take in specific circumstances.

Constructive Controversy

Sturges Health Care, a large, urban integrated healthcare system, was engaged in a review of its business strategy for the coming 3-5 years. The organization was located in a city of 1.5 million people. The care delivery system included 1 hospital, located in the south of the city, 12 clinics, and 425 employed physicians, NPs, and midwives.

Another integrated system, Marquette Health System, located in the northwest portion of the city, was a strong competitor. Sturges had established 2 clinics in this quadrant of the city, but they were not attracting many patients. Moreover, the patients seen at these 2 clinics were frequently resistant to using the Sturges hospital in the southern part of the city. They usually wanted to be hospitalized at Marquette's hospital, which was located in the northwest quadrant of the city, closer to Sturges' 2 clinics and closer to the homes of most of the patients using those clinics.

The discussions of the Strategy Task Force were led by Sturges' CEO. The participants were the executives who reported directly to the CEO plus 5 others who had special knowledge of the marketplace or who were especially prominent in the organization, including 2 highly influential clinicians who did not have management positions.

After 2 meetings of the Task Force, 3 principal options were identified: (1) redouble efforts to recruit patients for the 2 clinics in the northwest quadrant of the city and continue to use only the Sturges hospital, (2) continue to recruit patients for the 2 northwest quadrant clinics and contract with another hospital in that area (but not Marquette's hospital), to be used for patients not wishing to travel to the Sturges hospital, and (3) decrease the size of the 2 clinics in accordance with the numbers of patients using them—even to the point of closing them—and use only the Sturges hospital, abandoning the northwest quadrant to the competitor, Marquette, and concentrating instead on increasing market share throughout the rest of the city.

There were 13 people on the Task Force. The CEO formed 3 sub-groups of 4-5 people, one sub-group for each of the 3 options. Each sub-group was asked to build the case for the option assigned to it. At the same time, each sub-group was assigned a second option to critique. The sub-groups each met separately twice, and the whole Task Force then met to hear presentations for and against each of the 3 options. At that point, there was general agreement to eliminate option 1. The CEO then formed another small group to explore whether elements of options 2 and 3 might be combined to form an even more promising strategy. Eventually, the Task Force reached consensus on a variant of option 3.

This leadership team used a decision-making method known as *constructive controversy* (Tjosvold, 1998). The hallmark of this method is that discussion of options is deliberately designed to cover all the known options, to focus on the issues rather than on personal rivalries or competition among the participants, and to strongly encourage consensus formation. This method seeks to avoid uneven consideration of options and to construct creative choices that combine the best elements of multiple possibilities.

Devil's Advocacy

Another technique for increasing the likelihood that options will be evaluated critically is the appointment of a *devil's advocate* to critique either a particular point of view or all points of view on a specified topic. The devil's advocate is not expected actually to believe that the view she or he opposes is unsound. The expected negative advocacy is artificial but thorough and explicit. This technique can be used in management teams as well as clinical teams that are planning the management of complex disease problems requiring several modalities of treatment. However, it is not advisable to appoint someone as the regular devil's advocate for all matters considered by a given team. In this situation, the comments of the devil's advocate tend over time to be discounted as the other team members come to see the advocate as simply playing a role without any conviction (West, 2012, p. 145). An alternative to appointing a particular devil's advocate for a given viewpoint or topic is to encourage all team members to serve as devil's advocates whenever they see a disadvantage to any particular option being considered. This approach encourages more critical thinking and provides a conversational mode that enables team members to offer criticisms with little risk of personal attack. If someone begins his or her comments by saying "Let me be devil's advocate for a moment," he or she is serving notice that the criticism offered is not necessarily one that the speaker believes. In addition to decreasing risk for the critics, this approach permits team members to voice criticisms in a way that avoids the backlash that might be provoked if the criticisms were perceived as personal attacks on team members with opposing views.

Encouragement of Minority Viewpoints

An especially useful habit for team leaders to cultivate is *encouragement of minority viewpoints.* Many of the roadblocks to good decision making occur because team members with unique pieces of information or unique insights do not speak up or speak with little conviction. This problem occurs with suppression of novel ideas by fear, with the hidden profile phenomenon, and sometimes with groupthink. Effective meeting chairpersons, whether team leaders or other team members serving as chairs, should be always mindful of minority viewpoints and attentive to signs—often present in facial expressions or body posture—that someone in the team has a minority viewpoint that she or he is reluctant to express. Sometimes it is appropriate for the chair to note the clues to an unvoiced viewpoint and then to follow up after the meeting in a setting where the person who did not speak up will be more comfortable discussing his or her views. Repeatedly encouraging reluctant team members to voice their views will foster creativity in the whole team and avoid rushes to premature decision making.

Negative Brainstorming

Finally, *negative brainstorming* is a procedure for providing a final check on the quality of a particular decision. The procedure calls for the team, having tentatively selected an option for action, to engage in formal brainstorming to surface as many reasons as possible for *not* taking this course of action, including unintended, undesirable effects that might result from the action. The exercise is entirely hypothetical, that is, team members are not expected to limit their objections to ones that they regard as sound. Instead, they are expected to present any and all drawbacks that they can imagine. The list of potential objections to the contemplated action is then discussed in the team in order to reach an agreement about whether any of the objections are sufficiently substantial to warrant modifying or dropping the team's choice. Negative brainstorming is also discussed in Chapter 10 on creativity.

CONCLUSION

Many decisions in healthcare teams are appropriately made by individuals without any reference to other members of the team. These decisions are not team decisions. The purpose of this chapter is to explain team decision making, that is, decision making by the whole team or a portion of the team. Clinical decisions are made by clinical teams. Management decisions are made by management teams and by clinical teams functioning as management teams.

There are 4 basic methods for making decisions in teams: (1) decision by strong central authority, (2) voting, (3) unanimous agreement, and (4) consensus. Some of these methods include sub-types, for example, voting includes plurality rule and majority rule. The difference between unanimous agreement and consensus is that unanimous agreement requires positive affirmation of the decision by everyone on the team while consensus requires only that everyone on the team accepts the decision even if they do not agree with it.

Team decision making is subject to several pitfalls, for example, distortions caused by personality characteristics and by status differences within the team. Several well-studied group psychological phenomena can interfere with decision making, including the hidden profile phenomenon, group polarization, and groupthink. Most of these problems have effective solutions although some can be very difficult to detect or correct.

Beyond the solutions for common pitfalls, there are several other methods available to optimize team decision making. These methods include using evidence, constructive controversy, devil's advocacy, encouragement of minority viewpoints, and negative brainstorming.

Having covered this important topic for team leaders as well as other team members, we are ready to move on to a second particularly important component of leadership, namely, fostering creativity within the team.

REFERENCES

Alfaro-Lefevre R. *Critical Thinking, Clinical Reasoning, and Clinical Judgment: A Practical Approach.* 5th ed. St. Louis, MO: Elsevier Saunders; 2013.

Argyris C. *Overcoming Organizational Defenses: Facilitating Organizational Learning.* Boston, MA: Allyn and Bacon; 1990.

Christensen C, Larson JR, Abbott A, et al. Decision making of clinical teams: communication patterns and diagnostic error. *Med Decis Making.* 2000;20:45-50.

Cochrane AL. *Effectiveness and Efficiency: Random Reflections on Health Services.* London, UK: The Nuffield Provincial Hospitals Trust; 1972.

Díaz B. *The Conquest of New Spain.* Baltimore, MD: Penguin Books; 1963.

Dicenso A, Guyatt G, Ciliska D. *Evidence-Based Nursing: A Guide to Clinical Practice.* St. Louis, MO: Mosby, Inc.; 2005.

Diehl M, Stroebe W. Productivity loss in brainstorming groups: toward the solution of a riddle. *J Pers Social Psychol.* 1987;53:497-509.

Gray JAM. *Evidence-Based Healthcare: How to Make Health Policy and Management Decisions.* 2nd ed. Edinburgh, UK: Churchill Livingstone; 2001.

Groopman J. *How Doctors Think.* New York, NY: Houghton Mifflin Company; 2007.

Hastie R, Kameda T. The robust beauty of majority rules in group decisions. *Psychol Rev.* 2005;112:494-508.

Janis IL. *Victims of Groupthink.* Boston, MA: Houghton Mifflin Company; 1972.

Kassirer JP, Wong J, Kopelman R. *Learning Clinical Reasoning.* Baltimore, MD: Lippincott Williams & Wilkins; 2010.

Kovner AR, Fine DJ, D'Aquila R. *Evidence-Based Management in Health Care.* Chicago, IL: Health Administration Press; 2009.

Main EC, Walker TG. Choice shifts and extreme behavior: judicial review in the federal courts. *J Soc Psychol.* 1973;91:215-221.

París AP, Saleta HG, de la Cruz Crespo Maraver M, et al. Blind randomized controlled study of the efficacy of cognitive training in Parkinson's disease. *Mov Disord.* 2011;26: 1251-1258.

Straus SE, Richardson WS, Glasziou P, et al. *Evidence-Based Medicine: How to Practice and Teach It.* 4th ed. Edinburgh, UK: Churchill Livingstone; 2011.

Thompson LL. *Making the Team: A Guide for Managers.* 4th ed. Upper Saddle River, NJ: Prentice Hall; 2011.

Tjosvold D. Cooperative and competitive goal approach to conflict: accomplishments and challenges. *Appl Psychol.* 1998;47:285-342.

Tjosvold D, Feld RHG. Effects of social context on consensus and majority decision making. *Acad Manage J.* 1983;26:500-506.

West MA. *Effective Teamwork: Practical Lessons from Organizational Research.* 3rd ed. Chichester, UK: John Wiley & Sons, Ltd.; 2012.

Fostering Creativity in Healthcare Teams

Chapters 9-11 deal with key processes in healthcare teamwork. These processes are important for all team members, but they have special importance for the team leader, who guides their development in the team. Chapter 9 covers decision making. This chapter examines the process of fostering creativity in teams. Chapter 11 deals with managing conflicts.

Creativity is the generation of novel ideas, plans, and solutions to problems. A related concept, innovation, commonly is used to refer to the application of creativity in the form of a new product or service. With some exceptions (Mitchell et al, 2012, p. 5), creativity typically is not listed as a required characteristic for teams and members of teams in interprofessional team care (Canadian Interprofessional Health Collaborative, 2010; Interprofessional Education Collaborative Expert Panel, 2011). This is problematic, given that creativity can add value to almost every healthcare team. Exceptions might include template teams, where members count on each other to fill predefined roles reliably without deviation, and time does not permit the team to devise new creative approaches to their work. But even in template teams, responses to surprises, mistakes, and unpredicted challenges require a degree of creativity. Also, template teams are often composed of professionals drawn from a pool such as the pool of nurses and technicians in a surgical suite. These pools can be organized to do creative work.

The need for creativity is particularly salient for problem-solving teams, including virtually all management project teams and leadership teams as well as clinical teams that wrestle with customized treatments provided to patients who differ in ways that affect their clinical needs. Quality improvement project teams, in particular, often are charged with devising creative ways to improve outcomes or save resources. For such teams, there is a strong argument that creativity should be a required competency.

Creativity in healthcare teams also can go far in avoiding some common team pitfalls, enumerated in Chapters 6 and 9. Premature consensus and groupthink, 2 common hazards, are less likely in creative environments. Another hazard for teams, fear that suppresses the expression of novel ideas, by definition is avoided in teams that encourage creativity.

Creativity is a mysterious capability, to some degree. However, scholars of innovation and creativity have introduced several useful concepts that sharpen awareness of relevant team processes so that team structure, culture, and processes can be shaped to be more supportive of creativity. In addition, there is a wide range of formal tools for helping to generate team creativity. These concepts and tools are covered in this chapter.

FOUNDATIONAL ISSUES AND CONCEPTS

Shawn Jackson, MSN, PNP, a pediatric nurse practitioner, was particularly excited about Wednesday's quality improvement project team meeting. Mr. Jackson worked in a clinic closely associated with a community hospital.

The goal of the quality improvement team was to devise a new approach to patient education (and family education) for adolescents with type 1 diabetes, with the ultimate aim of improving blood sugar control among adolescent diabetic patients in the clinic. The team members were Jerry Pierce, MD (who served as chair),

Mr. Jackson, Anna Zasky, MSN, PNP (another nurse practitioner), a health educator from the hospital's Patient Education Center, a pediatric nurse, and the mother of an adolescent patient with diabetes. (The team was seeking an adolescent diabetic patient to participate but so far had not found a patient who was willing to join.)

Mr. Jackson was very interested in diabetic education for adolescent patients. He had read widely on the topic, and he subscribed to several e-mail exchanges and blogs in which new developments in the field were discussed. He was particularly interested in the rapidly growing field of self-management education for teenagers with diabetes and other chronic diseases. Self-management education enables diabetic patients to adjust their daily insulin doses, levels of exercise, and diets in accordance with their own observations and judgment.

As the team meeting began, Ms. Zasky got right to the point. She said that she had reviewed the educational materials available from 4 diabetic education programs that had strong national reputations. The materials from Martin Drew Diabetes Center in California, she said, were superb. She reported that the materials were innovative, visually pleasing, and well tailored to teenagers. For several years, Ms. Zasky had been the informal leader of the clinic's diabetes education activities. She was confident of her knowledge and skill in this arena, and in fact she had enabled the clinic to provide far better diabetes education than it had ever provided before. In speaking of the materials from the Martin Drew Center, she said that she hoped the team would approve the use of these materials because they were the best in the country. Continuing the use of the clinic's current materials, she said, would mark the clinic as out-of-date.

Dr. Pierce said that he also had reviewed the Martin Drew materials and that he strongly supported Ms. Zasky's proposal. He invited other comments on the proposal.

Mr. Jackson was familiar with the Martin Drew Center, which ran a conventional diabetes education program, providing patients with information and technical skills such as finger-stick blood glucose testing and administration of insulin by injection. The program had no component of self-management education. Mr. Jackson had no doubt that the teaching materials from Martin Drew were excellent. However, the overall education program at Martin Drew was not innovative. Mr. Jackson would have liked the team to consider a more cutting-edge approach to diabetes education, but he said nothing.

Team versus Individual Creativity

Team creativity is different than individual creativity. For example, a team of creative individuals may not be a creative team if individual creativity is stifled by nonsupportive decision making and problem-solving processes. The same point applies to creative team leaders: having a creative leader does not ensure a creative team, unless the leader implements processes that support team creativity. The preceding vignette illustrates the quandary of many creative individuals in teamwork settings. Mr. Jackson's individual creativity was stifled by team processes that did not invite participation and the widespread sharing of ideas. Team leader Dr. Pierce pre-empted creative suggestions by announcing that he strongly supported Ms. Zasky's preference for one option. Dr. Pierce actually may be a quite creative person, but, even if he is, his creativity was not enough to elicit a high level of team creativity.

Teams that would benefit from greater creativity should strive to improve creativity in both individual members and in team processes. In one study of hospital leadership teams, researchers found that both innovative individuals and innovative team processes predicted the overall level of innovation on the team, reporting that the *quality* of the innovation (radicalness, magnitude, and novelty) is more related to individual member characteristics, while the overall *level* of innovation is more related to team processes, such as participation and commitment to team goals (West and Anderson, 1996). Both individual and team-level creativity are important. A team with processes that are "creative-friendly" still depends on individuals to come up with the ideas that then are processed by the team. And, as the introductory vignette illustrates, teams with creative individuals need support through appropriate leadership, team processes, and norms.

Potential for Creativity in Individuals and Teams

All individuals (and teams) have the potential to be creative and innovative. Novel and useful ideas are not the purview of a select few individuals or teams. This recognition is important in stimulating creativity, since many individuals label themselves as noncreative and behave in accordance with that self-fulfilling prophecy. Some observers go so far as to suggest that there is only one major difference between people who exhibit creative tendencies and those who do not: people with creative behaviors regard themselves as creative (Quinn et al, 2011, p. 289).

There are some personality traits that make creative thinking more likely or more natural. For example, the personality trait of openness has been linked to creativity (King et al, 1996). Openness is an indicator of imagination, originality, aesthetic sensitivity, attentiveness to inner feelings, preference for variety, and intellectual curiosity (McCrae and John, 1992). But regardless of personality, behaviors that enhance creativity can be stimulated, learned, and increased. Among those individual behaviors are questioning, observing others, experimenting, and networking. All of these behaviors encourage individuals to stretch their minds and make connections across seemingly unrelated questions, problems, or ideas. Associations across seemingly unrelated ideas are the basis of creativity (Dyer et al, 2009). Other experts urge individuals to develop outward interests, to diversify their searches for solutions to problems, to practice creativity, and to be adaptable—willing to drop their preset ideas and engage new ones (Boynton et al, 2011). Again, the point is that creativity is a competence that can be learned by individuals. Individual creativity requires hard work and a strong knowledge base; it does not happen by luck or chance. The empirical evidence on creative achievement concludes that individuals have not been able to make generally recognized creative contributions to a domain unless they have mastered the relevant knowledge and skills in the course of a long preparatory period (Ericsson and Lehmann, 1999, p. 706).

Creative Realism

There is rarely, if ever, a need for teams to pursue creativity just for the sake of it. Novelty that derives from nonconformity, lack of discipline, blind rejection of what already exists, and simply letting oneself go has been referred to as *pseudocreativity* or *quasicreativity* (Cropley, 2006, p. 392). As noted earlier, creativity is linked to innovation, where innovations are the implementation of creativity in the form of useful new products or services. Creative individuals and teams may generate hundreds of ideas to solve a problem, while only one (or none) may emerge as an innovation. Most organizations establish boundaries on the performance-enhancing expression of creativity—sometimes overtly and sometimes by implication. Without those boundaries, creativity can be a burden rather than a value-add to team performance. If ideas are completely unconnected to current realities and knowledge, they are not implementable. Thompson (2003, p. 97) and others describe the optimal level of creativity as *creative realism*. Teams should strive for creativity that generates original but realistic ideas. In contrast, *creative idealism* is the generation of highly original but highly unrealistic ideas.

Types of Thinking

Three contrasts in the way that people and groups of people process information are useful in understanding the nature of creativity: critical versus creative thinking, divergent versus convergent thinking, and exploration versus exploitation.

Critical versus Creative Thinking

Critical thinking is the cognitive search for one answer to a problem through logical thinking and mathematical processes. It traditionally is emphasized in Western cultures, and it anchors most of the sciences that underlie the healthcare disciplines. Creative thinking begins with the same one problem, but generates numerous possible solutions (de Bono, 1970).

Most healthcare professionals exhibit strong critical thinking ability. They are rewarded in the extensive educational process of their professions largely for critical rather than creative thinking.

Problem solving by teams requires both creative and critical thinking, and creative thinking tends to be underemphasized. In healthcare interprofessional teams, creative thinking often needs to be expanded relative to critical thinking.

Convergent versus Divergent Thinking

The contrast between convergent and divergent thinking conveys similar messages. Convergent thinking means narrowing down alternatives quickly and logically, in the search for one right answer or solution (Cropley, 2006). It assumes that there is one right answer or solution. Convergent thinking leads to a single-best answer, with no or little ambiguity.

Divergent thinking involves producing multiple or alternative answers. It requires making unexpected combinations, recognizing links among remote ideas and themes, and transforming information into unexpected forms. Convergent thinking generates orthodoxy, while divergent thinking generates variability (Cropley, 2006).

Researchers have found that individuals are better than teams at divergent thinking, while teams are better than individuals at convergent thinking. The finding is counterintuitive to many individuals (Thompson, 2003). Teams do less well at divergent thinking because of the social pressures for conformity—members want to be approved of by other members. Individuals are more removed from the pressure to conform when they are left alone. Therefore, a collection of separate individuals can generate a larger quantity of creative ideas than a team of the same individuals. (In addition, several other social processes detract from the team's productivity on the creativity dimension, as discussed below in relation to brainstorming.) Teams do better at convergent thinking than individuals, however, because more minds are focused on the search and logic required to find an answer.

Experts argue that teams need both divergent and convergent thinking—typically sequenced with divergent thinking first, followed by convergent thinking. Convergent thinking is required to make the ideas generated by divergent thinking more fact based and reality based. Convergent thinking helps teams recognize promising solutions, see limits, be aware of weaknesses, and weigh feasibility of ideas.

Exploration versus Exploitation

Exploration versus exploitation provides another useful dichotomy in thinking about individual and team creativity. Exploration involves searching for new possibilities through experimentation, discovery, and innovation. Exploitation involves refining and extending existing products and services. Exploration, then, requires more creativity.

Organizational scientist James March noted that in general organizations have a tendency to focus on the exploitation of known alternatives rather than the exploration of unknown ones. Such organizations increase the reliability of organizational performance more than the average level of performance (March, 1991, p. 85). Organizations that focus too much on exploitation are likely to find themselves "trapped in suboptimal stable equilibria" (March, 1991, p. 71). The equilibria are suboptimal if the environment of the organization (for example, its customer base, technologies, or competition) is changing in ways that require the organization to produce different goods and services rather than becoming more reliable at producing existing goods and services. The dilemma can be summarized as the need to balance short-term efficiency with long-term effectiveness in a changing environment.

Like organizations, many teams focus on exploitation because its returns are positive, proximate, and predictable, while exploration is risky and its returns often are negative. Consider the trend toward patient-centered care over the past 2 decades or so. Healthcare organizations and teams face decisions about whether to continue doing business as usual or to introduce innovations such as e-mail communication with patients. Exploration of the new space of patient-centered care creates team learning, both positive and negative. In settings where competition and technology and patient expectations are driving the shift to patient-centered care, such learning through exploration is critical to the long-term success of healthcare organizations and teams. One interesting implication of the tendency to exploit rather than explore, noted by March (1991, p. 86), is that rapid socialization of new members may hurt the team, as the development of knowledge may depend on maintaining an influx of the naïve and ignorant. For purposes of team learning, relatively slow socialization of new members, as well as moderate turnover in membership, is preferred.

In summary, there are arguments for improving exploration, divergent thinking, and creative thinking in virtually all teams. All are paths to improved creativity. Yet too much exploration, divergent thinking, and creative thinking has dangers of its own, so a balance must be maintained.

There are specific practices that teams can employ to improve creativity in their work. We classify these into: (1) practices that embed creativity in team culture, and (2) tools that improve team creativity.

BUILDING A TEAM CULTURE OF CREATIVITY

Elk Valley Rehabilitation Hospital is a leader in its region on measures of quality and service. That was not always the case, as the hospital drastically improved patient satisfaction and recovery times (following mistakes or errors) over the past decade.

The Quality Council of the hospital was a major reason for the hospital's improvement in quality outcomes. The Council had originated and driven the idea of team-based care, for example. Not all of the Council's ideas worked, but several of them, like team-based care, did.

Meetings of the Quality Council were fast-paced and engaging. The Council chair, physiatrist Gary Kopek, MD, really enjoyed pushing the envelope on innovation. He always brought a light bulb (encased in a plastic cube) to the meetings, as a symbol of his commitment to innovation.

Today the Council was welcoming new member Casey Wilhoit, MHA. Ms. Wilhoit was administrator of the facility's transitional care unit, which she had transformed from a drab and depressing wing with a demoralized staff into a national trend-setter. The Council had expanded its membership to make room for Ms. Wilhoit. Dr. Kopek welcomed her warmly, noting that "You were selected because you aren't afraid to try new ideas. We want you to keep that up, whether we use your ideas or not. We like to think we're a really creative bunch and that we're responsible for the excellent quality outcomes that Elk Valley has enjoyed. We work hard to learn what works and what doesn't work. If you don't find that to be the case, let us know. We need some new blood—we don't want to rest on our laurels."

Today's topic was "what can we learn from the turnaround of our transitional care unit." Ms. Wilhoit looked forward to sharing her learning and to contributing new ideas to other areas of Elk Valley Rehabilitation Hospital.

How does creativity become embedded in the culture—the way we do things around here—of a team, as it apparently was for the Elk Valley Rehabilitation Hospital Quality Council? Organizational psychologist Michael West (2012, p. 168) provides a series of concrete steps for teams, beginning with setting a goal of creativity and selecting the right mix of members. Subsequent steps test the seriousness of the commitment to creativity through the hard work of changing team processes and norms to support creativity. The steps are listed in Table 10–1, with some modification and supplementation.

Table 10–1. Steps to build a team culture of creativity

Specify realistic creativity as a team goal
- Creativity is not easy to achieve
- Creative ideas need to be realistic

Select for and encourage diversity
- Appoint members with diverse perspectives and creative styles
- In permanent teams, strive for moderate levels of turnover
- Slow down socialization of new members

Build support for creativity in team activities and processes
- Build participation as a team norm
- Exhibit a positive attitude toward problem solving
- Say "yes, and..." rather than "yes, but..."
- Review and reflect on processes

Increase the base of relevant knowledge
- Study best practices
- Find *positive deviants*

Challenge the team
- Publicize high-performance standards
- Prepare members to expect that ideas often will not be used or implemented

Stop working
- Balance exploitation, critical thinking, and convergent thinking with their opposites
- Use humor and fun
- Employ formal tools for building creativity

Source: Based on West MA. *Effective Teamwork: Practical Lessons from Organizational Research.* 3rd ed. Chichester, UK: John Wiley & Sons, Ltd.; 2012:168.

Specify Realistic Creativity as a Team Goal

Countering the self-fulfilling prophecy that "we are not creative" is as important at the team level as it is at the level of the individual member. Achieving creativity as a team characteristic requires a conscious commitment to creativity or innovation as a team goal as well as norms and policies to support creativity. Team leaders are particularly important in this step. It is also important to establish that creativity is not easy to achieve, and that creativity has boundaries—it has to be realistic. In the vignette above, Quality Council leader Dr. Kopek states the team's commitment to maintaining excellent quality outcomes and claims that the team is creative and works hard. He links the team's creativity to measurable outcomes, all consistent with achieving realistic creativity as a team outcome.

Select for and Encourage Diversity

Diversity of perspective is a key to creativity at the team level. Indeed, this is one reason that interprofessional care is effective—by definition, diverse perspectives populate any interprofessional team. At the stage of selecting team members, this is a crucial design issue for teams that need creativity in order to perform well. Research finds that teams with diverse members in terms of background and perspective outperform teams with homogeneous members when teams perform tasks requiring creative problem solving and innovation. They generate more arguments, apply more strategies, detect more novel solutions, and integrate multiple perspectives (Thompson, 2003, p. 102). The opportunity to appoint members with diverse perspectives and creative styles generally falls to team sponsors and leaders, although team leaders and team members can lobby for creativity as a criterion for new members as well. Team sponsors in organizations searching for innovation in clinical processes are well served by seeking more creative participants as team leaders and members. In the Quality Council vignette, team leader Dr. Kopek sought out new member Ms. Wilhoit because of her reputation for innovation.

Earlier we noted the argument that slower socialization of new members, and moderate levels of turnover, help reinforce creativity in teams. Thompson (2003, p. 105) refers to *cognitive arthritis* which develops in teams that stay together for a long time without any change in membership. Researchers have found a negative relationship between repeat collaboration and creativity (Thompson, 2011, p. 225). The more that team members do the same task together, the more routinized the team performance becomes. This explains why low turnover can make the performance of a team better in one way—its errors are fewer. Highly stable teams are likely to be more reliable in the performance of their regular tasks, but less creative. New members in a team shake up the routine. And when new members enter a team, they not only bring a new perspective. They also can motivate existing members to revisit their own ideas and behaviors. In the vignette, Dr. Kopek hopes that Ms. Wilhoit will add some new blood to the team, perhaps to counter the possibility of cognitive arthritis.

Build Support for Creativity in Team Activities and Processes

After creativity is set as a team goal and an appropriate mix of individuals is on the team, the work of sustaining creativity in team activities and processes begins. Participation as a team norm is particularly important to creativity. People who have influence, interact frequently, and share information are more likely to invest themselves in team outcomes and offer ideas for new and improved ways of working. Leaders who require that ideas flow through them (a hub-and-spoke communication model) may feel threatened if ideas come from others on the team. In such settings, members will learn to self-censor their ideas, creating a collusive pattern in which leaders solicit input but do not receive any (Dye and Garman, 2006, p. 178). Another barrier to full participation is the tendency of physicians or other professionals with higher relative power or status to dominate discussions, thus repressing others' contributions, as noted in Chapter 9.

Team members who are particularly creative may have little patience with helping other team members to understand how they arrived at their ideas. Creative members must recognize that as team members, they are responsible for bringing others along.

Support for creativity includes having a positive attitude toward problem solving. Creativity is fueled by the faith that solutions exist and can be discovered. An underlying current of optimism invites openness and participation. Challenges are viewed as opportunities for creative action rather than worries to resolve. This is related to the notion of psychological safety, mentioned in Chapter 6. It can be risky for team members to suggest new ways of working, and a nonthreatening and supportive environment is important.

One common mnemonic device for supporting participation and psychological safety is the practice of thinking or saying "yes, and..." rather than "yes, but..." when responding to the ideas of others. Teams can explicitly establish this practice as a norm in discussions that are in the idea-generation phase.

To fight routinization of team processes, review and reflection on team decision-making and problem-solving processes can be helpful. Having an outside facilitator observe meetings and monitor participation and encouragement can be useful for teams that find themselves stuck in a routine.

Improve the Base of Relevant Knowledge

As discussed above, creativity is more likely to emerge when it is informed by facts and knowledge about an issue. Thus we added this step to West's suggestions for building a culture of creativity. Team members cannot be expected to be creative about things they know nothing about. Educational sessions to improve learning, share best practices, and explore how other teams are handling similar issues are useful. In the vignette above, Dr. Kopek's effort to transfer some of Ms. Wilhoit's knowledge from her experience in revitalizing the transition care unit to the Quality Council represents an improvement in the team's knowledge base. Team members who connect with other experts by travel to conferences, study, and other means should transfer their relevant learning to the team.

Knowledge about many knotty healthcare issues can be gathered by studying *positive deviants.* Positive deviance is a change management methodology which begins by identifying the small minority of individuals or groups who are handling a problem extremely well—the positive deviants (Pascale et al, 2010). For example, suppose a quality improvement project team is searching for ways to improve hand washing compliance by clinicians. Relevant knowledge would include information on teams or units that have high compliance, and understanding whether the experience of those positive deviants can be transferred to one's own setting.

Challenge the Team

As noted earlier, embracing creativity requires openness to new ideas, but not to any and every idea. This requires that openness be balanced with demanding criteria that are performance related. Otherwise, ideas go unchallenged, and there is little forward movement—anything goes. Teams that enjoy being creative can get caught up in the excitement of doing something new, for its own sake. Like most good practices, the pursuit of creativity can be taken too far.

Leaders need to set high standards for quantity and quality of creative ideas. Researchers have found increased idea generation when team members have information about other members' activity levels, when performance standards are set high, and even when it is simply announced that members will see a list of all ideas at the end of the session (Thompson, 2003, p. 105).

As noted in Chapter 6, a safe team climate is not the same as a comfortable climate if team members respond to comfort by becoming complacent and giving less than their best efforts. Among teams of scientists, for example, research shows that innovation is high when the atmosphere within the team is warm, supportive, but intellectually demanding (West, 2012, p. 157). Mining creativity requires that teams progress to synthesizing and acting on new ideas, rather than letting them sit. This final step can be viewed as convergent thinking, after a period of divergent thinking—both are necessary. For this reason, members need to be prepared, that is, they need to know that their creative ideas will not always be used or implemented. Rejection of most ideas is an expected part of the pursuit of creative realism. This understanding encourages team members to keep generating ideas without the guarantee of adoption.

Stop Working

Another guideline is to devote formal team time to creativity. The advice to "stop working" is tongue-in-cheek; work to "stop" refers to the traditional view of work as critical thinking, convergent thinking, and exploitation as opposed to work that involves creative and divergent thinking and exploration. The formal delineation by the leader of a shift in thinking is sometimes helpful; for instance, "Why don't we relax now and blue sky some possible solutions instead of critically assessing them."

To the extent that fun and humor stimulate creativity, though, the "stop working" adage has some literal meaning. Humor and fun fuel creativity. Making sure that meetings and social activities are fun encourages a creative culture. A positive social climate contributes to the freedom that members need to be open without fear of embarrassment or sanction. In the preceding vignette, Dr. Kopek set the stage for fun by bringing his symbol of creativity—the encased light bulb—to Quality Council meetings.

Stop working also can mean turning to formal tools to stimulate creativity, such as those discussed below. While busy team members may be irritated to be spending precious time using formal methods, often use of the tools symbolizes a serious commitment to creativity development, as well as producing positive results.

TOOLS TO SUPPORT TEAM CREATIVITY

The staff of Redborough Clinic, Wyndham Health Services, was restive. Wyndham Health Services was a large multispecialty group practice in a metropolitan setting crowded with other group practices competing for new patients. Statewide quality reporting statistics had been released earlier in the week, and Wyndham ranked in the lower quartile on diabetes care and several other measures of quality. Within the Wyndham organization, the Redborough Clinic had one of the lowest scores for diabetes care. Particularly troublesome was the distressingly low percentage of type 2 diabetes patients who had been tested in the past year to determine their hemoglobin A1c levels. National guidelines recommend that patients with type 2 diabetes have the test performed every 6-12 months.

Paul Pedersen, DO, an internist, was responsible for quality improvement in the Redborough Clinic. He called a meeting of staff who were most involved in diabetes care to discuss ways to improve performance as measured by adherence to the guideline recommendations. Attending the meeting in addition to Dr. Pederson were J. Stanley Wirth, MD, an endocrinologist; 2 general internists; 3 RNs; the Redborough Clinic administrator; and 2 clerks who helped patients with scheduling.

Dr. Pedersen opened the meeting with a request for ideas about improving compliance with the testing guideline. "The floor is open," he announced. "Who has an idea?" Dr. Wirth immediately jumped in with his favorite suggestion, one he had been pushing for years. He recommended that patients' insulin prescriptions would not be refilled if they had not had an A1c test done in the past year. A chorus of disagreement followed from one of the general internists and 2 of the RNs. They said that patients should not be deprived of insulin because it was not safe for the patients, and they speculated that patients whose refill requests were refused would simply go to another clinic. The other general internist then questioned the validity of the data used in the quality reporting program, and an RN sarcastically suggested they "move the clinic to a part of the town with a more educated population." One of the RNs stated, "We have worse problems with getting diabetic patients to pay attention to their high blood pressure problems. Why aren't we talking about those?" The 2 clerical staff members remained silent. The conversation was so chaotic that one of the RNs started to smile—although no one else knew why. After 15 minutes, Dr. Pedersen had heard enough. Saying "We'll just have to try harder," he asked 2 members of the team to meet to create a list of ideas for the whole team to consider at the next meeting. The team then moved on to discuss another disappointing aspect of its reported performance in treating patients with diabetes.

A plethora of tools and methods for improving creativity can be applied in team meetings and beyond. Following are a selection of several tools, with brainstorming and variations on brainstorming being the most prominent. Formal brainstorming is a tool that would have allowed Dr. Pedersen in the vignette efficiently to get more ideas on the table for improving the rate of hemoglobin A1c testing.

Brainstorming

Brainstorming is a focused discussion with systematic encouragement of creative thinking around an issue or question. Brainstorming enables widespread participation in discussions that are directed at innovation and creative problem solving. Formal brainstorming more systematically encourages group members to generate many ideas without worrying about whether they are good or bad ones. Approximations of brainstorming often are used informally in meetings when managers ask all participants for creative ideas about tackling a problem or pursuing an opportunity. Dr. Pedersen attempted to use informal brainstorming in the vignette above.

In organizations where participation in meetings typically is highly structured or routinized, formal brainstorming is an option for breaking the routine. Signs of routinized discussions include heightened predictability of the content of member contributions (for example, one member typically may suggest that the team will just have to work harder, as Dr. Pedersen did in the vignette) and a pattern of the same participants dominating discussions, with little participation from others. The lack of participation from the

2 clerical staff members in the vignette may be indicative of that sign of routinization.

Brainstorming as a formal method of generating ideas typically includes the following steps:

1. Introduce the question or issue and review guidelines for brainstorming, such as:
   - All ideas are welcome
   - No evaluation of ideas during the brainstorm
   - The more ideas the better
   - Do not worry about duplicate ideas
   - Suspend judgment
   - Be concise
   - Include the unusual and strange (West, 2012, p. 167)
2. Display the central question or issue on a flipchart or elsewhere.
3. Offer a brief quiet period for team members to collect their thoughts and jot down ideas.
4. Ask for ideas and record them on a flipchart or elsewhere as they are offered. A separate recorder may perform this task. Do not accept comments that are evaluations of ideas. Use encouragement to invite more ideas.
5. Allow for lulls in activity; it is not uncommon for good ideas to emerge after periods of silence.
6. Offer one last chance for additional ideas, including ideas from the recorder. End the brainstorm.
7. To facilitate next steps, ask for clarification of ideas if needed, and number the ideas so that they can be referred to easily.

Table 10–2 displays an abbreviated summary of these steps.

Table 10–2. Steps in team brainstorming

Introduce the question or issue and guidelines for brainstorming
Display the question or issue
Offer a brief quiet period
Ask for ideas and record them
• Do not accept comments that are evaluations of ideas
• Use encouragement to invite more ideas
• Allow for lulls in activity
Offer one last chance for additional ideas
Ask for clarification of ideas

During the brainstorm, suggestions of new ideas are not censored unless they are offensive. Unlike the discussion in the vignette, negative responses are not allowed during the initial flow of ideas. Assessment of ideas is deferred so as not to interrupt the focus on creative thinking. Unlike many group discussion techniques that discount or dismiss new ideas before they are discussed, brainstorming considers all suggestions that are offered. In formal brainstorming, a leader or assigned member records ideas for all to view. It is important that the recorder write exactly what has been said, if possible, paraphrasing only if necessary. Paraphrasing should be checked with the contributing member for approval.

Assessment and prioritization occur only after an extensive list of ideas has been developed by brainstorming. Those steps can proceed with varying degrees of formalization, after the brainstorm. The nominal group technique, outlined below, offers one way to formalize the prioritization process.

In a formal brainstorming session, the leader or facilitator plays a vital role, as team members are normally alert to their cues to focus, concentrate, and contribute ideas. Positive reinforcement of participation from the team leader and from teammates is important. The leader also monitors conversation to make sure that assessment of ideas is held until the brainstorming is finished. Because ideas are not solicited in round robin fashion there is a risk that some team members may be reluctant to offer suggestions, or that aggressively verbal members will dominate the session. The leader's management of participation is critical for the success of brainstorming. In the preceding vignette, Dr. Pedersen did a poor job of monitoring participation. In particular, the 2 clerical staff members should have been solicited for input on ideas to improve patient and clinician attention to assuring that annual hemoglobin A1c tests are obtained.

Limitations of Brainstorming

Researchers have found little empirical support for the hypothesis that team brainstorming fosters creativity compared to having the same number of individual working independently (Thompson, 2003, p. 100). In fact, nearly all controlled investigations have found that team brainstorming is less efficient than solitary brainstorming, both in terms of quantity and quality of ideas. One research group concluded, "the long-lived popularity of brainstorming techniques is unequivocally and substantially misguided" (Mullen et al, 1991, p. 18). Yet its continuing popularity suggests that brainstorming has subtle positive effects, such as building group trust, solidarity and optimism, and that it is superior to many existing team processes. Also, it may be that generating ideas in a group setting makes their eventual implementation easier because it engenders support for the ideas (even if they are fewer or less novel than they would have been if generated by individuals working alone).

Among the reasons that team brainstorming sometimes disappoints are the following: social loafing, production blocking, conformity, and downward norm setting (Thompson, 2003, pp. 100-102). (Social loafing is discussed in Chapter 1; production blocking is discussed in Chapter 9.) Avoidance of conflict is another possible reason for limited participation in brainstorming. Social loafing is increased because if ideas are not being judged, team members are more likely to loaf. Production blocking occurs because individuals working alone can enjoy uninterrupted flow of thought, while in a team they have to wait their turn to speak. Production of new ideas is blocked by the waiting-to-speak step and by the diversion of attention caused by listening-to-others-speak. Conformity pressures arise because people in groups tend to give more conventional responses than when they are alone due to the desire to conform to group norms. Downward norm setting refers to the tendency for the lowest performers in a team to pull down the average. Participants in brainstorming tend to match their performance to that of the least productive member. All of these forces can overwhelm the intuitive potential of brainstorming in teams. These constraints are particularly powerful in stifling participation by introverts, who often think more creatively when alone rather than in group settings (Cain, 2012).

Brainstorming, by itself, is constrained by the fact that better ideas often emerge through debate and criticism. Criticism can draw out and drive new ideas to become even better ideas. If every idea is right, as is the initial working assumption of brainstorming, there is no incentive to incorporate the perspectives of others.

Another reason that brainstorming can fail is that participants may be uninformed, and, if so, the quality of their ideas may be poor. As noted earlier, creativity requires a strong base of knowledge and experience. This limitation applies to individual as well as team brainstorming. A final limitation of brainstorming relates to its simplicity. Because brainstorming requires participants to focus on one issue, idea, or topic, the question must be thoughtfully worded, and interrelated issues cannot be addressed. Complex questions should be discussed in less structured forums that allow for interdependent issues to be raised.

Team brainstorming can be tweaked to address many of its shortcomings. The limitations of brainstorming covered above suggest several improvements that teams can make in the use of brainstorming. First, challenge the team to meet high standards. Brainstorming is as much work as it is fun, and social loafing should be discouraged. Second, allow more silent time for individual brainstorming prior to team brainstorming. Asking members to think about their ideas prior to meeting with one another (and to record their ideas on paper) takes advantage of individual creativity. Finally, make sure that brainstorming is followed by convergent thinking, so that creative realism rather than idealism is the outcome. This requires allowing enough subsequent time to process the ideas developed during the brainstorm.

Brain-Writing and Brain-Netting

Brain-writing is a variant of brainstorming that accentuates the major value of brainstorming, which is generation of a large quantity of ideas, irrespective of quality (West, 2012, pp. 163-164). In brain-writing sessions, each team member generates 5-10 ideas on a blank sheet of paper, without identifying themselves on the paper. This process addresses the problem of production blocking, noted above, and it also reduces the pressure to conform, due to its anonymity. The papers are placed in the middle of the table and then distributed randomly. Each member continues writing more ideas on the sheet she or he receives, with encouragement to build on the ideas already developed. Redundancy of ideas is reduced by the sharing of the sheets of paper. Another benefit of brain-writing is that all team members do not have to be present at the same time, as the process can be allowed to extend over multiple meetings or days.

A convenient alternative to brainstorming and brain-writing is electronic brainstorming or brain-netting. A digital file to which all members have access can be posted on a website, and team members can add their ideas to those of their colleagues. This creates a convenient record and removes the roadblock sometimes caused by scheduling problems. The digital record then can become an important source of team memory that can be accessed for other needs in the future.

Negative Brainstorming

Negative or reverse brainstorming applies the brainstorming method to the question, "What could go wrong?" By speculating on causes of negative outcomes, the process forces team members to consider offsetting actions that they may not have considered previously. For example, a discussion about shortening appointment times could include negative brainstorming around "what could go wrong if appointment times are cut by 10%?" Negative brainstorming is also discussed in Chapter 9 on decision making.

Table of Elements Brainstorming

Table of elements brainstorming is an extension of brainstorming in which a problem is broken into separate components, with brainstorming applied separately to each component of the problem. Components then are combined, and options are chosen from among the various combinations of components to derive new ideas. West (2012, pp. 165-166) gives the example of devising a social event for a team. The task is broken into 5 components: (1) people (who should attend), (2) place (where should it happen), (3) activities, (4) time, and (5) purpose. Brainstorming occurs around each component, after which discussion is used to develop consensus on an event. Ten or 15 minutes devoted to the activity can generate hundreds of ideas.

Nominal Group Technique

Like brainstorming and brain-writing, the nominal group technique attempts to achieve more equal participation of all members of a group. Both techniques are designed to prevent selected individuals from dominating group input, but the nominal group technique does so even more systematically. Unlike brainstorming, the nominal group technique also produces a set of priorities or rankings that reflect the structured input of all participants. The steps in the technique are as follows (Delbecq and Van de Ven, 1971):

1. The team discusses the process and objectives of the nominal group technique. A specific issue or question is identified. The specific issue is displayed in writing so that all can see it.
2. Ideas are generated and written down by each team member independently and silently. This step equalizes the opportunity for participation.
3. Ideas can be collected round robin style orally, or in writing. The facilitator distributes or posts a written collation of the responses. Again, this ensures participation by all team members.
4. The list of ideas is discussed and ideas are clarified and assessed, with a sharing of pros and cons. The provider of the idea may or may not choose to defend it.
5. Ideas are numbered for voting. Voting on the quality of ideas occurs. The facilitator requests that all members of the group privately prioritize the ideas using an agreed-upon set of criteria. There are several ways to vote (Fallon et al, 2013, pp. 329-330). One system gives each participant 5 cards. Participants then list their top 5 ideas, 1 per card, and rate the priority of each from 1 (low) to high (5). The facilitator collects the cards and tallies and posts the scores. The highest scores are the ideas most favored by the group. If desired, the discussion and voting process can continue for another round to winnow the list even further. Another system has participants vote on each idea. This approach becomes cumbersome when a large number of ideas are being evaluated. A third system asks team members to designate the 3 most appealing ideas and the 3 least appealing ideas. The least appealing for the team as a whole are removed from consideration, and the process is repeated until the team members reach a consensus about the most appealing idea or ideas.

The nominal group technique produces a quantitative ranking of priorities that is more tangible than the feelings expressed during traditional team discussions and brainstorming. However, the ordinal ranking system (if it is used) in the nominal group technique does not allow fine distinctions in preferences to be expressed. Rating each idea on a 1 to 100 scale has the potential to identify more precise differences, though the need for such fine distinctions does not commonly occur.

The Delphi technique is a variant of the nominal group, in which individuals do not interact face-to-face. This is an attractive option for teams that have difficulty meeting face-to-face because of scheduling problems. All of the communication is handled through questionnaires and feedback, which can be computerized. Cycles can take several days to complete, however, so speed is not a feature of the Delphi technique (Delbecq et al, 1975, pp. 83-107).

Scenario Planning

Scenarios are descriptions of possible futures. In scenario planning, a range of futures from worst case to best case is outlined, along with a *status quo* assumption scenario that is based on past trends and planned changes. Scenario planning opens participants' eyes to their abilities to shape the future. Standard forecasts of the future based on past trends do not use enough imagination to discover how circumstance might change. The purpose of constructing scenarios is not necessarily to predict the future, but to gain a better understanding of the forces that influence the future and, in light of those forces, the range of actions that are possible. This understanding sets the stage for considering more creative ideas about actions that might be taken to benefit from the forces identified or to abide by the constraints imposed by those forces. Scenario planning can be preceded by brainstorming in order to systematically generate lists of key forces driving change, which can increase the breadth of scenarios (Chermack et al, 2010).

For example, consider the example of the patient-centered care movement noted earlier. Team members could consider scenarios of no change in team services, incremental changes (the most likely path), and radical innovation. What would be the likely impact of each scenario on team outcomes, such as timeliness of care, efficiency, and safety? Discussions of the scenarios might influence the team to speed up or slow down its implementation of patient-centered care policies and processes.

Trained Facilitators

Facilitators with experience in team brainstorming and other tools can be excellent resources for healthcare team development. Team leaders who are reluctant to use formal methods for stimulating creativity due to their own style or inexperience can test new methods by using external facilitators. Some research supports the notion that teams using facilitators to encourage productive idea generation maintain high levels of productivity in subsequent sessions without facilitators (Thompson, 2003, p. 105). Teams can learn the techniques through guided practice.

Other Tools

There is a long list of other methods for stimulating creativity in those teams that have especially strong needs for creativity (Scholtes et al, 2003, pp. 8-1 to 8-12). Improvisation and role playing are among those methods. For example, team members could act out a meeting with an external party, such as an administrator, requesting new resources for the team's work. Ideally, newly improvised ideas for making the case for new resources would emerge during the role play. Other methods include mind mapping and design storyboards, which are methods for presenting ideas visually. Mind mapping software is available for visualizing increasingly complex tasks. Seeing relationships and ideas stimulates different thought patterns that may be more creative. For instance, a team within Kaiser Permanente, the Innovation Consultancy, has tried to improve the capture of the essence of patient-professional interactions using photographs, pictures, and stories (McCreary, 2010). Changes in physical arrangements and discussion formats in meeting rooms, such as fishbowls, conversation cafes, and celebrity interviews, can loosen up traditional team meetings and produce unexpected and powerful outcomes (McCandless and Lipmanowicz, 2012).

CONCLUSION

Most healthcare teams, whether they are interprofessional or not, could benefit from higher levels of creativity. This is particularly true for management and clinical teams searching for better and more efficient ways to deliver healthcare services. Creativity requires divergent and creative thinking and exploration rather than exploitation. Creativity can be embedded in team culture by defining it as a goal, selecting diverse team members, supporting creativity in team processes, challenging the team to achieve realistic creativity, developing the knowledge base, and making time for creative decision-making processes. Formal tools for pursuing creativity include brainstorming and its variants, scenario planning, and the use of trained facilitators.

REFERENCES

Boynton A, Fischer B, Bole W. *The Idea Hunter*. San Francisco, CA: Jossey-Bass; 2011.

Cain S. *Quiet: The Power of Introverts in a World That Can't Stop Talking*. New York, NY: Crown Publishers; 2012.

Canadian Interprofessional Health Collaborative. *A National Interprofessional Competency Framework*. Vancouver, BC, Canada: Canadian Interprofessional Health Collaborative; 2010. http://www.cihc.ca/files/CIHC_IPCompetencies_Feb1210.pdf. Accessed September 20, 2012.

Chermack TJ, Bodwell W, Glick M. Two strategies for leveraging teams toward organizational effectiveness: scenario planning and organizational ambidexterity. *Advances in Developing Human Resources.* 2010;12:137-156.

Cropley A. In praise of convergent thinking. *Creat Res J.* 2006;18:391-404.

de Bono E. *Lateral Thinking: Creativity Step-by-Step.* New York, NY: Harper and Row; 1970.

Delbecq AL, Van de Ven AH. A group process model for problem identification and program planning. *J Appl Behav Sci.* 1971;7:466-492.

Delbecq AL, Van de Ven AH, Gustafson DH. *Group Techniques for Program Planning: a Guide to Nominal Group and Delphi Processes.* Glenview, IL: Scott, Foresman and Company; 1975.

Dye CF, Garman AN. *Exceptional Leadership: 16 Critical Competencies for Healthcare Executives.* Chicago, IL: Health Administration Press; 2006.

Dyer JH, Gregersen HB, Christensen CM. The innovator's DNA. *Harv Bus Rev.* 2009;87(12):61-67.

Ericsson KA, Lehmann AC. Expertise. In: Runco MA, Pritzker SR, eds. *Encyclopedia of Creativity.* Vol 1. San Diego, CA: Academic Press; 1999:695-707.

Fallon LF, Begun JW, Riley W. *Managing Health Organizations for Quality and Performance.* Burlington, VT: Jones and Bartlett Learning; 2013.

Interprofessional Education Collaborative Expert Panel. *Core Competencies for Interprofessional Collaborative Practice: Report of an Expert Panel.* Washington, DC: Interprofessional Education Collaborative; 2011. http://www.aacn.nche.edu/education-resources/IPECReport.pdf. Accessed January 29, 2012.

King LA, Walker LM, Broyles SJ. Creativity and the five-factor model. *J Res Pers.* 1996;30:189-203.

March JG. Exploration and exploitation in organizational learning. *Organization Science.* 1991;2:71-87.

McCandless K, Lipmanowicz H. *Liberating Structures.* 2012. http://www.liberatingstructures.com. Accessed July 12, 2012.

McCrae RR, John OP. An introduction to the five-factor model and its applications. *J Pers.* 1992;60:175-215.

McCreary L. Kaiser Permanente's innovation on the front lines. *Harv Bus Rev.* 2010;88(9):92-127.

Mitchell P, Wynia M, Golden R, et al. Core principles and values of effective team-based health care. 2012. Discussion Paper, Institute of Medicine, Washington, DC. http://www.iom.edu/tbc. Accessed February 24, 2013.

Mullen B, Johnson C, Salas E. Productivity loss in brainstorming groups: a meta-analytic integration. *Basic Appl Soc Psych.* 1991;12:3-23.

Pascale R, Sternin J, Sternin M. *The Power of Positive Deviance: How Unlikely Innovators Solve the World's Toughest Problems.* Boston, MA: Harvard Business Press; 2010.

Quinn RE, Faerman SR, Thompson MP, et al. *Becoming a Master Manager.* 5th ed. New York, NY: John Wiley & Sons; 2011.

Scholtes PR, Joiner BL, Streibel BJ. *The Team Handbook.* 3rd ed. Madison, WI: Oriel Incorporated; 2003.

Thompson L. Improving the creativity of organizational work groups. *Academy of Management Executive.* 2003;17(1): 96-109.

Thompson LL. *Making the Team: A Guide for Managers.* 4th ed. Upper Saddle River, NJ: Prentice Hall; 2011.

West MA. *Effective Teamwork: Practical Lessons from Organizational Research.* 3rd ed. Chichester, UK: John Wiley & Sons, Ltd.; 2012.

West MA, Anderson NR. Innovation in top management teams. *J Appl Psychol.* 1996;81:680-693.

Managing Conflict in Healthcare Teams

Marion Blackwell, NP, a nurse practitioner, was finishing her work after a long day at the medical practice of Owen Andersen, MD, an allergist. The practice had just converted from paper records to electronic health records, and there was an unusual degree of anxiety and confusion in the air. The practice included 2 registered nurses (RNs), 2 licensed practical nurses (LPNs), and 2 clerical staff, and only one of those 6 was really "on board" with the new record system. All of the clinical staff carried portable computers from patient room to patient room during a transition period while permanent work stations were being installed. There were several occasions where results of in-house laboratory tests, such as spirometry (which measures the volume and flow of air during inhalation and exhalation) and records of allergy shot administration were not entered into the electronic record because a nurse had left a portable computer in another room or had technical problems with a computer. Nurses were sometimes duplicating entries of test results because they were unsure who was responsible for entering the results. The clerical staff members were having trouble locating electronic records for many patients due to electronic "filing" bugs, particularly for patients who had changed their last names over time. Most patient appointments were running late as a result. One of the clerical staff members told Ms. Blackwell that they should lengthen the time slots for routine appointments, at least until the new system was working more smoothly.

In the past, Dr. Andersen had not been particularly interested in hearing complaints from the staff. His personal style in facing adversity was stoical, and Ms. Blackwell guessed that Dr. Andersen likely preferred to just "plow ahead." Ms. Blackwell had a good working relationship with Dr. Andersen, but she couldn't decide whether to push him to take the time to "air out" the problems the team was having with the new system.

As with all social activity, teamwork processes commonly are fraught with conflict or with opportunities for conflict. In Chapter 6, effective teams are described as surfacing and processing conflict when appropriate. In Chapter 7, team members are said to need competencies in constructively addressing conflicts with other teammates and in facilitating team management of conflicts they observe.

Conflict resolution refers to the process of ending a conflict. *Conflict management* is a broader term, referring to optimal use of conflict to move the team forward toward its goals. Conflict management does not necessarily imply conflict resolution. In fact, conflict management sometimes means stimulating productive conflict, in addition to or instead of focusing on resolution. In this chapter, we use the term *conflict management* rather than *conflict resolution*. Conflict management "involves designing effective macro-level strategies to minimize the dysfunctions of conflict and enhancing the constructive functions of conflict in order to enhance learning and effectiveness..." (Rahim, 2002, p. 208). *Learning* and *effectiveness* are key words in the preceding statement.

In the case of the medical practice described earlier, conflict management includes thinking about the potential constructive functions of conflict as well as dysfunctions. If the members of the medical group described in the opening vignette are to improve patient care, it would be better to surface conflict concerning the electronic health record than to ignore it. If so, managing the conflict would mean addressing any important issues that are raised by the office staff. The practice team members could learn more about how best to implement the electronic health record, and Dr. Andersen could seek recommitment to the goal of improving patient care through implementation of the electronic health record.

According to the Canadian Collaborative interprofessional healthcare competency framework (described in Chapter 7), conflict management encompasses 8 distinct competencies: (1) value the potential positive nature of conflict, (2) take constructive steps to address conflict, (3) know common sources of conflict, (4) know strategies to deal with conflict, (5) set guidelines for addressing conflict, (6) work to resolve disagreements, (7) establish a safe environment for diverse opinions, and (8) allow all members to feel their viewpoints have been heard (CIHC, 2010, pp. III-IV). In this chapter, we cover those topics but in a more condensed format. Team members need to (1) understand causes of conflict, (2) distinguish types and stages of conflict, and (3) know and apply methods of managing conflict appropriate to different types and stages.

CAUSES OF TEAM CONFLICT

There are well-known patterns that make the emergence of conflict predictable in many teamwork activities and settings (West, 2012, pp. 191-193). These are summarized in Table 11–1. First, conflict in teams frequently emerges due to role ambiguity among team members—a lack of clarity or understanding of who does what, or real overlap in roles. For example, 2 team members may expect each other to follow up a team meeting with a communication to a patient, when in fact neither conducts the communication.

A second common source of team conflict relates to disagreements over goals. Such conflict may be due to the absence of a clear vision or clear goals, with individual team members substituting their own differing perceptions. Or, again, individual team members may have real differences in the goals they prefer for the team. This source of conflict is particularly apparent on interprofessional teams, because each profession brings different values and expectations for patient care to the team, as described in Chapter 3. An example is the preference of one team member to involve more family members in a team discussion, which may not be perceived as practical (or desirable) by other team members.

Conflict escalates when critical resources are scarce. For example, suppose 6 clinical professionals on a patient care team share the services of one clerical staff team member. If financial circumstances change such that the team only can afford a half-time clerical staff member, the 6 team members are more likely to engage in conflict over who gets the available time from the half-time clerical staff member.

Differences in perceived status or rank are potent sources of conflict on interprofessional teams. If members treat each other differently based on status,

Table 11–1. Sources of team conflict

Source of Conflict	Description
Role ambiguity	Lack of clarity or understanding of who does what, or real overlap in roles
Disagreements over goals	Absence of clarity or agreement on vision or goals
Scarcity of critical resources	Key resources, such as equipment and staff, are scarce
Differences in perceived status	Members treat each other differently based on status
Task interdependence	Interdependent members must rely on other members, and things do not always go as planned
Personal preferences	Team members may dislike other members for their personal characteristics, such as religion, political views, appearance, or behavioral idiosyncrasies

resentment on the part of the lower status member is likely to result. Lower status members are less likely to participate fully in team activities, or they may even work against team goals. Higher status members are more likely to devalue the contribution of the lower status members. A net result is increased levels of conflict or potential conflict in the team.

Conflict escalates when tasks are more interdependent, based on the simple fact that interdependent members must rely on other members, and things do not always go as planned. A team member who needs the input of another team member before making a recommendation for treatment, for instance, may resent the delay caused by a colleague who is late providing the input. In particular, interdependence is high during handoffs—transfer of responsibility and information from one member to another—making handoffs a common source of conflict in interprofessional team care.

Finally, a host of additional causes of conflict can be classified as personal. Team members may dislike other members for their personal characteristics, such as personality, religion, political views, appearance, or behavioral idiosyncrasies. While these sources of conflict are not based on features of the team or on characteristics of individuals specific to their team roles, conflicts arising for personal reasons can affect team performance.

Several of these causal factors were interacting to create the potential for conflict in the allergy practice described in the introductory vignette. Role ambiguity around who enters the test results was evident. All of the staff members were not on board with the proposition that electronic records would improve the quality of patient care, a goal clarification issue. Differences in perceived status likely entered into staff members' reluctance to confront Dr. Andersen with their issues. Task interdependence meant that if one staff member had a delay, others often were affected. The personal preference of Dr. Andersen to "tough it out" through adversity likely was not in line with the feelings of some or all of the staff.

Given that virtually all interprofessional teams have built-in status differences, scarce resources, multiple professional backgrounds, interdependent tasks, and members with personal differences, it is no wonder that the potential for conflict is high in interprofessional teams. How should such conflicts be handled? When should conflict be stimulated rather than reduced? A next step is to differentiate among types and stages of conflict.

TYPES AND STAGES OF TEAM CONFLICT

Diego Jimenez, MBA, loosened his tie. This meeting of the emergency department (ED) process flow project team was going to be a long one. Mr. Jimenez had administrative responsibility for the ED and headed the team, which was charged with reducing patient waiting time in the ED. Two ED physicians, 3 RNs, and 4 other clinical technicians or clerical staff members were on the team. Trouble had been simmering between one of the staff members (a front desk receptionist) and one of the nurses for several meetings, but at this meeting it spilled out in the open, with the front desk receptionist accusing the nurse of being lazy. In addition, several team members seemed to be using the process flow project to make the case for new equipment, such as faster personal computers, rather than thinking more broadly about other causes of delay in serving patients. Finally, the team was having trouble deciding how to proceed next with data collection: short interviews with a sample of ED personnel, or written surveys of all personnel.

Types of Team Conflict

It is useful to identify types of team conflict because type of conflict is related to decisions about how to manage the conflict. Three types of team conflict are commonly distinguished: relationship, process, and task (Thompson, 2011, pp. 183-185). While conflict often is of multiple types or morphs over time from one type into a different type, the 3 categories help provide a context for considering (1) the value of the conflict for team learning, and (2) how and when to surface or resolve the conflict. Table 11–2 summarizes the types of team conflict and examples of each type.

Team conflict can occur among individual team members or among combinations of team members. At its simplest level, team conflict occurs between 2 individual team members, as it did between the receptionist and the nurse in the vignette. When conflict surfaces, though, other team members likely will take positions. Opinions on issues often coalesce around a small number of positions, so conflict often involves one coalition of members versus another, or conflict among multiple coalitions.

Relationship conflict is conflict over personal or social issues not related to the team task. It often is

Table 11-2. Types and examples of team conflict

Type of Conflict	Examples
Relationship	Disagreement with another team member's political views, religion, sexual orientation, or gender, racial, ethnic, or personality characteristics; disagreement with another team member based on experiences outside of the team
Task	Disagreement over appropriate therapy, team tasks, and goals
Process	Disagreement over team processes, such as decision making; disagreement over how tasks or goals should be accomplished

referred to by teamwork scholars as "emotional" or "affective" conflict. For example, team members may disagree about health policy or other political issues that are largely irrelevant to the team's work. Or, team members may have different opinions about professional appearance and dress. (In both cases, such conflict actually could be relevant to the team's work if it affects patient care or other team performance goals.) In the preceding vignette, the accusation that another person is lazy is tangential to the team task and therefore is primarily a symptom of relationship conflict. On the other hand, the accuser might consider the issue to be relevant to the team task, because laziness may contribute to delays in serving patients. Often, relationship conflicts do have some degree of relevance to team processes or team tasks.

Relationship conflict frequently is detrimental to team performance: as relationship conflict increases, team effectiveness decreases. In general, relationship conflict is best handled outside of the purview of the team. Experienced conflict handlers take their issues "outside of the room" and address them privately so that they do not interfere with team tasks. We say more about this in the following section.

Task conflict is conflict over the content of the work that is being done by the team. It is the most critical of the types of conflict for teams to monitor and process. One teamwork commentator (Wheelan, 2013, p. 27) argues that disagreement over goals and values largely is inevitable, and that conflict is necessary in order to create a climate where members feel free to disagree with each other. It is easier for members to develop trust in each other if they believe that they can disagree and will not be abandoned or hurt because they have different perspectives. An example of task conflict in the preceding vignette is the discussion of old equipment as a factor in patient delay. Some team members feel that new equipment would improve patient flow; others likely think it would be of marginal value. Another example of task conflict, on a patient care team, is disagreement about the appropriate therapy for a patient. Conflict over tasks ideally is depersonalized, and therefore also is referred to as *cognitive* conflict. Task conflict typically consists of arguments about the merits of ideas, plans, and therapies. Task conflict frequently is useful for teams because it leads to new insights and allows for efficient progress—everyone gets "on the same page" about the content of the team's work.

Process conflict is conflict over the way that the work of the team is being done, with the issue of role ambiguity—who does what—being a potent source of process conflict. An example is conflict over who should communicate a team decision to a patient, or when. Like task conflict, process conflict frequently can be useful in creating efficient movement forward in accomplishing a team's task, and it should be encouraged and surfaced up to a point. In the vignette, process conflict has emerged over the best way to collect data for the ED process flow team to review.

Together, task conflict and process conflict can be called *substantive* conflict, in contrast to relationship conflict, because they are conflict over the substance of the team's work—what to do and how to do it. Recalling the first vignette about electronic health record implementation, the potential conflict in Dr. Andersen's allergy practice involved both task and process issues, in that there was conflict over the value of the task of implementing the electronic record (task conflict), as well as numerous issues about how best to accomplish the task (process conflict). The relationship of substantive conflict to team effectiveness can be visualized in the shape of an inverted U: effectiveness increases with conflict levels, up to a point. After that point, effectiveness decreases. (See Figure 11–1.) Teams can be overwhelmed if every process or task issue invites disagreement, and if team members learn to argue over every issue on the team agenda. A certain level of constructive conflict, though, should be encouraged. It clarifies roles and goals, creates cohesion because members feel that their feelings are heard, and surfaces new ideas and viewpoints. When followed by actions

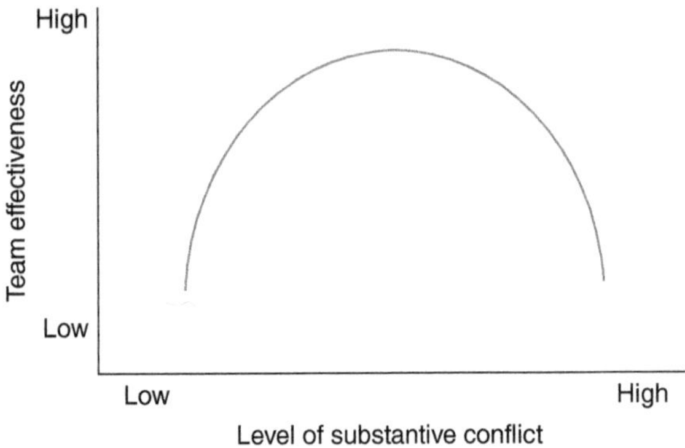

▲ Figure 11-1. Relationship of substantive conflict to team effectiveness.

to address problems, open disagreement promotes change and innovation (Reay et al, 2013). Hopefully Mr. Jimenez, in the preceding vignette, will be able to use the disagreements about task content and process to move the team forward.

Stages of Team Conflict

All types of conflict generally proceed through stages, from *anticipation* of the conflict on the part of one or more parties, to *awareness* of the conflict short of confirmation, to *discussion* which confirms that the conflict exists (or not), to open *dispute*. The stages can proceed almost instantaneously in the case of acutely erupting conflicts, or conflicts can simmer in the anticipation or awareness stages for months or years. Conflict can also stop at any of the stages.

In the case of the ED process flow team, Mr. Jimenez was aware of some bad feelings between front desk personnel and some of the nurses in the ED. Discussion and open dispute had not occurred in a formal setting, though, so it was difficult to judge its seriousness. Had he anticipated the conflict emerging in the team setting, Mr. Jimenez could have intervened to prevent it from being surfaced then, or he could have been more prepared to deal with the conflict when it did surface.

Inter-Team Conflict

In addition to intra-team conflict, the types and stages of conflict generalize to conflict among different teams. For example, in the same organization, multiple teams may be responsible for care to different populations of patients, and the teams may come into conflict over resources provided by the organization to each team. Or, teams that perform different stages of interdependent work for the same population of patients may fight over the appropriate scope and responsibility of each team. For example, teams in the primary care department of a large medical group may argue with teams in the orthopedics department about who should order diagnostic imaging services. The methods of managing team conflict described in the next section also can be applied to conflict among teams, although surfacing and resolving those conflicts may be more difficult because regular communication channels among different teams may be lacking. The organizational context for teams affects the way that conflict among teams is managed. The organizational context for teamwork is covered in Chapter 18.

Process and task conflict require team attention, as does relationship conflict that affects team performance. Methods to address conflict are covered next.

MANAGING TEAM CONFLICT

Jerry Nichols, NP, a gerontological nurse practitioner, headed to the weekly meeting of the home care team with a grimace on his face. In addition to Mr. Nichols, the team included an occupational therapist, a social worker, a physician assistant, and a primary care physician. The team leader was the primary care physician, Amy Bristol, MD. Other professionals, such as nutritionists, pharmacists, speech therapists, and home health aides, were invited to team meetings as needed, and patients and family members were also considered as team members.

The team does valuable work in these meetings, Mr. Nichols thought, but it meets too often. Weekly meetings are not necessary. Meeting every 2 weeks should be sufficient, as team members could e-mail or telephone others if there really were urgent business between meetings.

Although Mr. Nichols suspected that other team members also shared his concern, he did not know how to bring it up with the team's leader, Dr. Bristol. When Dr. Bristol joined the team a year ago, she had stressed how important it was to meet weekly "come hell or high water," in order to "stay ahead of the wave" and deliver the highest quality care.

Five Methods of Conflict Management

A quite common (overly common, many experts argue) method of managing conflict is *avoidance*. This is the first of 5 commonly discussed methods of managing conflict (Thomas, 1977). Avoidance is a frequent choice by busy healthcare professionals who are not comfortable with surfacing conflict (Skjørshammer, 2001). Drinka and Clark (2000, pp. 150-151) provide a long list of excuses (22 in number) that healthcare teams use to rationalize avoidance of conflict. Among common rationalizations are: the patient comes first (allowing a member to avoid addressing another member's concerns); procrastination; overoptimism (Everything is fine; I don't know what you are talking about); beepermania (the reader can guess how that one works); and too busy—no time. Team members may avoid conflict in the name of efficiency, but constructive conflict is actually a time saver (Lencioni, 2002, p. 203). Teams that avoid constructive conflict may revisit issues again and again without resolution and may be plagued with ongoing tension. Teams that avoid conflict may have boring meetings, ignore controversial topics, fail to tap into perspectives of team members, and waste time with interpersonal attacks. In contrast, teams that engage in constructive conflict have lively meetings, exploit the ideas of all team members, solve real problems more quickly, minimize the use of politics, and put critical topics on the table for discussion (Lencioni, 2002, p. 204).

Why is avoidance such a common response to conflict? Many people find conflict to be threatening, based on past negative experience or the belief that harmony requires keeping silent. Some cultures, particularly many Asian cultures, emphasize harmony and the avoidance of open conflict as a social norm. The emphasis on collaboration in interprofessional teams (imparted by books—including this book—and competency frameworks for interprofessional practice such as the US and Canadian frameworks covered in Chapter 7) reinforces the reluctance to surface conflict, as well. In fact, however, avoiding conflict can cause negative feelings to build and can deprive teams of relevant and important information and new ideas.

In the case of the home care team described earlier, if Mr. Nichols chooses to keep silent about his discomfort with the weekly meeting schedule, he is using avoidance to manage the situation. Maybe the weekly meeting issue is not important enough for Mr. Nichols to raise. Maybe he will not let the issue influence his performance on the team, and all will be well. But most likely, Mr. Nichols' frustration will influence his participation and performance, and avoidance is not a good solution.

Accommodation is an option as well. Accommodation requires that one party to the conflict give in to another party. An accommodative solution to the conflict in the vignette first would require that the conflict be surfaced. Mr. Nichols could talk to Dr. Bristol individually, for example, and the team leader then could decide whether to put the issue on the agenda for team discussion. Prior to responding to Mr. Nichols, Dr. Bristol might individually raise the issue with other key team members to assess their feelings. If Dr. Bristol then tells Mr. Nichols, "I think we're working well with the weekly schedule, so let's keep it that way," and Mr. Nichols agrees to drop the issue, he is being accommodating to the team leader. If Dr. Bristol concludes, "Jerry, you've got a good point, and I'll change the schedule as you suggest," the leader is engaging in accommodation. (In neither of those cases is the conflict formally processed by the team, though, so the accommodations are by the individuals involved rather than the team.)

A third option, *collaboration*, is the "gold standard" method of dealing with conflict. Collaboration has a specific meaning in the conflict management field (Quinn et al, 2011, p. 94; Thomas, 1977, 1988), narrower than the broad notion of collaboration as a teamwork competency. As a conflict management method, collaboration proceeds through (1) an airing of the multiple sides of an issue, (2) agreement on criteria for resolving the conflict, and (3) negotiation of a solution acceptable to all parties to the conflict. Collaboration is similar to "win-win" negotiation, popularized by Fisher and Ury in their classic book, *Getting to Yes* (1981). A key component of the win-win negotiation process is separating people from problems—depersonalizing the conflicts. The goal of win-win negotiation is to create new value for all parties, rather than having one party dominate the other parties, or leaving all parties dissatisfied.

Following is an example of collaborative resolution of the conflict about weekly meetings, described earlier. Team leader Dr. Bristol agrees to put the issue on the next meeting agenda. She begins the team discussion by noting that "our key interest here is quality of patient care, rather than convenience for ourselves, right—does everyone agree with that?" Following affirmation of that criterion for making a decision, several members of the team air opinions about the weekly meeting schedule, ranging from "we don't meet often enough" to "once a week is about right" to Mr. Nichols' opinion that once a week is too often. Mr. Nichols realizes that he is alone in his opinion. The team agrees by consensus (see Chapter 9) to continue the meetings every week, but agrees that if there is no pressing business, the meeting will be canceled. Mr. Nichols agrees to support the collaborative solution. The outcome is not much different than the outcome produced by avoidance or accommodation by Mr. Nichols, as no major change is made in the meeting schedule. However, Mr. Nichols does appreciate the possibility of having some meetings cancelled. Most importantly, Mr. Nichols now better understands and accepts the tenor of the team on this issue, and the team has acknowledged and listened to his frustration. Mr. Nichols remains committed to making the team work.

A fourth method of managing conflict is *compromise*, a close relative of collaboration. To achieve compromise, multiple parties (1) air their sides of an issue, (2) agree on criteria for resolution, and (3) negotiate a solution acceptable to all parties. The steps are identical to collaboration. Compromise receives second billing to collaboration, however, because the solution is less desirable to each party. No party gets what they originally want—by definition, each side gives up something from its original position, and no new, better solution is substituted. In contrast, with collaboration, a new and better solution is discovered. Admittedly, the distinction between collaboration and compromise often is more intellectual than practical, as new win-win solutions (resulting from collaboration) may still be viewed as less than optimal by each party in the same way that compromise solutions are viewed as less than optimal by each party.

Here is an example of a compromise solution to the weekly meeting issue: hold weekly meetings for 1 month, biweekly meetings the next month, and so on, producing 6 meetings instead of 8 meetings in every 2-month period. This might emerge in a team discussion if enough support for Mr. Nichols' position is expressed in the discussion. No side gets its original preference, so the sides split the difference. Neither side is fully satisfied.

When team members confront an issue but do not accommodate, collaborate, or compromise, *competition* is a fifth and final option for managing conflict. The members compete with each other, with one member a victor and the others losers. Teams that make decisions by competition typically employ political tactics. Political tactics use power, which typically derives from one's position (with the leader commonly holding more power), profession (with physicians commonly holding more power), or expertise (with more experienced or more highly educated professionals holding more power). An unspoken rule might be, for example, that the team leader makes decisions on most issues—she or he has position power. In a competitive solution to Mr. Nichols' quandary about weekly meetings, team leader Dr. Bristol would simply rebuff Mr. Nichols' request to have a team discussion of the meeting schedule, essentially winning that competition. To escalate the competition politically, though, Mr. Nichols could lobby other members to get the issue on the agenda. Dr. Bristol likely would relent if faced with enough pressure and would agree to a team discussion. A debate likely would ensue, and a team vote might seal the decision. The winners would celebrate (silently, hopefully) and the losers would be unhappy.

If powerful leaders or coalitions choose to exercise their power in competitive conflict resolution, the competition can demoralize and marginalize the other team members. Competition often is referred to as a forcing response to conflict, as resolution is forced on the other parties. The cultural norm of collaboration is strong in most settings and situations in healthcare delivery, however, which tempers the use of competition to resolve conflicts.

Balancing Inquiry and Advocacy

The 5 methods of conflict management can be arrayed by degree of *inquiry* and degree of *advocacy* involved. Competition requires the highest degree of advocacy for one's position, with avoidance and accommodation requiring little or no advocacy, and collaboration and compromise at the moderate level. Inquiry (soliciting and listening to the position of others) is highest for the compromise and collaborate methods (as well as the accommodate method) and is low for competition and avoidance. For thoughtful exchange, a balance of inquiry and advocacy is advised (Argyris and Schön, 1996, p. 117; Bolman and Deal, 2008, pp. 172-173). Labeled *Model II thinking*, combining advocacy with inquiry requires that participants openly express what they think and feel, while they actively seek understanding of other's thoughts and feelings. People suspend their assumptions, but they communicate their assumptions freely in open dialogue. Systems theorist Peter Senge notes that an emphasis on advocacy can be counterproductive, particularly when team members are not familiar with each other's work and experience. When team members are not in touch with the potential contributions of others, they need to inquire even more. Senge (1990, pp. 200-202) suggests that the competency of dialogue requires that people should follow 4 guidelines:

1. When advocating, clarify your own reasoning and encourage others to ask questions that explore how you arrived at a particular position. Encourage others to provide different views.
2. When inquiring, ask others to explain their assumptions and how they arrived at their conclusions. If you are making assumptions of your own about others' views, state your assumptions clearly.
3. If you arrive at an impasse, ask what additional information or logic you and the other parties might need to change your views. Ask if there is some way you might gather additional information.
4. If members are hesitant to express their ideas, encourage them to identify barriers. Design ways of overcoming those barriers.

Collaboration and compromise require high levels of both inquiry and advocacy, as proponents of positions are open and forthcoming about their own positions, and are able to see the other side, which enables them to feel good about compromise or collaboration. Team members who can listen with understanding rather than evaluation and who can accept the feelings of the involved individuals are able to contribute most to collaboration and compromise.

Situational Use of Conflict Management Methods

While collaboration may be a gold standard method of conflict management, its use is not ideal in all situations. Other options are gold standards too, given certain conditions. This is an important point, given the emphasis on collaboration in interprofessional work. Thomas (1977) notes that collaboration has been emphasized as an ideal in the study of organizations and management, and to be uncollaborative is not viewed positively in most settings. Yet behavioral choices surrounding conflict situations are much more complex than the one dimension of collaboration. Thomas notes that the alternatives of competition, compromise, avoidance, and accommodation also are positively viewed in the appropriate circumstances. Competition is associated with energy in the pursuit of excellence. Compromise is a cornerstone of practicality. Avoidance is associated with tranquility, peace, and diplomacy. Accommodation reflects values of humility, kindness, and generosity.

Table 11–3 lists some of the conditions that are suggestive of each of the 5 conflict management methods. Avoidance, while overused, is appropriate for issues that are trivial or require more information or a "cooling down" period before the issue is addressed. Accommodating others may make sense to build trust or to keep the peace when harmony is critical. Competing is useful for quick decisions, requiring a powerful leader or coalition to impose their will. Quick decisions imposed by leaders are critical in healthcare teams facing emergency conditions, particularly if the team members do not know and trust each other, as is the case for many template teams (see Chapter 2). Competing also is useful for distasteful decisions where the options are all unpalatable. Finally, for issues of important principle or moral issues, members may be unwilling to compromise or collaborate, requiring that competitive decision making ensue. For example, competition is often the ultimate way to get decisions made in the legislative arena.

The conditions for collaboration and compromise assure that they frequently are the clear preferences for managing team conflicts, however. Collaboration is needed when gaining commitment and is important to merge insights from people with different perspectives (Table 11–3). Such is usually the case with interprofessional team conflicts. Compromise is called for when differing goals are strongly held by equally powerful parties, and when the parties are not willing to collaborate or collaboration efforts have failed.

Managing Relationship Conflict

As stated in Chapter 7, all team members need basic competencies in managing conflict. This is particularly useful in the case of relationship conflict, as the conflict generally can be handled offline (outside the team) by the parties involved, rather than taking away from the team's work time. In the case of task or process conflict, members' knowledge and skills in conflict management make the team resolution process more efficient.

Table 11-3. Conditions for application of conflict management methods

Conflict Management Method	Conditions for Application
Avoiding	When an issue is trivial, or more important issues are pressing When you perceive no chance of satisfying your concerns When potential disruption outweighs the benefits of resolution To let people cool down and regain perspective When gathering information supersedes immediate decision making When others can resolve the conflict more effectively When issues seem tangential or symptomatic of other issues
Accommodating	When you find you are wrong—to allow a better position to be heard, to learn, and to show your reasonableness When issues are more important to others than yourself—to satisfy others and maintain cooperation To build social credits for later issues To minimize loss when you are outmatched and losing When harmony and stability are especially important To allow others to develop by learning from mistakes
Collaborating	To find an integrative solution when both sets of concerns are too important to be compromised When your objective is to learn To merge insights from people with different perspectives To gain commitment by incorporating concerns into a consensus To work through feelings that have interfered with a relationship
Compromising	When goals are important, but not worth the effort or potential disruption of more assertive methods When opponents with equal power are committed to mutually exclusive goals To achieve temporary settlements to complex issues To arrive at expedient solutions under time pressure As a backup when collaboration or competition is unsuccessful
Competing	When quick, decisive action is vital (for example, emergencies) On important issues where unpopular actions need implementing On issues vital to organizational welfare when you know you are right Against people who take advantage of noncompetitive behavior

Source: Adapted from Thomas KW. Toward multi-dimensional values in teaching: the example of conflict behaviors. *Acad Manage Rev.* 1977;2:487.

Team members can address relationship conflict in the 5 ways noted. Avoidance and accommodation of relationship conflict are common, particularly when teams are busy and when members are involved in large numbers of different teams. Personal differences may be ignored in the interest of getting the job done. Most professionals are able to accept working with others whom they personally do not like. They are willing to overlook personal differences in the pursuit of a common vision and goals. With permanent teams, though, personal differences can create lasting fissures, and may need to be addressed by the involved parties. Recall the earlier case of the ED project team in which a receptionist has accused one of the nurses of being lazy. Likely, such as accusation is not easily forgotten or ignored by either of the parties, and it will affect the 2 team members and other team members, who likely have opinions on the issue, in future interactions. Avoidance and accommodation are poor choices for handling it.

Compromise and collaboration are the most constructive ways individual team members can resolve differences. This requires that the involved parties have listening skills, such that they are able to validate the feelings of the other party. Managing one's emotions, and depersonalizing the conflict, are important skills. The parties need to set aside time, inquire and advocate, and reach a compromise or a creative, collaborative agreement. Or, team members can "agree to disagree," pledging not to let their personal agreement interfere with team effectiveness. In fact, "agreeing to disagree" can be labeled a collaborative solution from the standpoint of the team, because both parties feel that their viewpoint has been heard and validated, and they have committed to putting teamwork ahead of relationship problems. In the case of the receptionist-nurse relationship conflict, the team leader may be well advised to meet with the 2 parties and try to reach a collaborative agreement that will prevent future outbursts. The leader could suggest that these 2 parties meet on their own, without the leader. Or, one of the 2 parties may suggest an "air-clearing" meeting with the other, without leader intervention.

Probably most destructive to the team is the competitive approach to relationship conflict, when both parties continue to insist on advocating their own positions. In those cases, strong intervention by a team leader may be necessary. (If the team leader is party to the conflict, the team sponsor may need to be involved.) The team leader gives each party the platform for espousing his or her position, with a goal of establishing the facts. There are always two sides to every story. The leader works on separating facts and feelings. The leader then asks each member to commit to resolving the conflict, and to agree on an action plan. For more intractable conflicts or conflicts that the leader is uncomfortable addressing, an outside mediator can be engaged to go through the same process with the involved parties. In most large organizations, human resources departments provide such services.

In some cases, persistent or multiple relationship conflicts are driven by a particular individual who deliberately engages in behavior that is intimidating, humiliating, or abusive. Individuals who display this behavior pattern are often labeled "difficult." Chapter 17 presents methods for handling these individuals.

Managing Process and Task Conflict

Process and task conflict are team responsibilities, and members who are adroit at conflict management will make sure that important process and task issues make it onto the team's meeting agenda. In fact, these members will look for opportunities to surface issues before the issues create divisiveness or affect patient care or other team goals. This is particularly true, as noted earlier, for task conflict.

Conflict management of task and process issues begins, then, with identification of the issue itself—someone has to realize that parties are in conflict. This amounts to moving from the anticipation stage to the awareness stage. Second, the team needs to decide if the issue is worthy of formal team discussion time. Third, if the answer is yes, leadership must be committed to discussing the issue. Fourth, the issue is put on the team meeting agenda. At the meeting, steps to achieve compromise or collaboration are followed, as outlined earlier, beginning with an open sharing of perspectives on the issue. An action plan for addressing the issue is agreed on, with follow-up monitoring if appropriate. In the case of the weekly meeting issue described in the earlier vignette, a later evaluation of any compromise or collaborative solution would be expected.

Some observers of team processes (Edmondson and Smith, 2006) note that relationship conflict and task and process conflict often become intertwined—impersonal task and process issues intersect with personal issues; cognitive conflict can become intertwined with affective conflict. This can happen because people often attribute unflattering traits and motives to those who disagree with them on substantive issues. It is unrealistic to expect that task and process conflicts can be completely depersonalized. When relationship dynamics do enter a substantive conflict, Edmondson and Smith (2006) notice that (1) people start to repeat the same point over and over, (2) the discussion starts to get personal, and (3) substantive progress halts. For example, if Mr. Nichols in the earlier vignette were to say to Dr. Bristol, "You like to hold meetings because you like being in the limelight," he would be bringing a personal animosity into a conflict over a team process issue (the meeting schedule).

To keep team conflicts as depersonalized as possible, Edmondson and Smith (2006) recommend 3 practices:

1. When you find yourself getting upset with another team member, reflect on your own reactions and reframe the situation in order to cool down. Reframing involves considering that you may be missing important information held by the other party, rather than that the other party is simply wrong.
2. Acknowledge emotional reactions and relationship conflicts.
3. Build long-term trust into relationships so that they can survive temporary upsets.

The overall approach, then, is to be more aware and reflective about individual and team processes, including processes of communication during conflict. Debriefing of discussions, after the fact, in private with the involved parties or with the team as a whole, can help teams learn from critical blowups and emotional exchanges.

IMPROVING CONFLICT MANAGEMENT

Teams faced with levels of conflict that are too low or too high may find it necessary to implement longer-term strategies, ones that go beyond acute intervention around a specific issue. This is particularly important for true teams (see Chapter 2), which have stability of membership over time. The strategies for long-term improvement in conflict management fall into the categories of (1) team redesign and (2) team training.

Redesign of teams can have powerful effects on conflict. In Chapter 12 key design decisions are covered. They include decisions about team goals, membership, size, resources, interdependence, rewards, and norms of behavior. As discussed earlier in this chapter, all of these forces are related to the emergence of conflict. They are the root causes of many conflicts. Teams can be redesigned to raise or to temper levels of conflict. For example, more vocal individuals can be added to the team so that conflicts get surfaced more easily.

Because of the importance of design factors, many teams find it useful to periodically review team goals, priorities, and direction. Such reviews can prevent future conflicts from emerging. Evaluation of decision-making processes and delegation decisions can have a similar effect. Assessments can be automatically scheduled every 6 months or less, depending on team permanence. Particular attention should be paid to role clarification whenever changes to roles are made. Review of norms for discussion, including the need to respect the viewpoints of others, may be necessary periodically. In extreme instances, redesign can include removal of a team member who creates unproductive conflict or who is unable to manage conflict situations constructively.

Training on team processes or conflict management can improve the ability of teams to manage conflict, after the teams are designed appropriately. Training a team that has a design problem is counterproductive, as the root cause is not addressed. Training interventions could include the team building activities noted in Chapter 15. Teams interested in generating constructive conflict have an array of techniques available. These are summarized in Chapter 9, dealing with team decision making. They include constructive controversy, assignment of a devil's advocate, encouragement of minority viewpoints, and negative brainstorming.

Teams can directly discuss members' attitudes toward conflict and can work on communication techniques to keep discussions focused on solutions and away from relationship conflict. These techniques include delayed responding, listening for understanding, and respectfully summarizing contributions of others (Runde and Flanagan, 2010).

Self-awareness of conflict management style is useful for every team member. Some members may lack self-awareness as well as skills in handling conflict. Self-awareness can be increased by soliciting feedback or giving feedback on conflict management style in private or team discussions. Formal instruments to assess conflict management style are available from a variety of sources; these can form the basis for private feedback or team discussion. Two popular instruments are the Thomas-Kilmann Conflict Mode Instrument, which classifies mode by the 5 methods discussed in this chapter (avoiding, accommodating, collaborating, compromising, and competing), and the Kraybill Conflict Style Inventory, which identifies 5 slightly different styles (avoiding, harmonizing, cooperating, compromising, and directing). Some individuals have a particularly hard time participating in collaborative conflict management due to their highly competitive personalities. Off-site training for individual team members to enhance their ability to manage conflict is called for in some situations. Sometimes this is disparagingly referred to as "sending someone off to charm school." As with any form of behavior associated with deep-seated personality traits, change in conflict management style is difficult. But most people can learn new behavioral patterns that improve interactions in teams. It is worth a try for teams that cannot remove individuals from interdependent roles.

CONCLUSION

Improving conflict management in teams is a high-leverage intervention to increase team effectiveness, because frequently team members (1) avoid conflict and (2) do not have well-developed inquiry and advocacy skills. Moreover, team members often are unaware that they can improve their competence at conflict management.

On interprofessional healthcare teams, conflict or the potential for conflict is ubiquitous due to differing professional perspectives, limitations on resources, status differences, and task interdependence. Conflicts can involve relationship, task, or process issues. Relationship conflict generally inhibits team performance, while reasonable amounts of process and task conflict lead members to feel committed to the team and to clarify goals, roles, and processes. Team members can learn to employ the techniques of avoidance, accommodation, collaboration, compromise, and competition as appropriate, both in individual relationship conflicts and team conflicts. A balance of inquiry into the position of others and advocacy for one's own position is useful for advancing team conflict management. In instances where teams are seriously under- or over-conflicted, intervention in the form of redesign or training is recommended.

REFERENCES

Argyris C, Schön DA. *Organizational Learning II*. Reading, MA: Addison-Wesley; 1996.

Bolman LG, Deal TE. *Reframing Organizations*. 4th ed. San Francisco, CA: Jossey-Bass; 2008.

Canadian Interprofessional Health Collaborative (CIHC). *A National Interprofessional Competency Framework*. Vancouver, BC, Canada: Canadian Interprofessional Health Collaborative; 2010. http://www.aacn.nche.edu/education-resources/IPECReport.pdf. Accessed January 29, 2012.

Drinka TJK, Clark PG. *Health Care Teamwork: Interdisciplinary Practice and Teaching*. Westport, CT: Auburn House; 2000.

Edmondson AC, Smith DL. Too hot to handle? How to manage relationship conflict. *Calif Manage Rev*. 2006;49:6-31.

Fisher R, Ury W. *Getting to Yes: Negotiating Agreement Without Giving In*. Boston, MA: Houghton Mifflin; 1981.

Lencioni P. *The Five Dysfunctions of a Team: A Leadership Fable*. San Francisco, CA: Jossey-Bass; 2002.

Quinn RE, Faerman SR, Thompson MP, et al. *Becoming a Master Manager*. 5th ed. New York, NY: John Wiley & Sons; 2011.

Rahim MA. Toward a theory of managing organizational conflict. *International Journal of Conflict Management*. 2002;13:206-235.

Reay T, Goodrick E, Casebeer A, et al. Legitimizing new practices in primary health care. *Health Care Manage Rev*. 2013;38:9-19.

Runde CE, Flanagan TA. *Developing Your Conflict Competence: A Hands-On Guide for Leaders, Managers, Facilitators, and Teams*. San Francisco, CA: Jossey-Bass; 2010.

Senge PM. *The Fifth Discipline*. New York, NY: Currency Doubleday; 1990.

Skjørshammer M. Co-operation and conflict in a hospital: interprofessional differences in perception and management of conflict. *J Interprof Care*. 2001;15:7-18.

Thomas KW. The conflict-handling modes: toward more precise theory. *Management Communication Quarterly*. 1988;1:430-436.

Thomas KW. Toward multi-dimensional values in teaching: the example of conflict behavior. *Acad Manage Rev*. 1977;2:484-490.

Thompson LL. *Making the Team: A Guide for Managers*. 4th ed. Upper Saddle River, NJ: Prentice Hall; 2011.

West MA. *Effective Teamwork: Practical Lessons from Organizational Research*. 3rd ed. Chichester, UK: John Wiley & Sons, Ltd.; 2012.

Wheelan SA. *Creating Effective Teams: A Guide for Members and Leaders*. 4th ed. Los Angeles, CA: Sage; 2013.

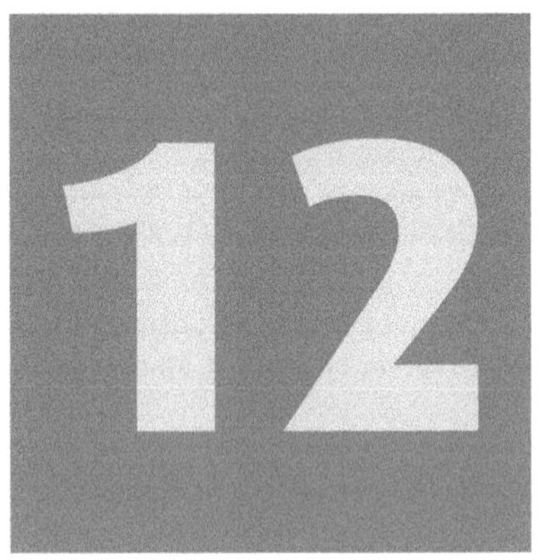

Sponsoring Healthcare Teams

Chapters 8-11 deal with team leadership and topics of particular importance to team leaders. This chapter moves one level higher in the organization to deal with team sponsorship, including the sponsor's most important responsibility, designing teams.

THE LEADER AND THE SPONSOR

As discussed in Chapter 8, the leader of a team creates the enabling conditions for the team, develops the team, and coaches it. But the leader does not create the team. The leader's role comes to life only after the team has been created. And for the team to exist, it must have been designed, that is, the purpose, initial composition, and leader of the team must have been designated by someone (or some committee) who has the authority to create the team. This designer-creator we call the *sponsor*. The sponsor also has functions to perform after the team has been designed, as discussed below.

The interaction between the leader and the sponsor is crucial to the team's success. Their linkage personifies the connection between the team and the larger organization. The leader represents the team in this linkage, and the sponsor represents the larger organization. The leader is accountable to the sponsor, and sponsor has duties of support and guidance to the leader. The leader is obliged to keep the sponsor informed about how the team is faring. The sponsor is obliged to keep the leader informed about conditions in the larger organization and beyond. The 2 roles are closely bound but distinct.

Only in very small organizations does the distinction between leader and sponsor collapse. For example, a freestanding medical practice of 4 urologists, physician assistants, and other staff is a single team. The team is the whole organization, and so the leader of the medical practice fulfills not only the leadership functions but also the sponsorship functions. If the urologists, physician assistants, and others were a department in a medical group, the sponsor would be another person in the larger medical group.

THE TEAM SPONSOR'S ROLE

The word *sponsor* has a variety of meanings in discussions of teams and management in general. Sometimes the word is used to imply that the sponsor provides funding for an endeavor. Sometimes the word is meant to imply that the sponsor represents the interests of a team or project within the circle of senior leadership in the organization. And sometimes someone is labeled *sponsor* because she or he has taken responsibility for an initiative or some other project. In contrast to all of these uses, we use the word *sponsor* to designate the person who supervises the leader. Yet, to say that the sponsor is the leader's supervisor is not quite accurate because the sponsor does not oversee, direct, or inspect the leader except in a very general way. The team sponsor's role is more similar to that of a coach or authoritative adviser than it is to the role of a conventional supervisor.

So, what does a sponsor, defined in this way, do? There are 3 elements to the role: (1) design the team, including the team's purpose and a few other key features; (2) evaluate the performance of the team; and (3) guide the team over time, normally by guiding the leader. These tasks are listed in Table 12–1.

Table 12–1. Tasks for team sponsors

1. Design the team
2. Evaluate the performance of the team
3. Guide the team

COMPETENCIES FOR TEAM SPONSORS

The 3 elements of the team sponsor's role serve well as categories of competencies for team sponsors. In order to design a team well, a sponsor must be able to establish its purpose, designate the composition of the team, and select a leader. Similarly, various competencies are necessary for effective evaluation and guidance of teams. When the team leader is performing well, many of the sponsor's functions are not performed by the sponsor alone. In these situations, effective sponsor-leader pairs take many of these actions jointly. The competencies for team sponsors are shown in Table 12–2.

Designing the Team

Sheamus Doyle, MD, was an ENT surgeon (ear, nose, and throat surgeon) at Clarkdale Clinic, a large referral center that attracted patients with unusual medical problems from across the western half of the United States. He often saw patients referred for vertigo, a particular form of dizziness. Arriving at a diagnosis and treatment plan for these patients usually requires the participation of an audiologist. Dr. Doyle worked with audiologists daily; they were regular collaborators. However, occupational therapists, neurologists, neurosurgeons, and radiologists were also needed for some patients, and bringing together these other professionals was more difficult because they were located in other departments, whose schedules and priorities were different from those of the ENT Department. Dr. Doyle thought it would be useful to establish a Vertigo Clinic.

He explored his idea with many other people at Clarkdale, and eventually the idea was presented to the Clinical Services Committee of the medical center, which included the Chief Medical Officer (CMO), Chief Operating Officer, and the heads of the major clinical departments. The idea was well received, and soon the Committee considered the question of where the Vertigo Clinic should be placed in the organization's management structure. The Committee decided that the new Clinic should be accountable to the Chief of Surgery, who was responsible for all surgical services. Alternatively, the Clinic might have been accountable to one or another of several people, including the CMO and the Chief of ENT Surgery. Part of the rationale for the choice of the Chief of Surgery was the rivalry between neurosurgery and ENT surgery in performing certain surgical procedures. The overall Chief of Surgery was well placed to manage any conflicts that might arise from this rivalry.

Yang Liu, MD, Chief of Surgery, was authorized by the Clinical Services Committee to establish the Vertigo Clinic. Not surprisingly, he appointed Dr. Doyle as its leader. Dr. Doyle was paired with an administrator to establish and run the Clinic. Together Dr. Liu and Dr. Doyle decided whom to invite to be members of the team: Dr. Doyle himself, a neurologist, a neurosurgeon, an audiologist, an occupational therapist, a physical therapist, a nurse with long experience in ENT, and the administrator for the new Clinic. These 8 people formed the new team. Dr. Doyle and Dr. Liu decided that a radiologist was not needed as a member of the team although most patients would have imaging studies done to investigate the causes of their symptoms. The team members would ordinarily be the ones to see the patients, but other clinicians would also work in the Clinic.

Table 12–2. Competencies for team sponsors

Design the team
1. Set the task
2. Establish the composition of the team
3. Appoint the team leader
Evaluate the performance of the team
1. Clarify the team's goals
2. Collect information
3. Assess performance against the team's goals and the characteristics of an effective team
Guide the team
1. Maintain a functional relationship with the team leader
2. Provide information and advice in keeping with the team's performance

Drs. Liu and Doyle also set the purpose of the Clinic. They decided to charge the team with diagnosing the causes of patients' vertigo and formulating treatments plans but not with providing treatment. They would refer patients elsewhere for treatment, sometimes to the ENT Department, sometimes to Neurosurgery, sometimes to Neurology, sometimes to Adult Medicine (primary care). Although the topic of decision making never discussed, Dr. Doyle understood that he was to use consensus for team making decisions. This model was routinely used at Clarkdale, and the use of strong central authority or voting did not even occur to Dr. Liu or Dr. Doyle.

Drs. Liu and Doyle jointly designed this new team although the final authority, assigned by the Clinical Services Committee, rested with Dr. Liu. The process of establishing the new clinic illustrates the components of designing a team.

Is a Team Needed?

Before a team is designed, someone must determine whether a team is actually needed. In the case of the Vertigo Clinic, this question was addressed by the Clinical Services Committee at Clarkdale Clinic. Clarkdale had been operating for decades without a Vertigo Clinic. Dr. Doyle proposed the formation of this new team, but was it really needed? Maybe a better choice would be to continue providing services for people with vertigo through the various relevant clinical departments without creating any new team. How should this decision be made?

As mentioned in Chapter 1, some tasks are not suitable for teams (Hackman, 2002, pp. 43-44). For example, novels, poetry, and symphonies are properly written by individuals. Authors and composers may request critiques by other people, but they do not partner with them in the creative work. Other tasks outside of the art world are also suitable for individuals to perform, for example, creating a vision for a new children's museum, crafting a proposal for the governance structure for a new philanthropic foundation, or designing buildings in a new architectural style. Individuals also perform better than teams in other less lofty tasks such as writing task force reports, political speeches, and book chapters. All of these tasks call for taking partially formed thoughts or dimly recognized feelings, synthesizing them, and expressing the newly formed ideas by using words, sound, or various visual means such as diagrams or sculpture. These are tasks that are performed well only within a single mind.

Individual effort is also appropriate for tasks that consist of decision making under time pressure and conditions of high uncertainty. When many factors pertain to a decision and these factors cannot be quantified, 2 (or more) people are likely to disagree or to make a joint decision only after long deliberation—even if their knowledge and values are very similar. Nonetheless, in some situations, a decision cannot be avoided and must be made in a short period of time. In these situations, a single decision maker is needed. Company presidents, political leaders, and military officers are examples of people who perform individual tasks of this second kind.

In contrast, a team is appropriate to a task when several individuals are needed to contribute expertise in different areas and to collaborate to achieve a goal. It is suitable for a team, rather than an individual, to perform a task if the task has both of the characteristics listed in Table 12–3:

1. To achieve the goal, the work must be done by individuals who possess knowledge and skills in different areas.
2. To achieve the goal, those individuals must work together interdependently, that is, as the work progresses, each individual must adjust what he or she does in response to what is done by other individuals.

A task that meets this twofold test has met the minimum requirements for a task that is appropriate for a team. However, in order for the task to be highly appropriate for a team to pursue, it must have some additional characteristics, as discussed below.

The Vertigo Clinic met the minimal test of appropriateness for teamwork. Diagnosing and treating people with vertigo requires people with knowledge and expertise in different healthcare fields, so the first requirement was fulfilled. Dr. Doyle's efforts to create the team were triggered by his observation that

Table 12–3. Characteristics of a task suitable for a team to perform

The task requires different areas of knowledge and skill
Contributors need to work interdependently

achieving successful interaction of the different clinicians was very difficult under the prevailing arrangements. He sought to create a team so that the interdependent action of the various parties would flow more effectively and efficiently.

Having established that a team would be useful, one must also answer the question of whether the expense of the team is justified. Using a team is sometimes more expensive than having the work done by individuals working with lower levels of collaboration. More administrative time may be required if a team is created. Clinicians' schedules may go unfilled if they spend time in a disease-specific clinic where open appointment slots cannot be used to serve patients with other problems. The person or committee deciding whether to establish a new clinical team needs to consider these financial issues as well as the question of whether a team would add benefits for the patients. Similar questions arise when considering whether to form new management teams.

Setting the Task

The sponsor needs to be able to delineate a task that will engage the team in performing well. Simply stating a task clearly is not sufficient. The task needs to have certain characteristics in order to be motivating. For many clinical teams, the task consists of providing clinical care; it is obvious, motivating, and requires no discussion. For management teams, the selection and clear delineation of the task is usually more difficult, for example, when the task is the formulation of a business strategy or the improvement of an equipment procurement process.

The team's task needs to be significant in the eyes of the team members; and for the task to have this significance, the goal needs to be a complete piece of work (Hackman, 2002, pp. 95-105). For many tasks, doing part of the task is not sufficiently gratifying to the team members to motivate them or even to keep the team intact. For example, sorting surgical instruments to be sterilized is a poorly chosen task. Bundling this task together with related tasks, for example, sterilizing the instruments and assembling surgical equipment packs, enables the people doing the work to have a sense that they are contributing to good surgical care in some way that they regard as important.

The task also needs to be defined so that the team can have autonomy in pursuing its goal. If the team has this autonomy, it is more likely to experience a sense of responsibility for the outcomes of the team's work. Without this autonomy, the team may pull back psychologically, feeling that success in achieving its goal is driven by forces outside of its control. For example, a team that handles bed assignments for patients entering a hospital may disengage from their task if their decisions are repeatedly overridden by physicians or nurses who redirect patients from one area of the hospital to another to balance out workloads or simply for their convenience.

And the task needs to be designed so that the team's output can be evaluated. Of course, receiving feedback about progress and results enables the team to improve its performance. But the more fundamental consideration in task design is that feedback enables team members to know whether what they are producing is worthwhile. If they cannot answer this question for themselves, they are unlikely to be engaged for long. Team members have a need to know not only whether their particular task is completed but also whether they are producing value. Sometimes this need is met by making the task larger than first envisioned so that team members are involved in the process long enough to see the benefits of their efforts. For example, it might be tempting to move hospital nurses from ward to ward depending on immediate staffing needs. However, keeping nurses in the same ward most of the time enables them to follow patients through their hospital stays and to see their patients' short-term outcomes.

Ideally, the task also affords opportunities for team members and the whole team to deepen their knowledge and learn new skills (West, 2012, p. 30). Teams that provide these opportunities are likely to be more engaged and more enduring than teams that do not.

Drs. Liu and Doyle set the task for the Vertigo Clinic. (They set the task after they decided the team's composition, but the order could have been reversed.) The general nature of the task for the Clinic was clear without any discussion. The Clinic was intended to provide clinical service to people with vertigo. However, making the task explicit led to a realization that there was a choice to be made. The Clinic could provide diagnostic services only, or it could also provide treatment. Dr. Liu decided that the goal should be limited to diagnosis and treatment planning. A major factor in his thinking was the political risk that would be incurred if the Clinic also provided treatment. The head of the Clinic was going to be an ENT surgeon, Dr. Doyle. If the

Vertigo Clinic provided treatment, it might be regarded by the neurosurgeons as a biased mechanism for routing surgical cases to the ENT Department or perhaps to Dr. Doyle himself. Having the Clinic refer patients for treatment would mean that referrals would be distributed impartially unless the patient's clinical characteristics called for a particular surgeon or other physician. The pattern of referrals could be easily audited if questions arose. A question to be considered here was whether stopping with diagnosis and planning made the team's task too small to be regarded as significant in the eyes of the team members. Without any discussion, Drs. Liu and Doyle both knew that this task was substantial enough.

Establishing the Composition of the Team

The sponsor needs to be able to specify the initial composition of the team. Establishing the composition requires considering the technical knowledge and skills needed among the members, the teamwork competencies needed in the team, diversity within the team (of age, educational backgrounds, personality, and so on), and the size of the team (Hackman, 2002, pp. 115-129).

Knowledge and Skill: Technical knowledge and skill are obvious requirements in any healthcare team. Both Dr. Doyle and Dr. Liu knew that the team needed an ENT surgeon, a neurosurgeon, and a few others with well-defined capabilities. There was a question about whether a radiologist was needed as a direct team member, but this was quickly resolved. Settling these issues is ordinarily quite straightforward for clinical teams. For management teams, the decisions are often less clear. For example, a project team charged with investigating the feasibility of a new heart care center in a hospital could include a wide range of management personnel and clinical specialists. For both clinical and management teams, the key to determining the necessary skill mix is the nature of the work the team is expected to do.

Teamwork Competencies: In sharp contrast to technical skills, teamwork competencies are often ignored in composing clinical teams. Every team needs to have some members who are adept at working in teams. Without these competencies, the team is likely to have difficulty organizing its work, settling relationship conflicts, making durable decisions, and carrying out many other tasks. If it can be envisioned that one or more of the team members is especially incompetent at working in teams and is likely to be disruptive, the need for other qualified people is even more important. It is the responsibility of the sponsor, working with the leader, to assure that the proposed team membership will provide enough teamwork competencies for the team to function well. If not, someone tentatively chosen for the team because of certain technical skills may need to be dropped in favor of someone who has those skills as well as teamwork competencies. Of course, teamwork competencies are also important for management teams. But here there is ordinarily less difficulty in meeting the need since managers have commonly acquired some degree of facility in teamwork through their education or experience.

Diversity: Diversity within the team also needs to be considered. Some age diversity appears to improve team performance, but there is some evidence that extreme age diversity results in instability, that is, in higher rates of members leaving the team (West, 2012, p. 56). Diversity of educational backgrounds within a single profession may be helpful in some clinical teams, especially when the approach to patients with a given condition cannot be evidence-based because evidence is lacking and different approaches are taught in different medical schools, nursing schools, or other professional schools. Diversity of history in working together, however, is often undesirable in healthcare production teams (for example, emergency cesarean delivery teams) since teams composed of people who have worked together in the past perform established tasks better than teams composed of people new to each other, as discussed in Chapter 2. On the other hand, in teams that do creative work, some diversity of history in working together is beneficial, as discussed in Chapter 10.

Consideration of cultural and ethnic diversity is more complex. Cultural and ethnic diversity results in diversity of perspective, which boosts creativity in both clinical and management teams, as discussed in Chapter 10. However, for the purpose of assuring smooth internal operations of a team, a low level of cultural diversity is useful. Still, for clinical teams this consideration is fairly unimportant. The values and roles of clinicians are fully and firmly instilled during education and training, as discussed in Chapter 3. These values and roles are reasonably uniform within any single profession, and they tend to override differences in the clinicians' ethnicity or country of origin. In management teams, ethnic diversity may carry more risk for smooth operations. Seeking a balance between no diversity and extreme diversity would appear to be prudent because some degree of diversity fosters creativity, while too much diversity slows down decision making and development within the team (Hackman, 2002, pp. 122-124; Watson et al, 1993). And yet, one must also consider the population of patients served. A clinical team that serves a diverse patient population will be more effective if the team is also diverse, that is, if the team has diversity in race, language, and ethnicity that approximates the diversity in the patient population. Diversity would also benefit the administrative team of a healthcare institution serving a diverse population. Several different factors need to be considered in determining the extent of cultural and ethnic diversity that will be most suitable for a new team.

In many circles in health care, diversity of personality is believed to contribute to improved team performance. Self-administered questionnaires can be used by team members to characterize their behavioral styles and personality traits. There are many profiling tools available, including StrengthsFinder, Insights Discovery, DiSC, and the Myers-Briggs Type Indicator (MBTI). These tools are discussed in Chapter 15; they are often used in team building. Having a mix of personality types represented on the team, as determined by one or another of the profiling questionnaires, is thought by some to bring benefit by assuring that many different cognitive approaches and behavioral dispositions are put to use, resulting in heightened creativity, improved decision making, and better team performance. While it is plausible that teams would benefit from balance across different personality types, there is no evidence to support this belief (West, 2012, pp. 43-45, 55).

Team Size: Team size is a consideration of paramount importance, in large part because sponsors (and leaders) almost routinely err on the side of making teams too large. Adding more members to a clinical team can be tempting because more skills will be immediately available for performing the task. In the case of management teams, sometimes many people or departments seek representation on the team so that their interests can be protected or advanced. Keeping teams small is often difficult, but there are strong reasons for holding the line.

First, interpersonal relationships, coordination, and communication become more cumbersome as the size of the team increases. The number of dyadic (2-person) interpersonal relationships in a team increases geometrically as the size of the team increases (Figure 12–1). A team of 6 has 15 interpersonal relationships (15 different pairs of people). A team of 15 has 105 relationships.

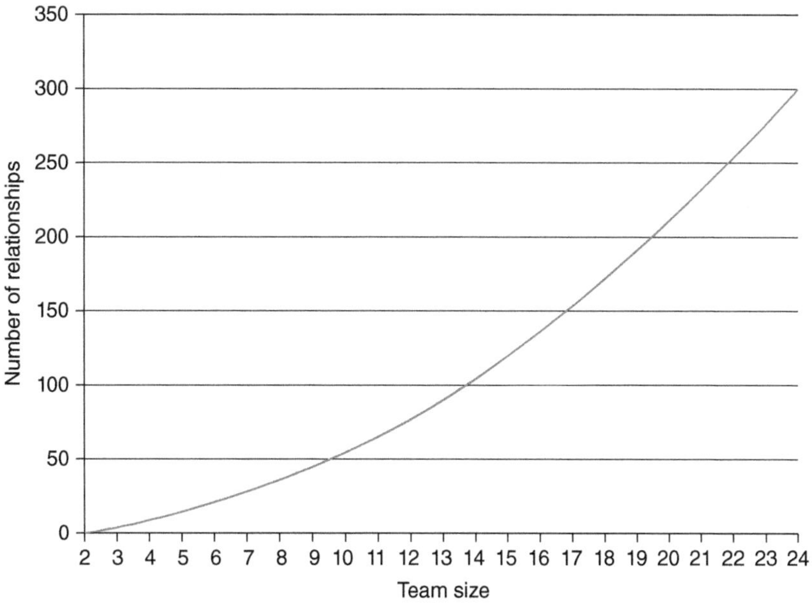

Figure 12–1. Effect of team size on number of dyadic interpersonal relationships.

Also, as team size increases, meetings become more difficult to schedule, meeting space becomes harder to find, and communication becomes more burdensome and less reliable.

Second, a large team has more difficulty functioning internally. It struggles more to achieve a common understanding of its purpose, to reach agreement, and to make decisions in general (Katzenbach and Smith, 2006, pp. 45-47). Large teams are more susceptible to groupthink (McCauley, 1998). They also experience disruptive relationship conflicts more often (Aubé et al, 2011). Because of these difficulties, they are vulnerable to establishing a hierarchy within the team, with subgroups operating independently of the whole—thus ceasing to be work teams and becoming instead small organizations of their own with policies and procedures replacing team decision making.

Third, the quality of deliberation deteriorates in teams larger than about 12. In teams of 12 or fewer, rapid, detailed analytical discussion is possible, enabling the team to consider multiple options carefully when they are making decisions. In larger teams, members are more likely to interrupt each other. Humorous critical remarks, even sarcastic remarks, are more common. Relationships are less immediately personal, and members are more likely to disrupt teamwork by jockeying for position in the informal status hierarchy of the team. These behavioral effects of larger team size make complex analysis and weighing of choices more difficult.

Fourth, larger groups are more prone to social loafing, as discussed in Chapter 1.

So, what size is best for a team? At the lower end, by definition, a team must have at least 2 members. With regard to the upper bound, different researchers give different answers. Although Hackman stated that teams can have various sizes, his short answer to the question was that ordinarily the best size is about 6 members (2002, p. 119). West says teams should generally have 6 to 8 members and rarely more than 15 (2012, pp. 28, 65). Katzenbach and Smith accept higher numbers, saying that teams can have 2 to 25 members (2006, p. 45). Thompson says that as a rule teams should have 9 or fewer members (2011, p. 35).

Of course, there is no single best size. The size of the team needs to correspond to the needs of the team. Some teams require more members because they require a wider variety of skills. Organizational politics sometimes dictate that several constituencies must be represented. Sometimes management teams, for example, planning teams, need to be able to proceed very quickly, necessitating very small teams of, say, 3-4 people. There is no general rule for determining team size, but team sponsors will be well served by remembering that "small is beautiful" and that the best size for a team is commonly smaller than the size first considered. If a team needs to be larger than 10 or 12 for political reasons or so that people with the necessary skills can be included, the sponsor (as well as the leader) needs to be aware that the team will have more difficulty in deliberation, in making decisions, and in other ways and that these difficulties will increase as the size of the team increases. If the size is more than 25 members, the team will not be functional. Below that size, skillful leadership and chairing of meetings can mitigate some of the difficulties.

In the vignette about the Vertigo Clinic, Dr. Liu, with Dr. Doyle's agreement, decided that the Clinic team would have 8 members (7 clinicians and an administrator), a workable number of members. He was aware that more than 7 clinicians would see patients in the Clinic, and Dr. Liu might have been tempted to include 2 ENT surgeons, 2 neurosurgeons, and so on. This would have been a mistake because the team would have become too large. Keeping the decision-making body for the Clinic to 8 members was characteristic of a good team designer.

Dr. Liu's possible temptation raises a final issue concerning team size. Some large groups appear to be teams when a sub-group is the actual team. The surgical intensive care unit (ICU) team described in Chapter 6 illustrates this point. The team consisted of the senior surgeon, the surgical residents and several others, including medical students. Someone observing the group on rounds might regard the whole group as a team, but in fact the medical students were not team members. Alternatively, one might say that they were peripheral or secondary members. In establishing many teams in health care, it is important to distinguish the *core members* from *peripheral members*. Core members can rightfully expect to participate in all team activities including, in particular, decision making. Peripheral members do not have the same rights although they usually participate in some activities and may be consulted about decisions. In the case of the surgical ICU, the medical students were peripheral members because of their lower status. In the Vertigo Clinic, the designated ENT surgeon, neurosurgeon, and so on constituted the team's core membership (8 people in total). The other clinicians seeing patients in the Clinic were peripheral members of the team even though their status was the same in the larger organization as the status of those on the team. The rationale for considering them to be peripheral rather than core members was that the team needed to be kept small in order to function well in managing the Clinic. Dr. Doyle expected the neurosurgeon in the core team to confer with any other neurosurgeons working in the Clinic when the team considered any decision that would affect the neurosurgeons significantly. And he expected the same of the neurologist, occupational therapist, and others as they related to other Vertigo Clinic clinicians in their respective fields.

Appointing the Team Leader

As part of designing the team, the sponsor also needs to be able to select an effective leader. As discussed in Chapter 8, the primary qualification to be a team leader is the possession of the competencies needed by leaders. In other words, the leader needs to be able to establish the conditions that enable the team to function well, to develop the team, and to provide coaching for team members about how they perform as team members.

As also discussed in Chapter 8, in a clinical true team the leader's particular clinical skill set is not relevant, and the leader need not be a physician, a nurse, or any other individual identified by his or her particular healthcare profession. (In contrast, as also discussed in Chapter 8, a clinical template team leader does not have the customary role of a team leader. A clinical template team leader is an operational manager, and some template teams require leaders who have a particular profession in order for them to be able to direct the operations of the team.) Regardless of her or his profession, the leader needs to garner the respect of the other team members, and normally this requires the leader of a clinical team to exhibit excellence in his or her clinical role, whatever that role may be. However, a mistake commonly made in choosing a clinical leader is to regard excellence in clinical performance as the foremost requirement for being a leader. Thus some superb physicians, nurses, and other clinicians are appointed leaders of their teams even though they cannot lead. Such appointments lower team performance, and eventually they usually cause distress for the leader as well as the others on the team. Despite these risks, the sponsor is sometimes severely restricted in selecting the leader because very few people (maybe only one) want to serve in the leadership role and have the necessary level of respect in the eyes of the other team members. In these situations, the appointment of the leader amounts to confirming a choice dictated by circumstances.

In management teams, of course, this confusion of clinical excellence with leadership excellence is not a problem. In management teams too, what matters is the leader's ability to lead.

Sponsors should consider a candidate's formal education relevant to leadership, but the possession of a management degree does not assure effective leadership. Many physicians, for example, earn Master of Business Administration degrees or other management degrees; and while the subject matter studied in the degree programs is helpful, it is not sufficient to make someone an effective leader. Most clinical leaders do not have management degrees, and they are not required. On the other hand, some experience in leadership positions, even in very limited roles such as chairing a committee or leading a time-limited project, is ordinarily necessary.

Personal attractiveness or charisma also is not necessary. Some experts on leadership argue, in fact, that the most effective leaders are not charismatic but are instead humble and self-effacing while also being extremely determined (Collins, 2005). Others would say that charisma is useful but not essential.

In short, a team leader needs to be able to lead. In assessing whether someone will be a suitable leader, sponsors can usefully consider whether the candidate has the competencies needed by a leader, discussed in Chapter 8. These competencies, listed under the headings of enabling, developing, and coaching, constitute a checklist for use in assessing potential leaders (Table 12–4). Not all potential leaders will have strength in all of the competencies listed. Often, in fact, especially when designing clinical teams, the best choice for a leader is deficient with respect to some or even many leadership functions. In that case, the burden of coaching is higher for the sponsor. Organized courses can also be useful, as discussed in Chapter 14. Many clinicians, however, do not have the time to pursue leadership courses or do not want to take the time. In that case, the sponsor needs to provide the necessary training informally or arrange for it. Unfortunately, finding the time to carry out this function is difficult for many sponsors.

Table 12-4. Checklist of competencies needed in a team leader

Enable the team

1. Establish and maintain a clear, common understanding of the team's goal
2. Establish shared responsibility, or, better yet, mutual accountability for achieving the goal
3. Assure that the team has sufficient authority to do its work
4. Establish interdependency of members
5. Assure defined membership for the team
6. Keep the team unified, that is, assure that there are no subgroups operating independently of the whole
7. Relate effectively to the team's sponsor and to the larger organization

Develop the team

1. Oversee recruitment, orientation, and team formation
2. Establish the team's values and behavior norms
3. Assure a common understanding of the team's approach to doing its work
4. Maintain sufficient hierarchy for the team to achieve its goal—and no more
5. Foster team identity
6. Assure a favorable social climate, including psychological safety
7. Assure that the team can carry out team-level operations effectively

Coach the team

1. Gather information on the performance of the team and individual team members
2. Evaluate performance
3. Provide feedback and advice

In appointing the leader, the sponsor must also make clear what means of decision making is acceptable, that is, whether the team is to operate using strong central authority or consensus or some other means for making decisions, as discussed in Chapter 9. The leader and the team may refine the basic approach over time, for example, using consensus most of the time but strong central authority in certain situations. However, the sponsor needs to let the leader know in general terms whether she or he expects the team to function using strong central authority or unanimous agreement or some means on the continuum between the two. Because of strong precedents at Clarkdale Clinic, Drs. Liu and Doyle assumed that the Vertigo Clinic would use consensus as its primary decision-making mode. In many senior management teams, the default mode is strong central authority with the team leader seeking extensive consultation with other team members. Sponsors and leaders often do not need to discuss this choice when a new management team is established because this approach is well established in the organization.

Self-managing teams, which are explained in Chapter 8, require the sponsor to take a different approach. If the team will be self-managing, no conventional leader is needed. In self-managing teams, the sponsor is the leader, but the sponsor does not function like an ordinary team leader because he or she does not interact with the other team members on a day-to-day basis. In establishing a self-managing team, the sponsor needs, first, to inform the team members of the goal and the initial membership of the team and, then, to make clear what authority the team has. For example, the sponsor might tell the team that it is authorized only to determine the means for achieving the goal. Or the sponsor might say that the team is also authorized to alter the team's composition or to modify the goal or both. It is normally assumed that decisions within a self-managing team will be made by consensus. After a self-managing team is established, the sponsor needs to follow its progress and provide guidance as he or she would for any other team.

Other Design Considerations

Team performance is influenced by design considerations in addition to the task, composition of the team, and choice of the leader. In particular, the reward system used and the values and behavior norms of the team have substantial effects on performance. These considerations are not discussed here because they are not primarily the responsibility of the sponsor. The reward system is usually set for the organization as a whole, that is, by leaders who are senior to the sponsor. The development of values and norms is part of the role of the leader. Still, the sponsor often has influence in both of these areas. The degree of influence varies by organization. In many organizations in which sponsor-leader relationships function well, the sponsor has substantial influence on how the leader establishes values and norms in the team. In very small organizations, for example, nurse-managed practices of 4-5 advanced practice nurses, the roles of the senior leader, sponsor, and team leader are commonly exercised by one person or by a committee of the whole, and so there is no assignment to different people of the responsibilities for setting the task, composing the team, establishing the reward system, and so on.

Design Requirements for Different Types of Teams

Although all teams need to have a specified task or goal, a defined initial composition, and a leader (or authorization to self-manage), the task of designing a team varies significantly depending on the type of team. (See Chapter 2 for an explanation of team types.)

True Teams: As explained in Chapter 2 (Table 2–1 in Chapter 2), true teams are stable teams. In other words, the individuals who comprise the team remain the same over long periods of time. Nearly all healthcare teams have a clear leader who participates in the day-to-day work of the team. In other words, self-managing clinical teams and self-managing management teams are unusual. If there is a clear leader, the design of the team follows straightforwardly the process described earlier. A minor change in the usual sequence is needed for self-managing teams, as indicated earlier.

A true team is a *clinical microsystem.* As defined by Batalden and colleagues, "A healthcare clinical microsystem is a small group of people who work together in a defined setting on a regular basis to create care for discrete sub-populations of patients" (Batalden et al, 2011, p. 3). Construing teams as microsystems encourages thinking of a team as a *system*, that is, as a functional unit whose parts interact to achieve the goal of the unit. The parts of the microsystem include the healthcare professionals, the patient, and the patient's family but also the information system, role definitions, communication routines, and care delivery processes. Microsystems are the building blocks from which clinics, hospitals, and all other healthcare delivery organizations are constructed. Thinking of a true team as a microsystem encourages the designers and developers of the team to pay attention to process engineering and continual improvement of the system. At the same time, the sponsor and leader need to view the team as a social enterprise with values, norms, interpersonal relationships, conflicts, and collective creative challenges that also need attention.

Template Teams: Designing template teams differs from designing true teams. For example, when the leadership in an emergency department (ED) designs a new template team to care for, say, patients with open head injuries, the designers are not appointing a particular person to be the leader or selecting individuals to be team members. Instead, they are defining the roles that comprise a template team, for example, a nurse in sterile surgical clothing to assist with immediate attention to the patient's head wound, a nurse in standard ED clothing to place an intravenous line and perform other tasks, an ED physician, a neurosurgeon, and so on. They may decide that the ED physician will routinely be the leader, or may leave this designation to the participating ED physician and neurosurgeon to decide each time a new head trauma template team is assembled. They will probably go further in specifying the means to be used in caring for the patient than would the designer of a true team. Template teams usually have little time to devise their own processes, and so it is useful for designers to specify routines for the first steps in care and for the communication of crucial information. For example, the designers may require the use of check-backs (discussed in Chapter 2) and other standardized communication procedures that are discussed in Chapter 14. These specifications of means go beyond the steps taken by the sponsor of a true team. As a consequence of the specifications, template teams are more rigid than true teams, and occasionally this rigidity may be a problem. Nonetheless, the roles and routines of template teams need to be reliable because the individuals comprising the teams change.

The designers of healthcare template teams are commonly not individual sponsors. More often they are pairs of people (for example, administrator-physician leadership dyads) or committees. In other words, the sponsors of template teams are often teams themselves.

A particularly important design consideration for template teams is the desirability of stable teams. In other words, sponsors should consider seriously and repeatedly how they can make their template teams more like true teams. When whole template teams can be scheduled instead of scheduling individuals into template teams, this approach should be used. When the pool from which template teams are assembled can be decreased in size, resulting in the same people working together more frequently, the pool should be decreased. Of course, a host of practical considerations will usually prevent sponsors from taking these actions; but when the opportunities arise, they should be taken. For example, if 4-person groups, each consisting of a scrub nurse, a circulating nurse, and 2 surgical technicians, can be kept intact to form the core of operating room teams, the teams will perform better—even if the surgeon and anesthesiologist are different each time the team assembles.

Another important difference between true teams and template teams becomes apparent when the original design is reviewed with the intention of improving it. Briefly, true teams improve their own designs, subject to oversight or approval by the sponsor. In contrast, template teams do not improve themselves because they do not persist long enough to pursue improvement and may never again be assembled with the same people comprising the team. Template teams are improved by the sponsoring person or committee or, more commonly, by a quality improvement project team that is chartered by the sponsor to make recommendations for changes. To function well in doing redesign work, the project team needs to include people who have been members of the template teams under review. For example, if the composition and routines of a hospital's emergency cesarean delivery teams were to be reviewed and updated, the group doing the work would not be any particular cesarean delivery team but would be instead a project team consisting of an obstetrician, a labor-and-delivery nurse, an administrator, and so on, all working under the aegis of the leadership in the Birth Center of the hospital.

Clinical Knotworks: Ordinarily there is no opportunity to design a clinical knotwork (defined in Chapter 2). Clinical knotworks are formed ad hoc when the needs of a patient require 2 or more individuals in one or more professions to collaborate in the care of the patient, for example, a family physician, neurologist, and health educator caring for a child with epilepsy and for the child's family. The team members make their arrangements in the course of interacting. There is no sponsor, and there is no advance planning. This fact of clinical life fairly often results in difficulties in communication and decision making.

However, any member of the team can take on a portion of the sponsor's role by seeking to clarify roles and communication routines, sometimes negotiating with other knotwork members about these issues. Beyond this avenue for planning simultaneously with the process of providing care, whole organizations can negotiate standard arrangements for working together in clinical knotworks, knowing that they will be forming knotworks in the future. This approach is discussed in Chapter 2. The resulting agreements for knotwork function are called *referral agreements* or *care agreements*. The effect of negotiating these agreements is to make knotworks function more like template teams by standardizing roles and communication routines. Recently the National Committee for Quality Assurance (NCQA) published draft standards for a new specialty practice recognition program (National Committee for Quality Assurance, 2012a, 2012b). Among the draft standards is a set of specifications for regular "referral process agreements" to be used by a specialty practice as it interacts with primary care practices and other specialty practices. These agreements call for explicit standardization of communication processes, including receiving information from a primary care practice for a given referral type and delivery of information back to the primary care practice. (There is no discussion of roles in decision making, long-term expectations for roles, or any other role issues, at least not in the draft standards.) The intent is to shift knotworks of specialty and primary care clinicians in the direction of template teams.

Advancing Team Design up the Design Hierarchy: A general principle emerges from these considerations of design as applied to different clinical team types (Figure 12–2). Since true teams have advantages over

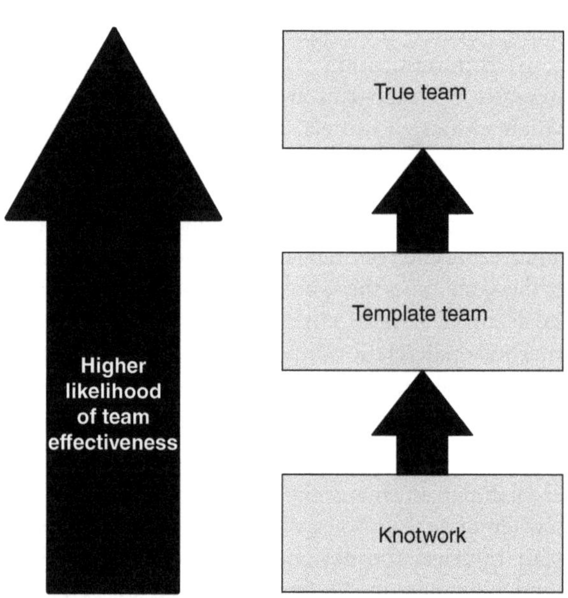

▲ **Figure 12–2.** Clinical team design hierarchy.

template teams and template teams have advantages over knotworks, sponsors and anyone else with influence in the design of clinical teams are well advised, when the opportunity arises, to move any template team in the direction of a true team and to move any knotwork in the direction of a template team and, if possible, to move any knotwork still further so that it takes on characteristics of a true team. For example, an ENT practice might standardize the roles and communication routines it uses when interacting with primary care practices whose physicians refer patients to the ENT practice. Better yet, the ENT and primary care practices might collaborate to establish the standardization. This action would convert unorganized knotworks into template teams. The ENT and primary care practices might then take a further step by pairing primary care physicians permanently with individual ENT surgeons, thus making these pairs stable over time as they would be in a true team.

Clinical Networks: Clinical networks are usually not deliberately designed but instead evolve in response to their members' wants and needs. However, deliberate design is possible. Sometimes 1 or 2 individuals will decide that a network would be useful for sharing clinical knowledge or doing clinical research. They will then craft a statement of the network's purpose and recruit members, maintaining a roster with contact information that is updated periodically. Over time, the network may become more formal with entry requirements, regular meetings by telephone or in person, and so on. Or the network may remain informal for many years, eventually dissolving as the members no longer find it useful.

Management Teams: Operational teams, project teams, consultative teams, and leadership teams are all true teams. (See Chapter 2 for an explanation of these team types.) Designing them is essentially the same as designing clinical true teams. There are a few differences, for example, the sponsor of a project team needs to specify not only the task for the team but the desired date of completion. Management template teams are rare. When they do exist, they are designed in the same way as clinical template teams. Management teams, especially project teams and consultative teams, are more often self-managing than are clinical teams although self-managing management teams are still unusual. Like their clinical counterparts, management knotworks and networks are ordinarily not deliberately designed although a management network is sometimes created by interested parties with a specified purpose and a target membership.

Evaluating the Team's Performance

Thomas Napier, MD, was the Chair of the Orthopedic Surgery Department in a multispecialty group practice. He had been appointed 2 years previously by the Chair of Surgery, Raphael Flores, MD. The Orthopedic Surgery Department consisted of 5 orthopedists, 3 physician assistants, 3 orthopedic technicians, 1 registered nurse, several certified medical assistants, and several front desk clerks.

All was not well in the Department. The most pressing problem was a series of postoperative infections caused by methicillin-resistant Staphylococcus aureus (MRSA), a bacterium that is untreatable with nearly all antibiotics and is thus a serious threat to patients' health. Also, the Department's scores on the Patient Experience Questionnaire used by the medical group had deteriorated over the past 9 months. In part, this deterioration appeared to be caused by the behavior of one particular orthopedist. His angry outbursts in the operating room were well known to the Chief of Surgery, and patients reported his dictatorial manner and refusal at times to answer their questions.

Dr. Flores had discussed some of these issues with Dr. Napier from time to time over several months. They discussed approaches to correcting the problems, and Dr. Napier had asked for advice about how to deal with the orthopedist who was generating complaints from both nurses and patients. After 6 months had passed, Dr. Flores asked to meet with Dr. Napier for an extended discussion of how the Department was performing and how performance might be improved. Prior to the meeting, Dr. Flores obtained postoperative infection data, patient experience data, surgical procedure counts for the 5 orthopedists, and data on several other topics. He also thought about how to present the information to Dr. Napier and how to encourage him to talk about how he might deal with the performance issues in the Orthopedic Surgery Department.

Once a team has been designed and begins to function, the sponsor needs to be able to evaluate the team's performance. The characteristics of effective teams are discussed in Chapter 6 (Tables 6–2 through 6–6 in Chapter 6). The sponsor's competency in evaluation consists of being able to assess the team's performance against the goals of the team and against the list of characteristics of effective teams, categorized under the 5 headings of structure, focus on the needs of patients, team orientation, collaborative work as a team, and team management. The topic of evaluation of teams is dealt with only briefly here. It is covered primarily in Chapter 13.

The first step in evaluating the performance of a team is to clarify the team's goals. In the case of the Orthopedic Surgery Department, the general goal is to provide excellent orthopedic care. Detail for this goal can be provided by using the 6 Institute of Medicine (IOM) aims, discussed in Chapter 6: safety, effectiveness, patient-centeredness, timeliness, efficiency, and equity. If a sponsor is evaluating a management team, she or he needs to be clear about the goal of that team. The goals of management teams vary widely. The goal could be, for example, to operate a clinical unit smoothly and efficiently or to formulate a strategic plan or to plan a hospital expansion.

In addition to their overall goals, both clinical and management teams usually are pursuing subsidiary, specific goals. For example, in the case of the Orthopedic Department, reduction of MRSA infections was a subsidiary goal of particular importance. In a management team, a subsidiary goal might be decreasing the cycle time for implementing electronic scheduling systems across several clinical departments.

The next step for the sponsor is to obtain information about the team. Ordinarily, the sponsor will expect to receive much of this information from the leader, but many other sources can also be used. In the case of the Orthopedic Department, Dr. Flores might want information on waiting times to get appointments, functional outcome information obtained from patients, survey information about work life obtained from people working in the Department, and so on. He is likely to want at least some information touching on each of the IOM 6 aims—with one exception. It is not likely that information will be available on equity because a single organization is not likely to be able to measure equity well unless it is extremely large. Equity is a consideration that pertains to populations, not individual episodes of patient care. Turning to the characteristics of effective teams, there are a total of 32 items across the 5 categories of characteristics discussed in Chapter 6 (Tables 6–2 through 6–6). Information will not be available on all of these items, and it is not necessary. Dr. Flores will need to inquire about any item which he has special reason to evaluate, for example, the social climate of the team. He had reason to be concerned about this issue because of what he already knew about the orthopedist who was misbehaving from time to time. It is not practical or necessary to obtain detailed information about all aspects of team performance. A part of the competency of the sponsor lies in maintaining familiarity with the team so that she or he can identify areas that need improvement and gather information pertinent to those areas.

Dr. Flores' third step will be to review the goals of the Department plus the characteristics of effective teams and, for each goal and characteristic of interest, to determine whether performance is satisfactory or appears to need improvement. This review of performance is often done by the sponsor and the leader together, and the sponsor usually relies heavily on the leader for information and for his or her assessments. A particularly important function of the sponsor in evaluation is to ask the right questions.

Guiding the Team

White Pine Medical Clinic was a multispecialty medical group with departments of internal medicine, pediatrics, and obstetrics and gynecology. In 1982, all 3 of these departments included advanced practice nurses as well as physicians. There were also a few specialist physicians in the group. Georgiana Morgan, MD, was the new head of the Internal Medicine Department. She had been appointed by Robert Wiebert, MD, president of the medical group, after John Larson, MD, the senior internist and former head of the Department, had decided he no longer wanted the position because he preferred to devote all of his time to seeing patients. (Dr. Larson regarded management as drudgery.)

Dr. Morgan was 34 years old and 10-15 years younger than 4 of the 10 other internists. When she became head of the Department, she faced an internal tussle between the internists and adult nurse practitioners (NPs). Ever since NPs had joined the staff, they were scheduled to see patients within a narrow range of medical needs, including Pap smears and other preventive services, diagnosis of respiratory symptoms such as cough or sore throat, and follow-up (but not initial assessment) of chronic conditions such as high blood pressure and diabetes. The NPs were pressing for removal of these restrictions. They wanted to see any patient with any healthcare need, and they readily acknowledged that some patients would be directed immediately to an internist or some other physician, for example, any patient with a high fever and a markedly tender abdomen or with a decreased level of consciousness.

Dr. Wiebert, the head of the group, was 63 years old and had practiced surgery for 32 years. When Dr. Morgan became head of internal medicine, Dr. Wiebert went to talk with her about the disagreement between the internists and the NPs. Dr. Wiebert was aware of the disagreement because one of the NPs had appealed to him to increase the scope of practice allowed to the NPs and because Dr. Larson had once vented his frustration about dealing with the disagreement. Dr. Wiebert asked Dr. Morgan what her views were on the issue. Dr. Morgan said that she thought the scope of practice should be widened but not so far as the NPs were requesting. Dr. Morgan said she thought that this was the appropriate way to handle the issue. Dr. Wiebert listened attentively and then advised Dr. Morgan to back the other internists in opposing the NPs' request—at least for the present. He said that Dr. Morgan would lose credibility with the other internists if she backed the NPs and that patients would perceive scheduling NPs to see any patient with any symptom as "cheapening the service."

In order to provide guidance effectively for a team, the team sponsor needs to be able to establish and maintain a functional relationship with the team leader and then provide information and advice in keeping with the team's performance.

Both Dr. Wiebert and Dr. Morgan were concerned with providing effective, safe health care to the Clinic's adult patients and with preserving reasonable tranquility among the NPs and internists. They were both well informed about what was happening in the department.

Dr. Wiebert had a good working relationship with Dr. Morgan. Dr. Wiebert was in fact Dr. Morgan's mentor, not merely the sponsor of her team. While sponsors often relate to team leaders as mentors to mentees, sometimes the sponsor simply provides occasional advice—advice that may or may not be accepted by the team leader. Dr. Wiebert was far older and more experienced than Dr. Morgan, making it comfortable for both of them that Dr. Wiebert relate to Dr. Morgan as her mentor and source of advice. If the team leader is older or more experienced than the sponsor, the leader may be less willing to accept guidance from the sponsor. Under those circumstances, the sponsor's responsibilities in providing guidance can be more difficult.

Nowadays Dr. Wiebert's advice would be seen by many physicians (and certainly by NPs) as excessively cautious, even reactionary. The attitudes of physicians and the general public in 1982 were different from what they are now. Judging Dr. Wiebert's advice 30 years later is difficult. In any case, in advising Dr. Morgan, Dr. Wiebert was exercising his competency as a guide for the Internal Medicine Department. A sponsor normally provides guidance for the team through the leader, not directly to the team as a whole. Dr. Morgan faced a difficult problem in managing the social climate of her new team. A decision involving several considerations was needed. Some might see the issue here as a purely political one—physicians vs NPs. But there was more at stake than a political victory for one side or the other. Dr. Morgan had very little experience as a team leader. She needed Dr. Wiebert's guidance.

This example of sponsor guidance concerns a reasonably complicated and hazardous situation. Other situations carry less risk. Sponsors can provide leaders with guidance on any issue pertaining to the team's achievement of its goals or the 32 characteristics of an effective team. Sometimes the sponsor and the leader have frequent conversations. Sometimes they simply have a chat from time to time.

Redesigning Teams

Timothy Paganni, MD, and Jane McAdams, MD, were academic pediatricians and investigators in a project funded by the National Institute of Mental Health. The project was partly a research project and partly a training program. The focus was attention deficit and hyperactivity disorder

(ADHD). The aim was to develop and evaluate new approaches to achieving coordination of schooling, pediatric care, and family support for children with ADHD. The project included 2 training programs, one for teachers and a separate one for parents and other family members of children with ADHD. The program for teachers was delivered over 7 weeks in the summer. The program for parents and families ran throughout the year.

Dr. Paganni was the project's principal investigator, that is, the team leader. Other participants were Paul Wang, PhD (Professor of Elementary Education), Ellen Poole, MSW (social worker specializing in family therapy), Steven Mitchell, PhD (child psychologist with special expertise in ADHD), Paj Moua (administrative assistant), and Diane Gowers (director of the training programs).

The whole group met monthly and covered a diverse agenda that included discussions of the long-term evolution of the project, methods for reaching out to schools, logistics for the training programs, grant renewal applications, and other topics. The meetings were going poorly. Dr. Paganni chaired the meetings, but he was not an able chair and often unintentionally frustrated the group by neglecting the clock and adding unexpected items to the agenda. Professor Wang had long experience with grant-funded projects, and over time he became more and more assertive to the point that Dr. Paganni thought that he was trying to usurp the role of principal investigator. Ms. Moua often raised important but very detailed questions about logistics for recruiting participants into the training programs, scheduling the training sessions, and other matters. Dr. McAdams was very impatient with these detailed discussions and often interrupted Ms. Moua to change the subject. Dr. Paganni was embarrassed by this behavior but did not know what to do about it.

The Chair of Pediatrics in the medical school was Joseph Boyle, MD. Although he would not have described himself as a sponsor, in fact he was Dr. Paganni's sponsor for the ADHD project. After hearing complaints from Dr. McAdams, Ms. Poole, and Dr. Mitchell over a period of 9 months, he sought a meeting with Dr. Paganni, and the 2 of them eventually decided to reorganize the project. There were several changes. The most important change was the division of the team into 2 parts. The project team was redefined to consist of Ms. Poole and Drs. Paganni, McAdams, Wang, and Mitchell. This team continued to meet monthly. Ms. Moua and Ms. Gowers also met monthly with Professor Wang to handle operational issues, and Dr. Paganni met every other week with Professor Wang to keep himself informed and assure coordination across the whole project. In addition, Dr. Boyle advised Dr. Paganni to meet with Professor Wang to air their frustrations with each other and to establish a more effective working relationship.

Strictly speaking, the competency to redesign a team is not a competency separate from design of the team, but it warrants special attention because the actions to be taken come after evaluation and usually require intervention, which is more difficult than designing the team initially.

Dr. Boyle tactfully redesigned Dr. Paganni's team, working with Dr. Paganni in the task. Dr. Boyle correctly perceived that the team had been poorly designed. Dr. Boyle's success in redesigning the team reflected his good working relationship with Dr. Paganni. The sponsor's first responsibility under the heading of redesign is to establish an effective relationship with the leader. In this case, fortunately, Dr. Boyle had established a good working relationship with Dr. Paganni long before any difficulties surfaced in the ADHD project.

As it happened, Drs. Boyle and Paganni had never discussed the original design of the project team. The team had been specified in the grant proposal, and Dr. Boyle signed off on the proposal with only brief consideration of it. The size of the team was workable; at 7 members it was not too large. The problem was that the team specification did not distinguish between core members and secondary members. The 2 pediatricians, professor of education, social worker, and psychologist were the core members. The program manager and administrative assistant were secondary members. Conferring equal status to everyone in the team had the effect of encouraging discussion of topics that were not central to leading the project. These topics were not engaging for all team members, and they were not suitable for discussion in project team meetings. It would have been possible to have Ms. Gowers and Ms. Moua continue to attend the meetings with a revised understanding that they generally should only listen and that they had no say in consensus formation. However, Drs. Boyle and Paganni agreed that this change would be awkward for Ms. Gowers and Ms. Moua and might alienate them from the project. So Drs. Boyle and Paganni settled for decreasing the team size and explaining the change privately to Ms. Gowers and Ms. Moua. As it happened, both Ms. Gowers and Ms. Moua were delighted at the change since they were frustrated with the conduct of the team meetings and had great confidence in Professor Wang to oversee the operations of the project. Professor Wang became the go-between bridging the leadership team and the staff.

This example of redesigning a team focuses on correcting a defect in team composition. In other situations, redesigning the team might consist of changing the definition of the task or changing the leader. When redesign is needed, the sponsor's responsibility consists of recognizing the need and taking action to alter the team. Sometimes the team requires redesign of features that are outside of the control of the sponsor. For example, the reward system in the organization may need to be changed if it does not adequately reward collaboration within the team. Also, more support for training may be needed from elsewhere in the organization. In these cases, the sponsor and leader need to decide whether they wish to try to persuade people with more authority to make the necessary changes.

HAZARDS FOR SPONSORS

The nurses on the pediatric oncology floor of the hospital were angry and demoralized. Susan Roberts, RN, MSN, had been appointed head nurse 18 months ago, succeeding a much loved head nurse, who retired after serving in the position for 12 years. The previous head nurse was extraordinarily gifted in dealing with people. She was approachable, insightful, and considerate. She was also firm in making decisions and always attentive to the interests of the patients and to the needs of the whole unit.

Ms. Roberts was different. Like her predecessor, she was confident, but she was also quick to make decisions and often did not welcome input from others. She believed that her duty was to run the unit in an orderly manner, handling issues promptly as they arose, without wasting time. She did not want to run a "support group for nurses."

Ms. Roberts reported to Mave Ryan, RN, PhD, the Chief Nursing Officer (CNO) of the hospital. Ms. Ryan had appointed Ms. Roberts as head nurse. They had known each other for several years but were not close friends. Soon after Ms. Ryan appointed Ms. Roberts, she learned that there was discord and distress among the nurses and other staff on the oncology floor. Ms. Ryan did not seek this information; it was provided to her by a few nurses of long tenure and by 2 of the pediatric oncologists. Ms. Ryan's unstated interpretaton was that the oncology nurses missed Ms. Roberts' predecessor. Anyone would have had difficulty in taking the place of the gifted and admired former head nurse. Ms. Ryan made no inquiries of her own and took no action. She did discuss the reported problem once with Ms. Roberts. At that point, they agreed that the unit would settle down in time.

After 18 months, matters had reached a crisis point. Seven of the 20 nurses in the unit had resigned or sought transfers to other parts of the hospital, and so had several of the nurse's aides and clerical staff. At last Ms. Ryan decided she needed to take action, but she did not know what to do. Ms. Ryan had high regard for Ms. Roberts, and some of pediatric oncologists had welcomed the quick decision making of Ms. Roberts compared with the former head nurse.

The CNO fell victim to a common hazard for sponsors, namely, inaction in the face of a team known to be functioning poorly. There was a plausible reason for discounting the early reports of trouble. A new team leader who follows a highly regarded former leader often has difficulty establishing her or his credibility and authority with the team members. However, Ms. Ryan clung to this interpretation too long.

Ms. Ryan did not fall victim to a more serious hazard, namely, failing to pay attention to the team for which she had sponsorship responsibility. In a well-understood hierarchy, which is common in nursing, simple inattention by a sponsor is not a frequent deficiency because responsibilities are clearly defined and attending to these responsibilities is a matter of well-established habit. Among physicians, inattention by sponsors is common. Because physicians have a less hierarchical culture, physician leaders often are uncomfortable with the fact that other physicians and their teams are accountable to the leaders. So they leave the teams to do as the team leaders think best with the result that the teams are inadequately tracked. While an organizational diagram for a large medical group can be drawn to show that the department chairs of pediatrics, obstetrics, and other departments are accountable to the medical director, in practice there is sometimes no accountability. This is a common failure of sponsorship and one which often causes distress for physician leaders because the physician culture is at odds with the needs of the organization as a whole.

CONCLUSION

As defined in this book, the sponsor of a healthcare team is the person (or committee) who (1) designs the team, (2) evaluates its performance over time, and (3) provides guidance as necessary. The team leader is accountable to the sponsor, and the leader is almost always chosen by the sponsor. A sponsor needs to be competent in the performance of the 3 tasks that constitute his or her role. Design of the team includes setting the task, composing the initial team, and appointing the leader. The size of the team merits special attention because sponsors are often prone to form teams that are too large to be effective. Different team types have somewhat different design requirements. In particular, true teams can be assembled straightforwardly of named individuals while template teams are composed by specifying roles that will be filled by different individuals at different times. Evaluation of the team consists of judging its performance against its goals and against the list of characteristics of effective teams. The sponsor provides guidance of the team through the leader, with whom the sponsor must have an effective working relationship. The principal hazards for sponsors are delay in addressing a team that is functioning poorly or, worse, inattention to the performance of a team.

Effective sponsorship is essential to good teamwork. Unfortunately, sponsorship is often undeveloped or even unrecognized in clinical settings, especially among clinicians who are functioning in a hierarchy but prefer to think that they are not. In management circles, sponsorship is a routine function.

REFERENCES

Aubé C, Rousseau V, Tremblay S. Team size and quality of group experience: the more the merrier? *Group Dyn.* 2011;15:357-375.

Batalden PB, Nelson EC, Godfrey MM, et al. Introducing clinical microsystems. In: Nelson EC, Batalden PB, Godfrey MM, et al, eds. *Value by Design: Developing Clinical Microsystems to Achieve Organizational Excellence.* San Francisco, CA: Jossey-Bass; 2011:1-46.

Collins J. Level 5 leadership: the triumph of humility and fierce resolve. *Harv Bus Rev.* 2005; 83(7/8):136-146.

Hackman JR. *Leading Teams: Setting the Stage for Great Performances.* Boston, MA: Harvard Business School Press; 2002.

Katzenbach JR, Smith DK. *The Wisdom of Teams: Creating the High-Performance Organization.* Collins Business Essentials ed. New York, NY: HarperCollins Publishers; 2006.

McCauley C. Group dynamics in Janis's theory of groupthink: backward and forward. *Organ Behav Hum Decis Process.* 1998;73:142-162.

National Committee for Quality Assurance. *Specialty Practice Recognition (SPR) Draft Standards: Overview.* Washington, DC: National Committee for Quality Assurance; 2012a. http://www.ncqa.org/LinkClick.aspx?fileticket=IpfezpVL_Bw%3D&tabid=938. Accessed August 18, 2012.

National Committee for Quality Assurance. *NCQA's Specialty Practice Recognition (SPR) 2013.* Washington, DC: National Committee for Quality Assurance; 2012b. http://www.ncqa.org/LinkClick.aspx?fileticket=HA4nI5Q57Ys%3D&tabid=93. Accessed August 18, 2012.

Thompson LL. *Making the Team: A Guide for Managers.* 4th ed. Upper Saddle River, NJ: Prentice Hall; 2011.

Watson WE, Kumar K, Michaelsen LK. Cultural diversity's impact on interaction process and performance: comparing homogeneous and diverse task groups. *Acad Manage J.* 1993;36:590-602.

West MA. *Effective Teamwork: Practical Lessons from Organizational Research.* 3rd ed. Chichester, UK: John Wiley & Sons, Ltd.; 2012.

Evaluating Healthcare Teams and Team Members

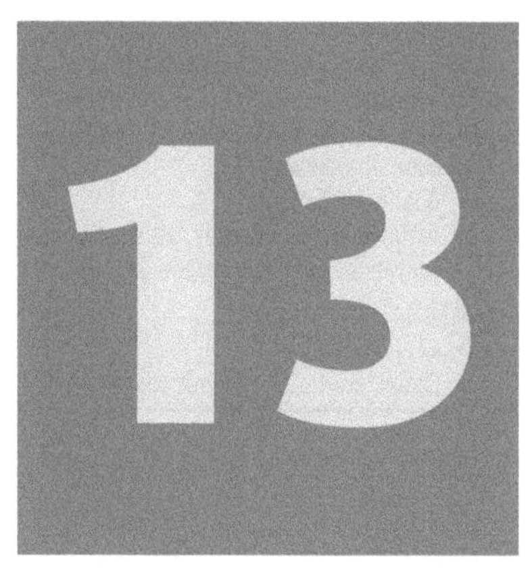

"How are we doing?" is a question that should be on the permanent agenda of teams of all types. This question underlies the content of this chapter, which covers evaluating teams. The ensuing chapters in this section (Chapters 14-17) present an array of ways to improve and develop teams. Improvement efforts are better planned and evolve more effectively if team members, leaders, and sponsors have an accurate and up-to-date grasp on how the team is performing. This applies to individual members in their teamwork, as well as to the team as a whole. In Chapter 13 we first present ways that individual team members can be evaluated; we then turn to several options for assessing teams as a whole.

EVALUATION OF INDIVIDUALS AND TEAMS

Team leaders, sponsors, and members have a wide variety of options for evaluating individuals as team contributors, as well as evaluating overall team effectiveness. Such teamwork evaluation efforts often occur within the context of broader job performance evaluations of individuals and teams in organizations. These evaluations are summarized (in a simplified manner) in Table 13–1. Individuals typically are evaluated, first, on the basis of goal achievement—the extent to which they meet objectives set in their workplace. For example, individuals may have goals to deliver services to 20 patients per day on average or increase patient satisfaction ratings by 10% or decrease inventory wastage by 10%. In some work settings, individual evaluation also includes competency assessment, listed in Table 13–1 as a second barometer of individual performance. For individuals who contribute to teams, an important part of competency assessment is the degree to which they exhibit teamwork competencies. A third common evaluative measure of individuals is the degree to which they have the education, training, and credentials to perform competently in their role. Such assessments might lead to a recommendation of training for a team member (see Chapter 14).

As discussed in Chapter 12 on team sponsors, whole teams generally are evaluated on the basis of: (1) goal achievement, and (2) whether the teams have the characteristics of effective teams. In Chapter 12, an example of a whole-team evaluation process was presented in the case of an Orthopedic Surgery Department, whose leader and sponsor reviewed the team based on the goals of the orthopedic surgery team and the 32 characteristics of effective teams. Goals of clinical teams generally include all of the Institute of Medicine aims (safety, effectiveness, patient-centeredness, timeliness, efficiency, and equity), while other goals are specific to the task at hand. Goals of management teams vary depending on the assigned task.

In this chapter, we focus on the highlighted dimensions of Table 13–1—evaluation of the teamwork competencies of individuals and the characteristics of effective whole teams. These topics generalize across individuals and teams, independent of the goals of the specific individual or team.

INFORMATION FOR INDIVIDUAL AND TEAM EVALUATION

Types of Information

A wide variety of information can serve as a basis for individual and team evaluation. Commonly, team

Table 13–1. Types of evaluation of whole teams and individuals

Evaluation of Individuals
- Goal achievement
- Teamwork competencies, other competencies
- Education, training, credentials

Evaluation of whole teams
- Goal achievement
- Characteristics of effective teams

leaders develop judgments about individual teamwork competencies and whole-team characteristics by observing interactions and behaviors in the team and obtaining information about impact on patients, colleagues, coworkers, and the overall organization.

Qualitative information comes from observation of qualities that cannot be measured numerically; this information may contain a high degree of subjectivity. Qualitative information relevant to individual teamwork competencies and whole-team effectiveness may come from praise or complaints from patients or fellow teammates, observations by team leaders of accomplishments or problems with individuals or teams, or sudden changes in team member behavior for the better or worse, for example. As a source of qualitative information, direct observation is far superior to secondhand reports, and reports from trusted sources are superior to reports from sources of unknown reliability.

Quantitative information measures quantities or other measurable properties with metrics. Commonly, quantitative information comes from ratings by supervisors, team leaders, sponsors, members of teams, and those served by teams. Quantitative information can be collected in a systematic, quantitative, and regular manner in order to monitor individual teamwork competency and overall team effectiveness. Instruments to collect quantitative information can vary widely in reliability and validity, as discussed later. Use of measurement instruments with established high reliability and validity are important in maintaining the legitimacy and utility of evaluation efforts.

Type and frequency of collection of information depend on the nature of the feedback and the nature of the team, particularly its permanence and stability of membership. Many permanent teams review indicators of progress toward goals at their regularly scheduled meetings; for example, a clinical team may monitor patient satisfaction measures as they are updated monthly. Outside experts or consultants are useful in providing another perspective. Stable teams should strive to have regularly scheduled evaluations of team members and the whole team as a basis for improvement. Evaluation of individual competencies and team characteristics in template teams and knotworks is likely to occur less regularly and less frequently, but in many cases it can be helpful to individual team member growth and development. Team members who work solely on one team are likely to have teamwork contributions regularly assessed by both qualitative and quantitative means as part of overall job performance evaluation. At the other extreme, team members who work on multiple teams can benefit from collation of information on their performance on the multiple teams, typically by a supervisor or sponsor who has formal authority over the multiple teams. Or, individuals can request performance feedback for their self-development.

Many individuals resist evaluation of their performance by others, as discussed later. As a result, some researchers advise working on whole-team assessment first, then individual assessment of each other's strengths and weaknesses. The rationale is that it is easier to critique the team than individuals in terms of emotional comfort (Heinemann, 2002, p. 14). The important step is having team members "step outside the team" to objectively evaluate its performance. With that preparation, members are able to evaluate their own performance more objectively and effectively.

Sources of Information

Evaluative information for whole teams and for individual team members typically is collated and delivered by the team leader or sponsor, or multiple team leaders or sponsors if the individual is on multiple teams. Often it is collated from multiple sources, and sources are kept anonymous if possible.

Multirater feedback comes from more than one source, with the traditional one source being the team leader. With *360-degree feedback*, information is solicited from those who are the individual's supervisors, peers, subordinates, and patients or other clients. In some cases, a list of knowledgeable raters can be codeveloped by the individual and the team leader. An advantage of 360-degree or multirater evaluation is the dilution of any one individual evaluator's bias. As noted earlier, typically the source of feedback is not identified, if possible. Performance appraisers give poor performers higher ratings when they give face-to-face feedback as compared to anonymous written feedback (Thompson, 2011, p. 64).

Human imperfections and the realities of implementation limit the utility of multirater evaluation, however. Individuals may collude to give high ratings to each other; raters may fear retaliation for honest comments if anonymity is compromised; team members unpopular for reasons other than performance can suffer; and team members may not understand the "big picture" (Thompson, 2011, pp. 54, 61-65). Inflation bias arises from empathic buffering and fear of conflict. Empathic buffering is reluctance to transmit bad news to a poorly performing teammate, which makes the bearer of news feel badly as well. Preference to avoid conflict is particularly acute if the other party is expected to respond defensively. Homogeneity bias means that appraisers rate others who are similar to themselves more favorably than those who are different from them. Halo bias holds that when a rater knows one positive (or negative) fact about someone, the rater tends to perceive newly acquired information about that person as conforming to the perceptions acquired earlier.

Determining who should participate in evaluating other individuals and whole teams is important. Core members who have sufficient knowledge of each other and team characteristics should be included. If peripheral members are not included, they may feel marginalized. If peripheral members do not possess enough information to make accurate judgments, though, their input may bias the information. Other individuals may neglect to provide input because they devalue it; requiring responses, however, can create animosity and biased responses as well. The more diverse the team, the greater the need for working on design of evaluation instruments, as members will vary by reading level, comfort with questionnaires, and comfort with different formats. Team members should actively participate in the design of evaluation instruments.

Confidentiality of sources is an important issue as well. Raters will be concerned about whether their responses will identify them (as a result of specific information provided in their response) and whether supervisors of the person being rated will have access to their identities. In many cases, it is preferable that supervisors have access to identities of raters, in order to forestall vindictive and unconstructive comments or ratings that a rater may otherwise direct at a personal enemy. If raters are totally anonymous (to both the person being rated and that person's supervisor), enemies of the reviewed person (or those who covet the reviewed person's job) may distort their reports, criticize by innuendo, or simply invent false reports—all without fear of being held accountable. A supervisor may be able to filter such comments if he or she knows the source.

EVALUATING INDIVIDUAL TEAMWORK COMPETENCIES

Robert Platt, RN, MSN, a clinical nurse specialist in the oncology unit at Gibbs Hospital, prided himself on being an expert clinician. He had been an "A" student in nursing school, and his preceptors in school and subsequent employers praised his knowledge base as well as his comfortable and engaging manner with patients and their family members. Mr. Platt was a fervent believer in patient rights and patient involvement. For example, frequently he would query patients and family members for their feelings about therapies, discharge dates, and other issues, sometimes urging them to question the recommendations made by other clinicians.

Mr. Platt worked on 3 different clinical teams comprised of combinations of oncologists, nurses, pharmacists, and others. He carried his passion for patient rights into case discussions in the 3 clinical teams he worked with. He frequently spoke about patient rights with great energy and at length. One team, in particular, challenged his opinions about patient rights. That team included a philosophical nemesis of Mr. Platt's, Terry Briese, MD. Dr. Briese was famous for goading other clinicians into arguments about patient involvement, with Dr. Briese professing that the less patients know, the better. The arguments often interfered with team discussions and team progress. Mr. Platt felt that sometimes Dr. Briese just wanted attention and that his beliefs weren't really as extreme as he pretended. The team leader showed little interest in breaking up the arguments and never had counseled Mr. Platt or Dr. Briese about their behavior in meetings.

Healthcare professionals are educated and socialized into individualistic professions, where personal knowledge and expertise in clinical or management practice is the main barometer of their achievement (see Chapter 3). Some professions, such as healthcare administration and pharmacy, build more teamwork into their training and education than other professions do. But individual performance review dominates the educational, training, and work experience of virtually all healthcare professionals. The growth of team-based clinical care and the increasing use of cross-functional teams in management are challenging this tradition, both in formal performance reviews by employers and in evaluations used by team leaders and members to improve their teams. It is becoming more common that job performance assessments of individuals include measures of contributions to team processes and outcomes. Such assessments become part of an employee's human resources file and are used in promotion and merit review decisions. For individuals employed full time on one team, assessments of contributions to the team can be a significant component of overall job performance reviews. For individuals working on more than one team, supervisors can collate performance feedback from the different teams to be used in job performance reviews. Even if such evaluations are not part of an employee performance review system, team leaders can use individual evaluations for developing and training purposes on their teams.

Why Evaluate Individual Teamwork Competencies?

The obvious reason to evaluate individual teamwork competencies is to provide a baseline for improvement and development, particularly in light of the inadequate training on teamwork that most professionals receive in their education and socialization. Leaders and sponsors of teams who are interested in improving team performance need to examine individual competencies as a root cause of team effectiveness and ineffectiveness. Team leaders driven to exercise the competency to assure that the team can carry out team-level operations effectively (see Table 8–3 in Chapter 8) can benefit from assessing individual member's teamwork competencies. In Chapter 7, we also pointed out that a basic competency of all team members is to be able to hold other team members responsible for their contributions (in a respectful way). Individual team members need to be able to evaluate others in order to fulfill their commitment to the team as well.

Yet many team members, like Mr. Platt and Dr. Briese and other members of the oncology team in the preceding vignette, receive little evaluative feedback about their teamwork competencies. Team sponsors, leaders, and members often are content to function in the absence of feedback.

Resistance to Individual Evaluation

The lack of individual evaluation of teamwork contribution on the oncology team in the preceding vignette is not surprising. Individual evaluation is seriously underutilized in healthcare teams, for several reasons. First, individuals in general are uncomfortable giving negative feedback to others. For this reason, individual team members often give (and receive) either no feedback or only positive feedback. They receive little in the way of constructive suggestions for improvement. Second, team leaders in healthcare frequently lack training and experience in individual performance evaluation, which exacerbates any natural inclination to avoid conflict or avoid giving bad news to others. Third, most individuals, including team leaders, do not like to be evaluated, and they assume the same for others. Projection of this bias decreases the likelihood of feedback provision even more. Another interesting assumption that works against the desire to evaluate is the *extrinsic incentives* bias, which states that people believe that others are more motivated by extrinsic factors (for example, pay and status) and less motivated by intrinsic factors (for example, personal accomplishment and learning new skills). People motivated by extrinsic factors are more likely to devalue the opportunity to grow, learn, and develop provided by feedback—they are satisfied with extrinsic rewards (Thompson, 2011, pp. 61-62). Believing this, a team leader is less likely to think that feedback will improve the behavior of others.

In addition, receiving feedback is problematic for many. Thus attention needs to be paid to improving team members' competency in hearing and acting on feedback. Several individual biases interfere with our ability to receive feedback accurately (Thompson, 2011, pp. 65-67). Egocentric bias (we give ourselves more credit than others do) explains why people feel underappreciated, no matter how positive the evaluation they receive. Interestingly, efforts to counter egocentric bias, for example, by praising the efforts of others, can backfire by decreasing motivation. Positive feedback can also decrease intrinsic motivation relative to extrinsic motivation, particularly if extrinsic rewards follow from the positive feedback. For example pay-for-performance tends to make people less enthusiastic about their work. Individual response to feedback is affected by comparison to others, too, such that positive feedback is less meaningful if everyone else also receives it. Sharing information about team averages and variation helps individuals make accurate comparisons to others. Finally, individuals accept feedback better if they think that the information collection process and the criteria for performance are equitable and fair. A transparent and well-vetted evaluation process leads to greater acceptance of the results of that process.

Overcoming Resistance to Individual Evaluation

Teams should strive to highlight the opportunity to provide feedback to others as a sign of commitment to the team and a sign of respect for the contribution of other members. To avoid giving respectful feedback is to hamper team effectiveness. It takes courage to call other members on behaviors that might be harming team progress, particularly if one has a positive relationship with the other member that may be affected. Again, though, if team outcomes are important, team members need to accept the possibility that personal friendships may be negatively affected if they give feedback to a personal friend. Feedback from peers is particularly powerful in promoting change on interprofessional teams. As one organizational consultant puts it, "No policy or system approaches the fear of letting down respected teammates to improve performance" (Lencioni, 2002, p. 213). Leaders and team members need to remember that the team is more important than any individual contributor, and that a responsibility of leadership is to do the tough work of holding individuals accountable if they are dragging down team performance.

Individual Feedback as a Two-Way Learning Process

Individual feedback should be an initial step in an ongoing process of learning between the provider of feedback and the receiver. This is not obvious from use of the term *feedback*, which formally can connote a one-time, one-way provision of information from one party to another. A first step in effective evaluation is defining performance feedback as a 2-way process. The provider of feedback is responsible for listening to the response of the receiver and adjusting the feedback accordingly, rather than imposing it on the receiver. Feedback is a joint learning process, then. In productive feedback sessions, both parties learn something.

Team leaders need to make sure that individual members' strengths and weaknesses are evaluated and the feedback is shared with them, whether it is done directly by the leader, sponsor, or a person delegated by the team leader. Such information will help the individual to improve weak competencies and sustain strong ones. It is not only good for the individual, but it enhances the team performance as well. In the earlier vignette, the oncology team is suffering because the leader is not providing individual feedback, and Mr. Platt and Dr. Briese are not contributing optimally to their team. Neither of the team members is providing respectful feedback to each other on their performance, either. Mr. Platt clearly was in need of feedback on his performance on the oncology team. His behavior was affecting team performance negatively, but his team leader was failing to take action. The team leader needs to understand Mr. Platt's position, as well. Hearing Mr. Platt's rationale for patient involvement might make his outbursts seem less baffling to understand and easier to address. In addition, the team leader needs to provide feedback to Dr. Briese. He needs a better understanding of Dr. Briese's reasoning and behavior in order to do so.

Instruments for Individual Evaluation of Teamwork Competencies

Individual feedback on teamwork competencies often is driven by specific incidents, such as the arguments between Mr. Platt and Dr. Briese in the vignette, and is given in the form of qualitative information. More formally, individuals can be rated by leaders or multiple raters, at regular intervals, on the range of individual member teamwork competencies. The instrument depicted in Figure 13–1 utilizes the list of teamwork competencies outlined in this book (see Chapter 7). Any list that covers the range of key competencies could be used, such as those models promulgated by the Canadian Interprofessional Health Collaborative (CIHC, 2010) and the Interprofessional Education

Name of rater: ______________________________ Date: ______________

In your opinion, to what extent does team member ____________ exhibit the following competencies?

4 = almost always
3 = usually
2 = occasionally
1 = rarely
NA = not applicable, or insufficient information to evaluate

	1	2	3	4	NA
Patient Focus					
1. Respects the interests of patients and families, as defined by them					
2. Actively solicits and integrates the input of patients and families in the design, implementation, and evaluation of services					
3. Performs professional roles in a way that respects the different cultures of patients and families					
Team Orientation					
4. Actively contributes to the formation of commonly agreed values, goals, and processes for doing the work of the team					
5. Actively contributes to building team identity and a positive social climate					
6. Acknowledges shared responsibility for the outcomes produced and holds other team members responsible for their contributions (in a respectful way)					
7. Understands the characteristics of effective teams and common pitfalls for teams					
8. Understands the competencies of effective team members and his or her personal strengths and vulnerabilities relative to the competencies					
Collaboration					
9. Respects the other members of the team and those peripheral to the team (for example, front desk staff)					
10. Values the contributions of people in the various professions and is constantly attentive to how people in other professions can contribute to the care of the patient and other team goals					
11. Is able to explain her or his own education, professional values, role, and responsibilities in the team					
12. Understands the education, professional values, roles, and responsibilities of all of the other team members					
13. Works interdependently with other team members					
14. Communicates (for operational purposes) effectively with other team members					
15. Refrains from domineering or demeaning behavior that inhibits communication and the effective performance of others on the team					
16. Applies the principles and methods of evidence-based practice					
Team Management					
17. Actively contributes to the selection and orientation of new members of the team					
18. Actively contributes to both the operational effectiveness and social health of the team					
19. Actively participates in the evaluation and improvement of the team's performance					
20. Actively participates in team building, training, and process improvement activities					
21. Actively contributes to the prevention and management of conflict in the team					

▲ **Figure 13–1.** Individual teamwork competency evaluation.

Collaborative Expert Panel (IECEP, 2011), discussed in Chapter 7. Or, a subset of competencies that are particularly important or troublesome for a team could be targeted, such as the 8 competencies covering collaboration listed in Figure 13–1. Several guidelines for delivering evaluative information to individuals follow.

Putting Individual Evaluations to Use

A relatively well-developed set of guidelines has evolved over the last few decades to assist team leaders and others in giving feedback (Fallon et al, 2013, pp. 185-186). Table 13–2 summarizes the guidelines, which begin with alerting the team member in advance of an evaluation session, and then delivering feedback in a private space. It rarely is useful to provide individual feedback in front of team peers—and potentially quite damaging. Individual feedback generally should be given in private, though there are occasions when public sharing of anonymous statistics or rankings of team members can help motivate better performance, because individuals may feel more peer pressure (thinking, perhaps, that anonymity can be pierced by perceptive teammates). Most team leaders benefit from the following adage: "praise in public; criticize in private."

The goal of individual performance assessment is to motivate improvement, so support and encouragement to achieve desired behaviors are preferable to threats. Exceptions would include individuals who have demonstrated they are not receptive to support and encouragement, and, as discussed later, some persistently low performers. After receiving feedback, the team member should be offered time to reflect and respond, and a joint action plan should be developed. Action plans can range from changing incentives to adding new demands with consequences for failure. For team members who are performing well, action plans can include aims for the individual to perform even better in specific areas. Finally, the team leader should search for ways to continue to motivate the member to improve her or his behavior. This can include checking in at regular intervals and exhorting or praising positive change or pointing out failure to change.

Other guidelines for giving feedback include anchoring it in observed behaviors (you were late for 2 of 4 meetings) rather than generalizing across all possible behaviors (you seem to ignore schedules) or assigning personality traits to behaviors (you seem to be the type who dislikes authority). Mixing positive comments with negative ones helps the receiver take in the negative information. In employee evaluations, some consultants suggest "sandwiching" criticisms in between positive comments.

On the receiving end, team members who most effectively receive feedback seek it out proactively, from both colleagues and team leaders. They view feedback as an opportunity to improve the quality of their performance. When receiving feedback, they fight the natural tendency to fight or flee—to defend oneself or not to hear the feedback. They consider the information, check out its credibility, and carefully respond to it. They learn from it. They work with the provider of feedback to develop an action plan. They ask for support and follow-up from the provider of feedback. Table 13–3 summarizes guidelines for receiving evaluative information from others.

Table 13–2. Guidelines for giving an individual evaluation

Provide lead time
Deliver feedback in a private place
Describe perceptions of the other person's behavior using specific examples
Provide feedback on both positive and negative behaviors
Be supportive and encouraging, focusing on desired behaviors
After giving feedback, give the recipient time to respond—listen
Agree on what the issue is
Agree on an action plan
Identify ways to make positive contributions to improving the team member's behavior
Follow up regularly

Different Levels of Performers

Team leaders who evaluate large numbers of team members or multiple teams may benefit from adopting different approaches for top, middle, and low performers (Studer, 2003, pp. 123-129). In general, the goal for top performing team members is to maintain their enthusiasm and contribution. They should be provided specific positive feedback about what they do well and their accomplishments. To sustain continued high performance, sharing information about the

Table 13-3. Guidelines for receiving an individual evaluation

Value feedback as a means to meet team goals and an opportunity for self-improvement
Listen for and appreciate the positive; do not focus on the negative
Expect and seek out feedback to improve and change
Sift, filter, and take time to consider the input
Decide if you can commit to change
Carefully respond to the input
Work with the provider of feedback to develop an action plan
Ask for support
Follow up with the provider of the feedback

whole team's success and its role in the larger organization (if applicable) and its future can be energizing. The leader can ask if there is anything that she can do to make the top performers' work even better. Middle performers can be praised and encouraged to improve as well. Studer suggests the sandwiching technique for middle performers—support-coach-support—to assure that the overall tone of the assessment is positive. Team leaders begin by reassuring these individuals that their contributions are valued, and thanking them for what they do well. Then, the leader can identify and discuss one specific area for development and end by reaffirming the good qualities of the individual and expressing appreciation.

Persistently low performers present the most difficult challenge. Confronting reality means not starting on a positive note but rather starting by observing shortcomings in behavior and the implications for team effectiveness. Low performers often offer excuses, claims of victimhood, and indignation, so these conversations can be difficult for team leaders. It is important to listen, but to insist on accountability and improvement. Being calm, objective, and clear about consequences if performance does not improve are all important to effective presentation of feedback. Assign small, achievable goals and then follow through and take action.

When team leaders ignore the responsibility to confront poor performers, middle and high performers gradually perceive the performance gap between them and poor performers as unfair. They slow down, pace themselves, and team progress slows down with them, negatively affecting the entire team.

While some team leaders can be too blunt and insensitive in delivering feedback, others can be too sensitive, avoiding confrontation and understating an employee's weaknesses. Both the team member and the team are better served by clear and open communication. If the problems are difficult to discuss, team leaders can seek support from human resources professionals to plan the evaluation meeting and role-play the session in advance.

Another tough evaluative assignment for team leaders is to deal with a team member who is persistently disruptive to team proceedings and resists constructive criticism. In Chapter 17 on troubleshooting, guidelines for dealing with the difficult team member are offered.

Who Gets Feedback?

Team leaders and sponsors should be included in the evaluation of individual contributions to team effectiveness. Ideally, team members periodically should assess their team leader's performance. Surveys of team members can provide ratings of desirable competencies of team leaders, such as the competencies of team leaders listed in Tables 8–2, 8–3, and 8–5 of Chapter 8. In practice, the evaluation of team leaders is rare, unless team sponsors are active in coaching the leader and evaluating the team as recommended in Chapter 12. Or, team leaders could request evaluation by team members for their own self-development.

Assessment of sponsors is even less common, as sponsors may not offer the opportunity. Team leaders could reflect on the sponsor's performance in relation to the tasks of sponsors discussed in Chapter 12. Sponsors should invite feedback from team leaders and those higher in the organization. Such feedback could go directly to the sponsor, or to the sponsor's supervisor. In any case, feedback from the team on strengths and weaknesses of individual team sponsors should be given. Chapter 18 describes organizations that infuse teamwork into the organizational culture and structure. In those organizations, effective sponsorship of teams is measured and rewarded.

We should note the difficulty of collecting and giving feedback to members of clinical template teams, who sporadically work on teams of variable composition. If the volume of team participation is high for a given template team member, surveys of the pool of potential template team members and all team leaders may provide enough information to give useful feedback to that template team member. If his or her volume of team participation is low, however, fellow team members and team leaders may be unable to offer informed evaluation of the member's competencies. In those settings, feedback from a leader likely will occur by exception, following a notable lapse in performance or a notable accomplishment on a given team. Thus, in a hospital surgical suite, providing feedback to the nurses and technicians can be accomplished using information collected from the whole pool of those working in the operating rooms. However, if the surgeons are members of a voluntary medical staff and operate at the hospital only occasionally, providing feedback on their teamwork competencies would be appropriate but difficult to achieve. Under these circumstances, the surgical medical director (if there is one) might provide occasional feedback based on unsolicited reports received about lapses in performance or about outstanding performance as a team member.

EVALUATING WHOLE TEAMS

Palliative care teams were new to Fellowship Medical Center, and Xiaohong Chang, RN, MBA, wasn't sure where they were headed. Ms. Chang was administrator of the inpatient services division of Fellowship Medical Center. Palliative care teams had been implemented a year earlier, and Ms. Chang had heard rumblings from several staff members about various problems.

In one case, the family members of a dying patient had been told by a home healthcare nurse that their family member would be admitted to the hospital to enable the care team to achieve control of the patient's pain. As the family understood the plan, the patient would return home in a few days. When one of the family members telephoned the Hospice Unit at the hospital to make arrangements for the patient's admission, a nurse told him that there were no beds available and that in any case a change in the patient's oral morphine dose should be tried.

In another case, a patient had decided that she did not want to be admitted to the inpatient service again—regardless of what happened. She was not in great pain and wanted to die at home. Her decision was recorded in the healthcare record and in several other places. She then developed what was later diagnosed as pneumonia. She became confused and was obviously having trouble breathing. A family member, who was distraught and in tears, telephoned the emergency department at the hospital. The physician who took the call (and who did not know the patient) arranged for an ambulance to go to the patient's home and bring her to the Hospice Unit for admission.

Ms. Chang did not know where to start in dealing with these problems. The palliative care teams were relatively low on her list of responsibilities in her administrative work. She wondered if evaluation of the teams was worth the time and trouble. If she did proceed, should she interview selected team members, or just the team leaders? Should she keep the interviews confidential? And how should members be judged on their competencies? Are there resources for doing such assessments?

Why Evaluate Whole Teams?

Teams cannot monitor teamwork effectiveness or progress toward goal achievement without some notion of how they are performing. As noted earlier, information about performance can be qualitative or quantitative. Quantitative measures are emphasized here, because despite their limitations (in particular, valid quantitative measures may not be available for some important outcomes) they enable corrective management intervention. Some observers of healthcare teams argue that measurement of both processes and outcomes, used to track and improve performance immediately and over time, is a basic principle of team-based health care (Mitchell et al, 2012).

Evaluation of whole teams ultimately is the responsibility of the sponsor to whom the team is accountable, as noted in Chapter 12 on sponsoring healthcare teams. In addition, team leaders need information on performance in order to carry out team-level operations. In Chapter 7, the responsibility for whole-team evaluation is noted for individual members as well, in the form of the competency to actively participate in the evaluation and improvement of the team's performance.

Resistance to Whole-Team Evaluation

While whole-team evaluation may seem noncontroversial, it is far from the norm. Most interprofessional healthcare teams have primitive and partial information about their performance. Members may participate in teams for many reasons other than a desire to work toward the teams' goals, for example, they may find a position on a team to be a source of status. Team outcomes may be unrelated to individual salary and promotions, with the effect that commitment to the team is decreased. Team performance may not be closely monitored by sponsors or patients or clients, such that teams can get away with poor performance. The occurrence of any of these difficulties suggests a lack of seriousness about teamwork. Team members in such teams may be willing to go along and collaborate to a point, but not to make sacrifices or experience inconvenience or hardship for the sake of achieving the team's goals. Lencioni says it best: "The ultimate dysfunction of a team is the tendency of members to care about something other than the collective goals of the group. An unrelenting focus on specific objectives and clearly defined outcomes is a requirement for any team that judges itself on performance" (2002, p. 216). On this dimension, there is substantial progress yet to be made in many interprofessional healthcare teams.

Instruments for Whole-Team Evaluation

There are a large number of academic and consulting firm sources for instruments for whole-team evaluation. Hundreds of quantitative evaluation instruments for teams are available. As a generalization, those developed by consultants tend to lack proven validity and reliability and tend to be shorter; those developed by academics tend to be longer and have better statistical properties. Many of the instruments were developed in business settings and are not as useful in healthcare settings. Some of the instruments put strong emphasis on measuring the extent to which the team contributes to the quality of work life of members and enhances their development, learning, and growth. While enjoyment of work by team members is included among the characteristics of effective teams in Chapter 6 (Table 6–6 in Chapter 6), the emphasis on benefits for team members is stronger in many other work settings.

Ideally, instruments measuring teamwork characteristics have solid anchoring in a conceptual understanding of what produces effective teams. This assures broad coverage of the key levers for improving team effectiveness. An instrument based on the characteristics of effective teams presented in Chapter 6, for example, would be categorized under the 5 headings of team structure, team focus on the patient, team orientation, team collaboration, and team management.

In addition, ideally an evaluation instrument has strong validity (accuracy) and reliability (consistency). There are several potential indicators of validity and reliability (Heineman and Zeiss, 2002; Valentine et al, 2012). Reliability frequently is judged by correlation among items measuring the same construct (internal consistency reliability), correlation among different judges (interrater reliability), and correlation among responses of the same judge at different times—typically using a short time interval so that the judge does not change his or her "true" responses (test-retest reliability). Validity commonly is assessed by comparing the results produced by using the instrument with the results of other assessments that are deemed to be accurate (concurrent validity) and the degree to which items measuring one construct diverge from those measuring other theoretically unrelated constructs (discriminant validity). Many teamwork evaluation instruments are proprietary, however, and many have not been formally assessed for reliability and validity. When assessed, most instruments do not meet standard criteria for reliability and validity (Valentine et al, 2012). A range of whole-team instruments used in health care (65 of them) is presented and evaluated in one source (Heinemann and Zeiss, 2002), although the source is somewhat dated. Another research group provides a more current statistical assessment of 35 surveys that can be used to assess teamwork in healthcare settings (Valentine et al, 2012).

Whatever instrument is used, collection of similar data over time, for comparative purposes, is particularly valuable. Longitudinal data are useful to provide team members, consultants, and sponsors objective data about improvement or decline in meeting standards of effective teams over time.

The Team Diagnostic Survey (TDS) is a popular tool for assessing how well teams are meeting conditions for effectiveness (Wageman et al, 2005). The TDS is proprietary, has established statistical properties, and has been in use for more than a decade. It is based on a theoretical model of team effectiveness (Hackman, 2002) with 5 sets of conditions for team effectiveness: the team is a real team (has a clear task, defined membership, clear authority, and stability over time), and the team has compelling direction, an enabling structure, a supportive context, and coaching available. In addition, quality of task processes on the team is measured by several items relating to how well members perform their tasks, and ratings of interpersonal relations on the team and individual well-being are included. Individual responses are averaged to produce team ratings. While the instrument is designed to be completed in 20 minutes, the large number of items (around 100) makes it less suitable for smaller or temporary teams.

The TDS is designed for teams of all types across industries. Interprofessional healthcare teams may benefit from instruments more customized to healthcare settings. One instrument customized for clinical healthcare teams is the TeamSTEPPS Team Assessment Questionnaire (Agency for Healthcare Research and Quality, date unknown). Figure 13–2 depicts the instrument, which is included in the TeamSTEPPS training program, described in Chapter 14 and sponsored by the Agency for Healthcare Research and Quality. Statistical properties of the Team Assessment Questionnaire are not available. The program has developed 2 other instruments for measuring teamwork climate in organizations as well as individual attitudes—the Teamwork Perceptions Questionnaire and the Teamwork Attitudes Questionnaire. Descriptions of the development and statistical properties of those instruments are available (American Institutes for Research, 2008, 2010; Baker et al, 2010).

Another instrument specific to health care delivery settings, the Clinical Microsystem Assessment Tool (CMAT), derives from quality improvement efforts based on the clinical microsystem as the unit of analysis. As discussed in Chapter 12, the parts of a clinical microsystem include the healthcare professionals, the patient and the patient's family, the information system, role definitions, communication routines, and care delivery processes. The CMAT includes 12 summary indicators of microsystem leadership, staff, patient focus, performance, and information resources (Foster et al, 2007; Johnson, 2003, 2010). One limitation of the CMAT's use in diverse interprofessional teams (as is the case for many instruments) is the relatively high level of literacy needed to accurately respond to it (Jukkala et al, 2011).

An option for larger healthcare organizations that have the statistical staff and resources is to customize an instrument to the organization's particular setting and needs. An advantage of this approach is that instruments developed by the organization are more likely to be embraced as "our" product, which can encourage utilization. Disadvantages are lack of benchmarking from nationally standardized instruments and (perhaps) less well-developed assessments of reliability and validity. For example, PeaceHealth, a 9-hospital integrated healthcare system in the Northwest United States, designed its own Team Development Measure (PeaceHealth, 2012). The instrument is based on a conceptual understanding of teams. It measures 4 components of effective teams (cohesiveness, communication, role clarity, and goals-means clarity), and how firmly the components are in place. Stages of team development are posited, as teams progress from developing cohesiveness to communication to role clarity to goals-means clarity. Statistical properties of the instrument are available, and it has been used in over 150 inpatient and outpatient teams. It is short (31 items) and customized to health care. Members anonymously rate each item on a 4-point scale from strong disagree to strongly agree. Averages for the 4 dimensions and their strengths yield approximate indicators of team development, from the pre-team stage to the fully developed stage.

Instruments targeted to specific areas of performance can be designed or are available. For example, a team concerned about the effectiveness of its meetings might draw value from the Team Meeting Assessment, a 27-item instrument for measuring team meeting effectiveness. It consists of simple questions such as "Everyone understands the purpose of the meeting," rated from 0 (never) to 4 (always). Academic reviewers highly rate its clear wording and easy readability, though it lacks testing for reliability and validity (Heinemann and Zeiss, 2002, pp. 152-154). Sources like *The Team Handbook* contain a meeting evaluation checklist and several other commonly used instruments (Scholtes et al, 2003, pp. C-13 to C-15). Another example of a targeted instrument is the Collaboration and Satisfaction about Care Decisions survey, originally developed for intensive care units and expanded in application to geriatric teams and others (Baggs, 1994). It is rated highly for its brevity and strong theoretical basis and statistical properties but has a high reading level, making it inappropriate for some staff (Heinemann and Zeiss, 2002, pp. 131-135). The Collaboration and Satisfaction about Care Decisions instrument is listed along with several other tools on the National Cancer Institute's Team Science Toolkit website, which collates resources for building teamwork in research teams (National Cancer Institute, 2012).

TeamSTEPPS

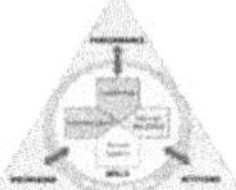

Team Assessment Questionnaire

INSTRUCTIONS:
This assessment is a statistical measurement of your impressions of team behavior as it relates to patient care in your current work setting. Please answer all 55 questions so an overall score may be calculated.

Facility ____________ Unit ____________ Date ____________

	Strongly Agree	Agree	Undecided	Disagree	Strongly Disagree
Team Foundation					
1. The team has a clear vision of what it is supposed to do.					
2. The team's activities are guided by a clear Mission Statement/Charter.					
3. The team's goals are closely aligned with the goals of the organization.					
4. The team has adequate skills and member resources to achieve its goals.					
5. Everyone on the team has a clear and vital role.					
6. The team has adequate meeting time, space, and resources to achieve all objectives.					
7. Team meetings are well attended by all team members.					
8. The team can measure its performance effectively.					
9. The team understands its customer requirements (internal and/or external).					
10. This team is promptly informed of changes in policy or new developments.					
11. The department or unit has clear expectations of this team.					
12. The team receives adequate training to function effectively.					
Team Functioning					
13. Team meetings are run efficiently.					
14. Everyone on the team participates at an acceptable level.					
15. This team works well together.					
16. This team works well with other teams/departments in the organization.					
17. The goals and objectives of this team will have a positive impact on the organization.					
18. The team is on a continuous improvement curve.					
Team Performance					
19. The team uses an effective short and long-term strategic planning process.					
20. The team meets its (internal and/or external) customer requirements.					
21. The team is productive.					
22. Team functioning doesn't interfere with getting my own job done.					
Team Skills					
23. The team members communicate well with one another.					
24. Constructive feedback is given by the team.					
25. Team members are familiar with each other's job responsibilities.					
26. The team uses effective decision making processes and problem solving skills.					
27. The team monitors and progresses the plan of care.					
28. The team can change or improve the way it goes about working on its tasks.					

Please continue on next page

▲ **Figure 13-2.** TeamSTEPPS team assessment questionnaire. *Source:* Agency for Healthcare Research and Quality. Available at: http://www.ahrq.gov/teamsteppstools/instructor/reference/tmassess.pdf.

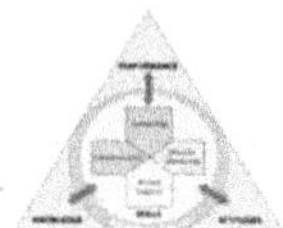

TeamSTEPPS

	Strongly Agree	Agree	Undecided	Disagree	Strongly Disagree
Team Leadership					
29. My boss/supervisor promotes participation by the team in key decisions.					
30. My boss/supervisor shares responsibilities with team members.					
31. My boss/supervisor is an effective leader.					
32. I share my ideas/suggestions whether or not my boss/supervisor agrees with my input.					
33. My boss/supervisor focuses on building team's technical and interpersonal skills.					
34. My boss/supervisor coaches and supports individual team members.					
35. My boss/supervisor promotes individual problem solving and intelligent risk taking.					
36. My boss/supervisor leads by example.					
Team Climate and Atmosphere					
37. Team members trust each other.					
38. Morale on this team is high.					
39. Team members support each other.					
40. There are no feelings among team members which might pull this team apart.					
41. The team resolves conflicts soon after they occur.					
42. I feel free to express my opinions.					
43. I have an influence on team decisions.					
44. Team members can openly discuss their own problems and issues.					
45. Team members show consideration for needs and feelings of other team members.					
46. Team members receive recognition for individual performance.					
Team Identity					
47. I know why I am on a team.					
48. I am pleased to be on a team.					
49. The team subscribes to a clear set of values.					
50. This team is fun to work with.					
51. No individual, group or gender dominates team activities.					
52. The team has a positive self image.					
53. The team recognizes the patient as a critical team member.					
54. The team is a safety net for patients.					
55. I am a member of a team in which the leader promotes teamwork.					

▲ **Figure 13-2.** (*Continued*)

Although the Toolkit has been devised for research teams, it also is useful for other healthcare teams.

Putting Whole-Team Evaluation to Use

John Squire, MD, was an obstetrician practicing at Gale River Memorial Hospital, a large suburban community hospital. The Labor and Delivery Unit where he delivered babies was among the best in the region. At least Dr. Squire thought so—until he saw the data. The new medical director for the unit, Joanna Miles, MD, showed the unit's obstetricians and nurses the hard truth.

Gale River was participating in a new consortium of 46 hospitals working together on improvement of obstetrical care. All participants had agreed to collect and share data using the Adverse Outcomes Index (AOI), a measure of quality in the outcomes of obstetrical care. Collecting the data was arduous and costly. Everyone at Gale River hoped that the effort and cost would be repaid in improved obstetrical care. Dr. Miles had just received the first comparative report from the consortium, which showed the performance of all 46 hospitals and how their performance numbers compared with one another.

Gale River's Labor and Delivery Unit was performing in the lower quartile of similar hospital units. The numbers were presented and discussed at a special meeting of the Department of Obstetrics and Gynecology (a portion of the voluntary Medical Staff). The obstetrical nurses and others working in the Unit were also invited. Some attendees were angry and attacked the data. Most of the attendees were downcast.

In addition, several units in the hospital had recently undergone assessments of teamwork in their clinical teams. The Unit had some glaring weaknesses—in communication and in levels of work satisfaction among the nurses and others employed by the hospital. These performance data were also presented at the Obstetrics and Gynecology meeting. Shirley Yoshida, RN, CNS (head nurse in Labor and Delivery) was dismayed.

In previous years, the Unit had reviewed some reports on quality, but the data were limited and consisted mainly of reports of rare, serious adverse events. Those reports were shared among obstetricians, the head nurse in the Unit, and senior hospital administrators—but not consistently and not more widely.

The major purpose of conducting whole-team evaluation within an organization is improvement. (In addition, team evaluations are used for rewarding team members, as discussed in Chapter 18 on senior leaders and organizations.) Evaluative information simply accumulates in computers and file cabinets unless it is acted on. Evaluative information on the Labor and Delivery Unit of Dr. Squire, Ms. Yoshida, and their colleagues had been selectively released in the past, and bad news often had been buried, for many years. Time would tell whether they would be able to use the new data to make improvements in obstetrical care.

Three steps in using whole-team evaluations counter the tendency to avoid evaluative information. First, make goals and standards transparent. This reduces ambiguity, which allows some members to claim confusion or ignorance about goals or commitments to the mastery of teamwork competencies.

Second, conduct regular, simple reviews of how things are going. Keeping the reviews regular demonstrates focus on the end results (goal achievement and characteristics of effective teams). The practice of reporting results (for example, in the preceding vignette the AOI results compared with other hospitals) reinforces the transparency principle initiated by the sharing of goals and standards. Review information should be shared with sponsors. In the case of the Labor and Delivery Unit vignette, the sponsor most likely would be the Vice President for Medical Affairs for the whole hospital. Joint review meetings between the teams and sponsors greatly increase the teams' chances of success (Scholtes et al, 2003, p. 2-22). Regular feedback about progress should be provided to the team and any sponsor. In the case of hospitals, these progress reports might also be submitted to a hospital-wide Quality Committee. These reports can be short and simple, with measures communicated in writing and discussion focused on team reactions and opportunities to change. Keeping the reviews simple minimizes the costs of conducting the reviews, in terms of both team members' time and mental energy. Consultants recommend avoiding the temptation to cancel team meetings devoted to performance improvement because there is nothing to report, since the purpose is to keep lines of communication open. The meeting reinforces the importance of monitoring results and the importance of the team to the sponsor (if there is one).

Finally, use the evaluative information for taking action. Use negative feedback to create action plans for improvement. Reward achievement of team goals and accomplishment of higher levels of the characteristics of effective teams. In team-based organizations, rewards can include money, promotion, and other job benefits and perquisites. In other organizations, rewards can be as simple as praise or public announcement of an accomplishment. Application of the information reinforces the value of collecting it.

Whole-team evaluation is part of a larger cycle of using measurement to canvass for suitable areas for improvement, setting goals, taking action using various means, and measuring again. The means for action include training (Chapter 14), team building (Chapter 15), and process improvement (Chapter 16).

CONCLUSION

Team leaders and sponsors have a wide variety of options for evaluating individuals as team contributors, as well as evaluating whole-team effectiveness. Evaluation efforts are critical to improving healthcare teams, as they provide a basis for training, team building, process improvement, and monitoring of goal attainment. Quantitative and qualitative sources of information are both useful, including feedback from peers to individual members and from patients and families. Individual feedback is one step in an ongoing process of learning between the provider of feedback and the receiver.

A large number of instruments for whole-team evaluation have been developed, with many customized to the healthcare setting. Ideally, instruments derive from comprehensive frameworks for team performance and have reasonable levels of reliability and validity, though this is often not the case. Putting whole-team evaluations to best use requires making goals and standards transparent, conducting regular evaluations, and using the evaluative information to take action.

REFERENCES

Agency for Healthcare Research and Quality. TeamSTEPPS team assessment questionnaire. http://www.ahrq.gov/teamsteppstools/instructor/reference/tmassess.pdf. Accessed October 20, 2012.

American Institutes for Research. *TeamSTEPPS® Teamwork Attitudes Questionnaire Manual.* Washington, DC: American Institutes for Research; 2008. http://teamstepps.ahrq.gov/TeamSTEPPS_T-TAQ.pdf. Accessed October 20, 2012.

American Institutes for Research. *TeamSTEPPS® Teamwork Perceptions Questionnaire (T-TPQ) Manual.* Washington, DC: American Institutes for Research; 2010. http://teamstepps.ahrq.gov/Teamwork_Perception_Questionnaire.pdf. Accessed October 20, 2012.

Baggs JG. Development of an instrument to measure collaboration and satisfaction about care decisions. *J Adv Nurs.* 1994;20:176-182.

Baker DP, Amodeo AM, Krokos KJ, et al. Assessing teamwork attitudes in healthcare: development of the TeamSTEPPS teamwork attitudes questionnaire. *Qual Saf Health Care.* 2010;19:e49. http://qualitysafety.bmj.com/content/19/6/e49. Accessed October 20, 2012.

Canadian Interprofessional Health Collaborative (CIHC). *A National Interprofessional Competency Framework.* Vancouver, BC, Canada: Canadian Interprofessional Health Collaborative; 2010. http://www.cihc.ca/files/CIHC_IPCompetencies_Feb1210.pdf. Accessed September 20, 2012.

Fallon LF, Begun JW, Riley W. *Managing Health Organizations for Quality and Performance.* Burlington, MA: Jones and Bartlett Learning; 2013.

Foster TC, Johnson JL, Nelson EC, et al. Using a Malcolm Baldrige framework to understand high-performing clinical microsystems. *Qual Safe Health Care.* 2007;16:334-341.

Hackman JR. *Leading Teams: Setting the Stage for Great Performances.* Boston, MA: Harvard Business School Press; 2002.

Heinemann GD. Teams in health care settings. In Heinemann GD, Zeiss AM, eds. *Team Performance in Health Care: Assessment and Development.* New York, NY: Kluwer Academic/Plenum Publishers; 2002:3-17.

Heinemann GD, Zeiss AM, eds. *Team Performance in Health Care: Assessment and Development.* New York: Kluwer Academic/Plenum Publishers; 2002.

Interprofessional Education Collaborative Expert Panel (IECEP). *Core Competencies for Interprofessional Collaborative Practice: Report of an Expert Panel.* Washington, DC: Interprofessional Education Collaborative; 2011. http://www.aacn.nche.edu/education-resources/IPECReport.pdf. Accessed January 29, 2012.

Johnson JK. Clinical microsystem assessment tool. 2003. http://clinicalmicrosystem.org/materials/worksheets/microsystem_assessment.pdf. Accessed October 20, 2012.

Johnson JK. The health care interdisciplinary context: a focus on the microsystem concept. In: Freshman B, Rubino L, Chassiakos YR, eds. *Collaboration Across the Disciplines in Health Care.* Sudbury, MA: Jones and Bartlett Publishers; 2010:19-41.

Jukkala AM, Patrician PA, Northen A, et al. Readability and usefulness of the clinical microsystem assessment tool. *J Nurs Care Qual.* 2011;26:186-191.

Lencioni P. *The Five Dysfunctions of a Team: A Leadership Fable.* San Francisco, CA: Jossey-Bass; 2002.

Mitchell P, Wynia M, Golden R, et al. Core principles and values of effective team-based health care. Discussion Paper. Washington, DC: Institute of Medicine; 2012. http://www.iom.edu/tbc. Accessed February 25, 2013.

National Cancer Institute. Team Science Toolkit Web site. Collaboration and satisfaction about care decisions. https://www.teamsciencetoolkit.cancer.gov/public/TSResourceMeasure.aspx?tid=2&rid=439. Accessed October 20, 2012.

PeaceHealth. PeaceHealth Web site. The team measure. 2012. http://www.peacehealth.org/about-peacehealth/medical-professionals/eugene-springfield-cottage-grove/team-measure/Pages/default.aspx. Accessed April 23, 2013.

Scholtes PR, Joiner BL, Streibel BJ. *The Team Handbook.* 3rd ed. Madison, WI: Oriel Incorporated; 2003.

Studer Q. *Hardwiring Excellence.* Gulf Breeze, FL: Fire Starter Publishing; 2003.

Thompson LL. *Making the Team: A Guide for Managers.* 4th ed. Upper Saddle River, NJ: Prentice Hall; 2011.

Valentine MA, Nembhard IM, Edmondson AC. Measuring teamwork in health care settings: a review of survey instruments. Working Paper 11-116; Harvard Business School; December 6, 2012. http://www.hbs.edu/healthcare/faculty-and-research/articles-and-papers.html. Accessed April 23, 2013.

Wageman R, Hackman JR, Lehman E. Team diagnostics survey: development of an instrument. *J Appl Behav Sci.* 2005; 41:373-398.

Training Healthcare Teams and Team Leaders

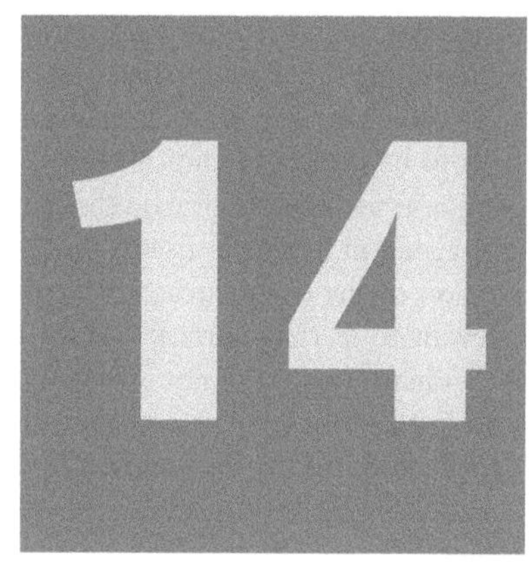

Section III (Chapters 13-17) covers the evaluation and improvement of performance by healthcare teams. The previous chapter deals with evaluation of both individual team members and whole teams. This chapter examines training. It is the first of 4 chapters covering action for improvement.

From time to time both team leaders and whole teams need training. Determining what training is needed by a team and the timing of the training is ordinarily the responsibility of the leader, as noted in Chapter 8. The sponsor also has a role in suggesting team training when he or she perceives a need. In addition, the sponsor may suggest training for the leader and sometimes may provide that training directly. And, of course, team leaders often choose to obtain training without being prompted.

In small organizations, for example, small medical groups, training can be provided informally through mentoring or coaching, or it can be purchased from outside sources. In large organizations, there is often a Human Resources Department with a training component, and large organizations also often purchase training from consulting or training firms.

TRAINING OF TEAM LEADERS

Three years ago, Nathan Mitchell, PharmD, was appointed head pharmacist in a 325-bed hospital in Michigan. Twenty-four other clinical pharmacists as well as 32 pharmacy technicians and other staff reported to him. Since taking the job, Dr. Mitchell had gradually come to believe that he would benefit from training in team leadership. Foremost on his mind was the distress he experienced in coping with occasional conflicts among the other pharmacists. He also wondered how best to structure his large group and whether he might be able to find a better way to make decisions so that the decisions would not be questioned and repeatedly revisited by the other pharmacists. And he hoped he could gain some insights into how to work more effectively with the nurses and physicians with whom he served on various teams in the hospital.

His boss, the Director of Clinical Operations, suggested that he attend a 3-day course in leadership, provided by a highly regarded national organization that trains leaders in many different fields. Dr. Mitchell considered her suggestion but decided that he really wanted leadership training that was specific to health care. He spoke further with his boss, and she suggested additional people who might be able to help him identify training that would be right for him.

What would be the best way for Dr. Mitchell to obtain the training he wanted? Leadership training is commonly conceived as training for people who will be leaders of institutions, for example, Chief Executive Officers and Chief Medical Officers (CMOs). Training for these leaders needs to include content on strategic planning, marketing, healthcare policy, finance, accounting, and other topics that are relevant to leading teams at a senior level in an organization. Institutional leaders often benefit from Master of Business Administration (MBA) and Master of Healthcare Administration (MHA) degree programs that cover this wide range of organizational management and leadership competencies. However, such programs may have limited value for people who wish to be leaders of clinical teams. While these degree programs include material on concepts of leadership and management, which is useful for team leaders, a large portion of the degree programs' content is not directly relevant to leading clinical teams. On the other hand, individuals who aspire not only to lead teams but also to lead institutions or departments within institutions will benefit from the degree program content that deals with broader organizational management and leadership topics.

For the clinical arena, Blumenthal and colleagues (2012) have usefully distinguished what they call *service leaders* from *frontline leaders*. Service leaders are leaders of departments, for example, the Neurosurgery Service, or leaders of other parts of an organization. Frontline leaders are clinical team leaders. The core of training for frontline leaders is training about how to work with other people. Clinical team leaders also need to know how to manage work processes and special projects pursued by teams (for example, quality improvement projects). Many team leaders oversee the management of processes and projects but do not do this work themselves. Other team leaders, especially template team leaders, need to be able to manage events directly.

Team leaders need to understand core concepts of team leadership and management. While there is no standard or generally recognized curriculum for training team leaders, the content to be covered consists essentially of the topics covered in this book. A suitable list of topics for team leader training is shown in Table 14–1. Organized courses covering only these topics are rarely offered. Commonly, however, these topics, or some of them, are included along with other topics more suitable for senior leadership training, for example, strategic planning and the other topics noted earlier. Many large healthcare organizations offer this training in-house. This approach has the advantage of being tailored to the specific organization where the trainees work. Such customization makes the training more engaging by providing content that is immediately useful to the trainees (Stoller, 2008). Leadership training is also available from the American College of Healthcare Executives, the American College of Physician Executives, the Center for Creative Leadership, and many other organizations, including universities. Again, most of these programs provide leadership training that is broader in scope than the training needed by team leaders who do not intend to be leaders of institutions or divisions or departments within institutions.

Table 14–1. Topics for healthcare team leader training

Topics
Introduction to work teams and types of healthcare work teams
Characteristics of effective healthcare teams
Team leaders
The role and competencies of team leaders
Hazards for team leaders
Team sponsors
The role and competencies of team sponsors
What support to expect from sponsors and senior leaders
Team members
Including patients and families as team members
Healthcare professionals' education, values, and roles (nurses, physicians, pharmacists, social workers, administrators, and others)
Competencies for healthcare professionals as team members
Developing teams
Communication in teams
Decision making in teams
Creativity in teams
Negotiation
Managing conflict
Evaluation of team performance and team member performance
Improvement of team performance, including systems thinking, process improvement, and change management
Training for team members
Team building
Troubleshooting team performance
Relating effectively to the larger organization

Perhaps in the future organized training will be available more often for individuals, especially clinicians, who seek training specifically as team leaders. Blumenthal and colleagues (2012) have called for inclusion of clinical team leadership training in graduate medical education. The recent Institute of Medicine (IOM) report on nursing appeals for teaching leadership at all levels of nursing education (Institute of Medicine, 2011, pp. 221-254). At present, for nurses as well as physicians, leadership training is only very rarely part of entry-level degree programs or residencies, but it is available to practitioners in various freestanding programs. In contrast, colleges of pharmacy have begun to include leadership training in their curricula. In 2009 the Argus Commission of the American Association of Colleges of Pharmacy called for the incorporation of leadership development into pharmaceutical education (Kerr et al, 2009). At least 2 universities have added leadership training to their curricula, one in its Doctor of Pharmacy (PharmD) degree program (Sorensen et al, 2009) and one in its residency program (Fuller, 2012). Of course, team leadership is a standard part of the curriculum for MHA and other degree programs for healthcare administrators.

Healthcare professionals who have not had the benefit of leadership training in person can acquaint themselves with the core concepts through online courses, which are offered by many universities. These courses often lead to a master's degree or a certificate in healthcare leadership, but some programs will permit students to take selected courses without enrolling in a degree or certificate program. In addition, of course, one can simply read. Table 14–2 contains a focused list of books and articles that team leaders will find useful.

Experiential learning with self-reflection and discussion is an important component of any organized leadership training program, whether it is offered in-house or by a training institution or university. Participants commonly report that this is the most valuable component for them. Both new and experienced team leaders benefit by interpreting their leadership experiences, using concepts of leadership obtained by formal study or reading on their own. Especially helpful is discussion with other leaders or, ideally, with a mentor who is an effective team leader. Self-reflection and discussion generate more clarity of understanding and new insights into how best to lead. At present, most team leaders learn how to perform well in their roles through reading, reflection, and discussion with other leaders or a mentor.

Dr. Mitchell, the pharmacist depicted in the preceding vignette, discussed various training options with several people and in the end decided to read on his own and seek mentoring from his boss and one other leader at the hospital.

Table 14–2. Beginning reading for team leaders

Freshman B, Rubino L, Chassiakos YR, eds. *Collaboration Across the Disciplines in Health Care*. Sudbury, MA: Jones and Bartlett Publishers; 2010.
Goleman D. What makes a leader? *Harv Bus Rev*. 1998;76(6):93-102.
Hackman JR. *Leading Teams: Setting the Stage for Great Performances*. Boston, MA: Harvard Business School Press; 2002.
Katzenbach JR, Smith DK. The discipline of teams. *Harv Bus Rev*. 1993;71(2):111-120.
Lencioni P. *The Five Dysfunctions of a Team: A Leadership Fable*. San Francisco, CA: Jossey-Bass; 2002.
Mosser G, Begun JW. *Understanding Teamwork in Health Care*. New York, NY: The McGraw-Hill Companies, Inc.; 2013.
Stone D, Patton B, Heen S. *Difficult Conversations: How to Discuss What Matters Most*. New York, NY: Penguin Books; 1999.
West MA. *Effective Teamwork: Practical Lessons from Organizational Research*. 3rd ed. Chichester, UK: John Wiley & Sons, Ltd.; 2012.

TRAINING OF TEAMS

Interprofessional Education in Professional Schools and Colleges

It would be desirable for healthcare professionals to begin their team training when they begin their professional education. Ideally the training would address teamwork within each profession and, more importantly, across different professions, that is, interprofessional teamwork. Unfortunately, in the United States, with very few exceptions, this training is not provided. There have been calls for interprofessional education for several decades, including recommendations from the Institute of Medicine (Institute of Medicine, 2003) and associated committees (Mitchell et al, 2012). Within the past 5 years, progress has been made, but the efforts are still at an early stage (Thibault, 2011). The need for interprofessional education is discussed further in Chapter 19.

Team Training Programs

It was 4:30 p.m. on a winter afternoon. Thirty-five people were assembled in a classroom at Trent Medical Center, a 400-bed, urban hospital. The group included surgeons, nurses, surgical technicians, housekeeping personnel, nurse anesthetists, anesthesiologists, and others. At the front of the room, Derek Cavadov, MD, the Chair of the Surgery Department was speaking to the group about teamwork. He and Mary Peterson, RN, an operating room nurse, collaborated in teaching the 3-hour session.

Four months earlier, Dr. Cavadov had approached the Chief Medical Officer of the hospital to request funds to hire a training firm to teach principles of teamwork to the surgeons, anesthesiologists, and staff at Trent. He and Ms. Peterson had then worked with 2 of the firm's trainers to customize the material for Trent. Dr. Cavadov, Ms. Peterson, and the trainers thought it would be important for the material to be presented by people with whom the attendees already had working relationships. The trainers coached Dr. Cavadov and Ms. Peterson and served as assistants in the teaching program, distributing materials during the teaching sessions and facilitating discussions when the large group broke into small groups to work on exercises that were included in the curriculum.

Dr. Cavadov and Ms. Peterson talked about safety in aviation and drew parallels between cockpit crews and surgical teams. At times they posed questions to the whole group and asked the participants to formulate answers in small groups, which then presented their views for discussion in the whole group. Over the 3 hours, the teachers covered material on communication, the role of the team leader, and other aspects of teamwork. Attendance was required, either as a condition of employment (for example, for the nurses) or as a condition of having privileges to perform surgery at the hospital. For the most part, the members of the class were attentive. At one point, a gynecological surgeon interrupted the flow of the presentation to say that her surgery team already performed very well and that she thought the time spent that afternoon would have been spent better in patient care—although she finished her statement with a mildly positive comment about the interesting stories of aviation accidents that the teachers had presented.

The session described in this vignette is being repeated throughout the United States in various forms. This session was a simple classroom lecture–discussion. Often role-playing or other similar group exercises are also used, sometimes using actors or life-sized dolls (mannequins) to simulate surgical emergencies. Several years ago, hospitals began to provide teamwork training with the intent of improving patient safety. This interest in providing teamwork training was generated by the Institute of Medicine report *To Err Is Human* (2000). Prior to this report, team training in US health care was rare. Despite the fact that healthcare team training is not yet routinely provided in professional schools, it is widely regarded as necessary for nurses, physicians, pharmacists, and others in clinical practice, and it is available from a number of sources.

TeamSTEPPS

A commonly used training option is the TeamSTEPPS program (King et al, 2008). This program was first developed in the Department of Defense and then adapted by the Agency for Healthcare Research and Quality (AHRQ) for general use in health care. The primary purpose of TeamSTEPPS, as stated by AHRQ, is to improve patient safety. It has been used extensively in hospitals across the United States. Underlying the training is a model of team function with 5 elements: team structure, leadership, situation monitoring, mutual support, and communication. Team structure includes essentially the same items that are listed in Table 6–2 (in Chapter 6), namely, team membership, a clear leader, and so on. Leadership in TeamSTEPPS emphasizes coordination of team members' activities and assurance of good communication. In other words, as we would describe it, leadership in TeamSTEPPS is more concerned with managing than leading—as is characteristic of leadership in template teams. Situation monitoring means active observation and interpretation of events occurring in the team's work setting, performed in order to be able to take appropriate action promptly. Mutual support is support by each team member for every other team member as a contributor to the team's success. One could say that the term *mutual support* is a gentle label for the actions that are sometimes required by mutual accountability. In other words, mutual support consists of team members helping other team members who cannot perform their assigned tasks because of problems with competence or excessive workload. In an earlier version of the model, mutual support was called *back-up behavior* (Salas et al, 2005). Finally, communication is the sharing of information among team members.

Several of the 5 elements of TeamSTEPPS training include specific action concepts and tools for use by a team. For example, the leadership module of the program includes information about running brief planning sessions called *huddles*. In these sessions, team members come together to assure that everyone on the team understands the team's current situation and plan. Sometimes huddles result in adjustments to the plan. The communication portion of the model includes 3 communication routines that are already widely used in hospital care: the *SBAR technique*, *call-outs*, and *check-backs*. *SBAR* (pronounced "ESS-bar") stands for "Situation, Background, Assessment, Recommendation." The abbreviation provides a sequence for delivering 4 succinctly stated items of information in situations where time is short and immediate action is required for patient care. The person delivering the SBAR message is expected to state the symptom or difficulty of the patient in question (the situation), then to provide the clinical background of the patient, then to state what he or she believes is the problem at hand (the assessment), and, finally, to recommend a course of action. The SBAR technique is particularly useful for nurses speaking to physicians about patient-care problems and recommending action. It can also be used by physicians providing information to each other or by social workers reporting information to nurses or by any pair of healthcare professionals serving the same patient in need of immediate attention. *Call-outs*, mentioned in Chapter 2, are audible statements of steps in a process or statements of action being taken. For example, the leader of a trauma resuscitation team might call out "Blood pressure 110/70" as a way of notifying the other team members that the patient's blood pressure has been measured and is within the acceptable range, or a nurse might call out "Unit of packed cells started" to let everyone in the room know that a blood transfusion with packed red blood cells has been started. *Check-backs*, mentioned in Chapter 6, are audible confirmations that information has been received or that requested action has been taken. For example, a nurse asked to administer a drug intravenously might state aloud the drug and the dose given, confirming to the rest of the team members that the administration of the drug has been completed.

TeamSTEPPS also includes content on change management in order to elicit support from frontline team members for widespread adoption of the teamwork principles that are covered in the 5 principal elements of the program. Actual use of the principles of change management falls to senior leaders in the organization rather than to the frontline team members to whom TeamSTEPPS training is directed.

AHRQ has developed an extensive array of training materials, for example, slides, pocket-sized memory aides, instructions for training exercises, and questionnaires used to measure team members' attitudes toward teamwork. These materials are in the public domain and are available without charge (Agency for Healthcare Research and Quality, 2012). The TeamSTEPPS team assessment questionnaire is discussed in Chapter 13. Various consulting and training firms have also elaborated on the TeamSTEPPS materials to produce additional materials, some of which are tailored to teams with particular purposes, for example, emergency cesarean delivery teams.

TeamSTEPPS is especiallly suitable for template teams. It is particularly appropriate for teams that must contend with high risk of injury to patients, must operate under intense time pressure, and must cope with turnover of personnel from one patient-care episode to the next. The method used in TeamSTEPPS for achieving improvement in safety is standardization of behavioral expectations and communication. As the use of huddles, check-backs, and other routines becomes habitual, everyone participating in the teams in a given department or hospital comes to expect these items of behavior, and any awkwardness in the new behavioral routines dissipates over time. The standardization enables successive template teams (for instance, surgical teams or resuscitation teams) to continue to behave in the prescribed manner even though team members change from team to team.

This standardization ordinarily would not be useful in true teams, where it would be constraining and artificial. Teams with stable membership operating without intense time pressure have the opportunity to develop more varied and nuanced behavior and communication processes.

However, several components of TeamSTEPPS have wide application, including application to true teams. For example, huddles can be used to advantage in many healthcare settings. Some primary care teams use a huddle every morning as the day starts. Interprofessional teams on rounds in a hospital can use huddles before seeing all patients or before seeing selected patients whose situations are especially complicated. Also, the SBAR technique can be used in almost any transfer of clinical information aimed at forming a plan, regardless of whether the planning is urgent or not. Call-outs and check-backs are useful in any team coping with time pressure and high risk, regardless of whether the team is a template team (for example, an emergency department team) or a true team (for example, a stable emergency rescue team that is called into action repeatedly over long periods of time).

Anesthesia Crisis Resource Management

The first medical specialty to engage in systematic team training was anesthesiology, beginning in about 1990. The model for this training came from aviation. In about 1980, responding to the need to decrease or eliminate commercial air crashes, airlines began to use a training method called *Crew Resource Management (CRM)* (Hamman, 2004). Pilots, flight attendants, and aircraft dispatchers participating in a CRM program learn teamwork skills such as communication, conflict resolution, and workload management. The teaching methods used include conventional classroom teaching coupled with exercises in handling simulated in-flight emergencies. Flight simulators provide an artificial cockpit space that mimics the real world—with familiar seats and other equipment, instrument panels, and even simulated views into the space ahead of and around the airplane. Carefully orchestrated disaster scenarios are conducted in the simulator. The scenarios are controlled by the instructors, who are able to provide the trainees with flight experiences such as loss of engine power, an electrical fire, and so on. The trainees practice working together to handle these unexpected events. The exercises include follow-up debriefing, feedback, and coaching.

Gaba and colleagues developed a method for training operating room teams in the same way that airlines train cockpit crews (Gaba et al, 2001). Fully equipped, fully functional, simulated operating rooms are used. The patients are elaborate mannequins constructed to mimic human anatomy and physiology with high or low blood pressure, normal or abnormal heart rhythms, an airway (throat) into which a tube can be inserted to provide oxygen to the lungs, and other bodily features relevant to the training exercises. Emergency scenarios are played out in the training venue. The events are videotaped, and the team members go through careful debriefing as a group after the exercise. The debriefings are led by trained instructors. The training method is called *Anesthesia Crisis Resource Management (ACRM)*. It is now widely used throughout the United States and Canada.

Simulation

ACRM has provided a precedent that has been adapted for use in many other settings in health care (Eppich et al, 2011). For example, CRM-like team training using simulation is now used in obstetrical units (Clark et al, 2010) and pediatric trauma teams (Hunt et al, 2007). In these settings too, life-like venues and mannequins are used to enable teams to learn teamwork skills and to be able to handle unusual adverse events. Hospitals and universities across the country have established simulation centers so that the quality of team training can be advanced.

ACRM and similar training programs have substantial benefits, but there are limits to the application of aviation CRM methods to health care. For example, while CRM training is relevant to care provided in intensive care units (ICUs), there are several differences between intensive care and aviation that call for differences in the approach used in the 2 settings (Reader and Cuthbertson, 2011). In ICUs, the decision makers commonly deal with multiple patient-care situations unfolding simultaneously while air crews (like surgical teams) deal with one situation at a time. And the work of ICU teams, including diagnosis, treatment, counseling families, and other activities, is more varied than that of aviation crews.

Use of simulation has also been extended to settings that are not characterized by high risk or the need for immediate action, for example, primary care. In some training programs, medical students, nurses, and social workers participate in simulations of interviewing patients or delivering bad news to patients and their families. Either real or simulated physician office rooms are used. Actors are cast as patients, using scripts. The actors are instructed to vary their behavior in specific ways that depend on what the students choose to do.

TeamSTEPPS, although based on teamwork principles that derive from CRM in aviation, does not have a simulation component. However, since TeamSTEPPS is in the public domain, some training firms have used the TeamSTEPPS program and added simulation exercises to it.

High Reliability Organizations

The aim of simulation training programs focused on safety improvement is to enable teams to emulate the performance of *high reliability organizations (HROs)* (Roberts, 1990). HROs are organizations that routinely function under demanding conditions and yet perform with extraordinarily low rates of mishaps. Examples are air traffic control centers, nuclear power plants, aircraft carriers, and electrical power grid operations centers. Weick and Sutcliffe have identified 5 traits that characterize HROs: (1) preoccupation with failure, (2) reluctance to simplify interpretations, (3) sensitivity to operations, (4) commitment to resilience, and (5) deference to expertise (Weick and Sutcliffe, 2001, pp. 1-23). HRO workers who are preoccupied with failure are not pessimistic; the phrase "preoccupied with failure" is misleading. Workers with this trait cultivate a thorough-going thoughtfulness about what *might* go wrong so that they can anticipate mishaps and either design them out of the system or recognize and correct them promptly. Reluctance to simplify interpretations means that the organization's members accept the complexity of its operations and avoid simplistic explanations of mishaps, thereby avoiding distortions in their understanding of events. Sensitivity to operations means that members of the organization pay close attention to what actually happens in their operations, noting minor unexpected events and changes in circumstances that might signal vulnerability to mishaps. This sensitivity at an organizational level requires psychological safety (explained in Chapter 6) for the individuals working in the organization because a sense of safety is necessary if people close to unexpected events and changing circumstances are to report their observations and voice their concerns, thus enabling action to be taken. Commitment to resilience means determination to identify mishaps promptly and to limit the damage or correct it. Deference to expertise does not mean deference to people with high status and high levels of expertise in their fields. It means deference to those people who have the most knowledge about the issue at hand. If the issue is surgical instrument sterilization, then the expertise lies with those who sterilize the instruments. If the issue is surgical technique, then the experts are surgeons. HROs do not tolerate decisions made by people with high rank who do not have knowledge of the particular areas affected by their decisions.

Although the concept of HROs pertains to whole organizations, all of the characteristic HRO traits are desirable in healthcare teams, especially teams that must contend with high risk and time pressure. And all of the traits are compatible with the characteristics of effective teams presented in Chapter 6. In fact, some of the characteristics of effective teams are necessary for a team to be highly reliable, for example, psychological safety and pursuit of systematic performance improvement.

The Joint Commission (which accredits and certifies healthcare organizations and programs in the United States) is a promoter of high reliability in health care. It hosted its fifth conference on HROs in 2012. The support of The Joint Commission for the concept of HROs is hastening the development of team training and the use of simulation centers.

Other Team Training Programs

Several other formalized team training programs have been developed over the past 10 years. Some of these programs have been summarized by Baker and colleagues (2005). With rare exceptions, they are especially suitable for template teams working in high-risk areas of hospitals such as operating rooms, emergency departments, obstetric departments, adult intensive care units, and neonatal care units. Some of the programs use simulation, and some do not. A list of several sources of training appears in Table 14–3. To date most organized healthcare team training has been centered on improving safety.

Of course, improving safety is not the only purpose of healthcare team training or simulation training. One training program that departs from the theme of training for high-risk care is the Geriatric Interdisciplinary Team Training (GITT) program (www.gittprogram.org; Reuben et al, 2004). Starting in 1995, 8 academic and clinical partnership groups began developing interprofessional training for advanced practice nursing students, social work students, and residents in internal medicine and family medicine. These groups

Table 14–3. Interprofessional healthcare team training programs used in the United States[a]

Geriatric Interdisciplinary Team Training (GITT): coordinated by The John A. Hartford Foundation, New York, NY
Healthcare Safety Solutions: offered by Healthcare Safety Solutions, Salem, OR
HTT: offered by Healthcare Team Training LLC, Fayetteville, GA
LifeWings: offered by LifeWings Partners LLC, Memphis, TN
Medical Team Management: developed and used by the US Air Force
MedTeams: offered by Dynamics Research Corporation, Andover, MA
Safety Management Systems: offered by Southern California Safety Institute, Torrance, CA
TeamSTEPPS: available from the Agency for Healthcare Research and Quality; training materials in the public domain

[a]This list is not comprehensive.

constitute a consortium and are supported by a national foundation. The aim of the program is to improve interprofessional care for elderly patients with complex medical problems. Initially the program focused mainly on training for students in professional schools (for example, nursing, medicine, and social work), but the training also has been delivered to healthcare professionals who are already in practice. For example, GITT training was used in Rhode Island to train geriatric teams at hospitals, community clinics, and a home health agency (Clark et al, 2002). GITT is noteworthy for being the only organized training program in the United States for interprofessional teams providing chronic care.

At this time, we (the authors) are unable to identify any organized team training programs in the United States that serve the full training needs of primary care true teams or specialty care true teams that provide both acute and chronic care. There are programs that provide medical groups and healthcare systems with help for disease management, clinical practice guideline implementation, and development of patient-centered medical homes (Peikes et al, 2012). Many of these programs are focused on clinical service for patients with a specific chronic disease, for example, asthma, diabetes, or depression. These programs deal with some aspects of teams, but they are more limited than GITT in their coverage of team function. For example, most of the programs do not deal with principles of communication, decision making in teams, conflict resolution, and interdependence. TeamSTEPPS does cover these particular topics, but TeamSTEPPS does not deal with several other topics that have value for true teams, for example, achieving agreement on values, team formation, achieving a favorable social climate, and developing team identity. And GITT, despite the breadth of its coverage of teamwork principles, is limited to team training for chronic care.

Customized Team Training for Special Needs

From time to time, hospitals, medical groups, and other providers of health care need to provide training for their own teams as part of instituting new processes or improving care processes already in place. These training needs are sufficiently specific that they cannot be met by purchasing standardized training packages from outside sources. Chapter 6 includes a vignette about a Department of Pediatrics that is dealing with a need to change the way patients are scheduled to see either pediatricians or nurse practitioners (NPs). The solutions under consideration in the vignette all involve having the front desk clerks use algorithms to decide which clinician a patient should see. If the algorithms are developed, the clerks will need training in order to use them.

When pursued with care, these occasions for in-house training offer important opportunities for developing a team. First, the training must to be carefully crafted so that different trainees receive the same instruction and message, both those in the initial group trained and those who join the team later. Training some team members and having them informally train other team members results in undesirable variation and error, as was noted years ago by Deming (1986, pp. 327-332). Second, delivery of the training is an excellent opportunity for team members to achieve a deeper common understanding of the team's purpose and the processes to be used by everyone to achieve the purpose. For example, if the Department of Pediatrics in the vignette were to institute the use of algorithms to improve its scheduling processes, both the desk clerks and the clinicians would benefit from participation in training on use of the algorithms. The clerks would learn how to use the algorithms and, in the process, would learn about different patient needs served by the Department of Pediatrics. The pediatricians or NPs serving as trainers would learn about how the clerks experience their work, including the ways that patients' symptoms are presented to them on the telephone and the difficulties that the clerks can be expected to encounter in using the algorithms. The algorithms might be revised in response to what is learned during training. Both the trainees and the teachers would gain a deeper understanding of how patients move through the care system. This deeper understanding would be likely to increase interdependency in the team and to enable both clerks and clinicians to make best use of each others' knowledge and skills.

Evidence for the Effectiveness of Team Training

There is by now ample evidence that improvements in team performance can be obtained through the use of team training in many different fields, including aviation, oil drilling, health care, and the military

(Salas et al, 2008a). With respect to health care specifically, there is evidence that TeamSTEPPS and similar programs can improve team performance. Sometimes the improvement has been demonstrated by assessing processes of teamwork and sometimes by measuring outcomes. For example, one academic surgery department experienced improvements in team performance with the use of TeamSTEPPS although performance deteriorated during follow-up observation (Forse et al, 2011). Use of the MedTeams training program in 6 hospital emergency departments resulted in improvements in team behavior, team attitudes, and clinical error rates (Morey et al, 2002). The Veterans Health Administration (VHA) Medical Team Training (MTT) program resulted in an 18% reduction in surgical mortality across 74 hospitals compared with a 7% reduction in mortality across 34 hospitals in a comparison group (Neily et al, 2010). While the MTT program was devised specifically for VHA and was unique, it was similar to TeamSTEPPS. It used training methods derived from CRM but did not use simulation.

A recent systematic review of studies on interventions to improve team effectiveness identified 32 studies of team training (Buljac-Samardzic, 2010). Many of the studies showed that team training brought improvements, especially in acute care. However, several studies did not demonstrate that training improved outcomes. Not surprisingly, team training is no panacea. Salas and colleagues (2008b) have identified 8 steps that will increase the likelihood that training will be effective. Among these steps are: (1) identify critical teamwork competencies and choose a training program or design a program based explicitly on these competencies; (2) do not use lecture–discussion teaching methods alone—use hands-on practice, including simulation if it is relevant and feasible; (3) use feedback, usually in the form of debriefing after practice exercises; and (4) evaluate the effect of the training by measuring results and report the results to the trainees, including changes in knowledge and attitudes and, when possible, behavior changes—and, better yet, changes in clinical outcomes.

CONCLUSION

Both team leaders and whole teams need training from time to time. Monitoring the need for team training is normally the responsibility of the team leader. Monitoring the need for team leader training is the responsibility of the sponsor although, of course, the team leader can opt for training without prompting.

Training for team leaders is available from many sources, although it is often packaged with training and education that is useful only for those who aspire to be institutional or department leaders, for example, education in strategic planning and finance. Large healthcare organizations often provide team leadership training in-house. Otherwise team leaders can pursue training from outside sources, through self-study, and by seeking mentoring that takes makes use of the team leader's own experiences in leading.

Team training in hospitals has become common over the past 10 years. Most team training now in use focuses on the needs of template teams and is aimed at improving patient safety. A good example of hospital training is the TeamSTEPPS program, promoted by AHRQ, which provides training materials without cost. At this point, most team training in health care derives from the methods of Crew Resource Management, devised in aviation for training pilots. Many healthcare team training programs use simulation, for example, ACRM. These programs help healthcare organizations to function like high reliability organizations, which operate under trying conditions with very low error rates (for instance, air traffic control centers). To date very little team training has been developed for primary care teams.

There is substantial evidence that team training can be effective in improving healthcare teamwork, especially in acute care settings. However, training is not always effective. Certain steps can be taken to increase the likelihood that training will be effective.

REFERENCES

Agency for Healthcare Research and Quality. TeamSTEPPS: National Implementation Web site. http://teamstepps.ahrq.gov/. Accessed August 25, 2012.

Baker DP, Gustafson S, Beaubien JM, et al. Medical team training programs in health care. In: Henriksen K, Battles JB, Marks ES, et al., eds. *Advances in Patient Safety: From Research to Implementation*. Vol. 4. Rockville, MD: Agency for Healthcare Research and Quality; 2005. http://www.ncbi.nlm.nih.gov/books/NBK20580/. Accessed August 26, 2012.

Blumenthal DM, Kernard K, Bohnen J, et al. Addressing the leadership gap in medicine: residents' need for systematic leadership training. *Acad Med*. 2012;87:513-522.

Buljac-Samardzic M, Dekker-van Doorn CM, van Wijngaarden JDH, et al. Interventions to improve team effectiveness: a systematic review. *Health Policy*. 2010;94:183-195.

Clark EAS, Fisher J, Arafeh J, et al. Team training/simulation. *Clin Obstet Gynecol.* 2010:53:265-277.

Clark PG, Leinhaas MM, Filinson R. Developing and evaluating an interdisciplinary clinical team training program: lessons taught and lessons learned. *Educ Gerontol.* 2002;28:491-510.

Deming WE. *Out of the Crisis.* Cambridge, MA: Massachusetts Institute of Technology Center for Advanced Engineering Study; 1986.

Eppich W, Howard V, Vozenilek J, et al. Simulation-based team training in healthcare. *Simul Healthc.* 2011;6:S14-S19.

Forse RA, Bramble JD, McQuillan R. Team training can improve operating room performance. *Surgery.* 2011;150:771-778.

Fuller PD. Program for developing leadership in pharmacy residents. *Am J Health Syst Pharm.* 2012;69:1231-1233.

Gaba DM, Howard SK, Fish KJ, et al. Simulation-based training in anesthesia crisis resource (ACRM): a decade of experience. *Simul Gaming.* 2001;32:175-193.

Hamman WR. The complexity of team training: what we have learned from aviation and its applications to medicine. *Qual Saf Health Care.* 2004;13:i72-i79.

Hunt EA, Heine M, Hohenhaus SM, et al. Simulated pediatric trauma team management. *Pediatr Emerg Care.* 2007;23: 796-804.

Institute of Medicine. *To Err Is Human: Building a Safer Health System.* Washington, DC: National Academy Press; 2000.

Institute of Medicine. *Health Professions Education: A Bridge to Quality.* Washington, DC: National Academies Press; 2003.

Institute of Medicine. *The Future of Nursing: Leading Change, Advancing Health.* Washington, DC: National Academies Press; 2011.

Kerr RA, Beck DE, Doss J, et al. Building a sustainable system of leadership development for pharmacy: report of the 2008-09 Argus Commission. *Am J Pharm Educ.* 2009;73(8), article S5.

King HB, Battles JB, Baker DP, et al. TeamSTEPPS: team strategies and tools to enhance performance and patient safety. In: Henriksen K, Battles JB, Keyes MA, Grady ML, eds. *Advances in Patient Safety: New Directions and Alternative Approaches.* Vol. 3. Rockville, MD: Agency for Healthcare Research and Quality; 2008. http://www.ncbi.nlm.nih.gov/books/NBK43686/pdf/advances-king_1.pdf. Accessed August 29, 2012.

Mitchell P, Wynia M, Golden R, et al. Core principles and values of effective team-based health care. 2012. Discussion Paper. Washington, DC: Institute of Medicine; 2012. http://www.iom.edu/tbc. Accessed October 9, 2012.

Morey JC, Simon R, Jay GD, et al. Error reduction and performance improvement in the emergency department through formal teamwork training: evaluation results of the MedTeams project. *Health Serv Res.* 2002;37: 1553-1581.

Neily J, Mills PD, Young-Xu Y, et al. Association between implementation of a medical team training program and surgical mortality. *JAMA.* 2010;304:1693-1700.

Peikes D, Zutshi A, Genevro JL, et al. Early evaluations of the medical home: building on a promising start. *Am J Manag Care.* 2012;18:105-116.

Reader TW, Cuthbertson BH. Team work and team training in the ICU: where do the similarities with aviation end? *Crit Care Med.* 2011;15:313-318.

Reuben DB, Levy-Storms L, Yee MN, et al. Disciplinary split: a threat to geriatrics interdisciplinary team training. *J Am Geriatr Soc.* 2004;52:1000-1006.

Roberts KH. Managing high reliability organizations. *Calif Manage Rev.* 1990;34:101-113.

Salas E, DiazGranados D, Klein C, et al. Does team training improve team performance? a meta-analysis. *Hum Factors.* 2008a;50:903-933.

Salas E, DiazGranados D, Weaver SJ, et al. Does team training work? Principles for health care. *Acad Emerg Med.* 2008b;15:1002-1009.

Salas E, Sims DE, Burke CS. Is there a "big five" in teamwork? *Small Group Research.* 2005:36:555-599.

Sorensen TD, Traynor AP, Janke KK. A pharmacy course on leadership and leading change. *Am J Pharm Educ.* 2009;73(2), article 23.

Stoller JK. Developing physician-leaders: key competencies and available programs. *J Health Adm Educ.* 2008;25:307-328.

Thibault GE. Interprofessional education: an essential strategy to accomplish the future of nursing goals. *J Nurs Educ.* 2011;50:313-317.

Weick KE, Sutcliffe KM. *Managing the Unexpected: Assuring High Performance in an Age of Complexity.* San Francisco, CA: Jossey-Bass; 2001.

Building Healthcare Teams

Chapters 14-17 address action for the improvement of team performance. The previous chapter covers team training. This chapter deals with building teams. Chapter 16 explores process improvement. Chapter 17 examines troubleshooting for teams.

Concurrent with the movement toward team-based activity in many sectors of work, including health care, more attention is being paid to mechanisms to improve the effectiveness of teams. As one researcher argues, "Effective teams do not simply evolve, but must be developed through team building" (Venneberg, 2010, p. 3). The history of team building has a checkered past, however, because there are so many diverse options for building teams and little evidence about which options are more likely to improve team effectiveness. For example, long-time healthcare team members no doubt have experienced team or organization retreats that meandered off course and failed to address critical issues. Healthcare professionals may harbor negative impressions of team building as a result. This makes it even more important that team building activities be carefully planned, evaluated, and integrated with overall team operations.

WHAT IS TEAM BUILDING?

Team building refers to activities that teams undertake to develop the capacity of the team to be effective. Although team building was initially designed to improve interpersonal relationships and social interactions within the team, the purpose of team building has evolved to include achieving results, meeting goals, and accomplishing tasks (Klein et al, 2009). Team building generally is stimulated by particular issues or problems, but it also can be pursued proactively to prevent problems. Additionally, the early stages of team development can be accelerated by team building activities. Among issues frequently addressed by team building are goal clarification, improvement in interpersonal relationships, role clarification, and specific task-related problems (Shuffler et al, 2011).

Conceptually, team building is a continuous process throughout the life of a team. When team building is viewed as an isolated event or activity, it is bound to fail. Any well-run team meeting contributes to building the team, in the sense that it reinforces participation, listening, interdependence, and movement toward team goals. Accomplishing a successful outcome builds the team. While those normal operational activities typically are not considered team building, they serve the same purpose. The specific activities designated as *team building activities* should be viewed as part and parcel of ongoing efforts to reach team goals. Even when a team building activity is focused on one specific team issue, team building should be considered an ongoing process rather than a quick, one-time fix. The length and content of one specific team building intervention is less important than a team's commitment, participation, and involvement in team building as a whole.

Team building is distinguished from team training, which involves instruction of team members on individual and team competencies. Team training for healthcare teams is covered in Chapter 14. Together, the activities of team building and team training have been referred to as *team development*. Like team training, team building can be the responsibility of either the leader or the team sponsor, and it can be conducted by existing team members or external facilitators, often arranged through a Human Resources department or some other central office of the sponsoring organization. We address choosing facilitators below, as well as the general question of when to engage in team building activities.

WHY AND WHEN TO USE TEAM BUILDING

Stan Richter, DPT, a physical therapist, mused about the just-ended meeting of the interprofessional long-term care patient management team. The team was large, with 12 members in addition to Dr. Richter—a primary care physician, 2 nurse practitioners (NPs), a clinic nurse, a home health nurse, a social worker, an occupational therapist, a dietitian, a recreation therapist, 2 healthcare aides, and a patient transport ambulance driver. His team was one of several in an innovative program developed by a consortium of provider organizations working with an insurance company. The teams were attempting to provide comprehensive care at a lower cost to frail elderly individuals who had spent time in nursing homes.

Team meetings were always interesting, although Dr. Richter wasn't sure whether the team leader, primary care physician Sara Keller-Jackson, MD, was going to be able to push the team to do anything new or risky. Team meeting time was dominated by information sharing about the new program. Dr. Richter felt that he barely knew several of the team members, despite having attended 7 team meetings. One of the NPs had missed the first 2 meetings, and she was not introduced when she began attending.

Dr. Richter knew the team was supposed to save money by keeping patients out of the hospital, but he wasn't sure that everyone in the team bought into the "program." He wondered in particular about the 2 healthcare aides, who rarely spoke. He really believed in the program, though, and he wanted the team to move faster to accomplish its goals. The team's work would be rigorously evaluated by the sponsor at the end of 1 year, and 3 months had already passed. He wondered if there was any way to move the team along faster.

Early in the life cycle of most permanent teams, building positive interpersonal relationships, a positive social climate, and team identity are particularly important. For this reason, many teams engage in team building exercises to introduce each other in their initial or second meeting. In the preceding vignette, Dr. Richter's concerns suggest that his team has not built the interpersonal relationships necessary for effective teamwork. In addition, Dr. Richter is worried that not all team members embrace a shared team goal, which is essential to team identity and success. The team is still early in its life cycle, however, so his impatience may be misplaced. On the other hand, the team is under pressure to produce in a relatively short period, and team building may help them get there.

Often, a team building intervention is put into place when a leader or some team members identify a problem or concern that is affecting team effectiveness. Possible symptoms of such team problems include a decline in productivity or other performance outcome, an observed lack of clarity in communication, or a level of hostility among team members. These areas of concern often are revealed by (as well as caused by) noticeable, growing differences among team members or differences between team members and their team leader (Dyer et al, 2007). Team building commonly is initiated by team leaders in response to conflicts or other signs of differences among team members.

To know why and when to use team building, it is useful to review the characteristics of effective teams. Table 15–1 depicts those characteristics, which are drawn from the discussion of effective teams in Chapter 6. Effective teams have appropriate structure, focus, orientation, collaboration, and management. Difficulties in any of those areas can cause teams to falter in meeting their goals. Some of those difficulties are beyond the reach of team building. For example, team building will not address ill-defined membership or ineffective sponsorship. However, ineffective teams or teams with difficulties often can benefit from team building. In Table 15–1, characteristics that are subject to improvement through team building are identified with a check mark. Most of the characteristics have to do with team focus, orientation, collaboration, or management. Team building is less relevant to the arena of team structure.

Teams that anticipate difficulties in advance, based on prior experience with particular team members or complex tasks or goals, can engage in preemptive team building. Other occasions for team building include arrival of a new leader, influx of new members, or a major shift in the task or goals of the team.

Table 15-1. Characteristics of effective teams influenced by team building

	Influenced by Team Building
Team Structure	
A shared goal, understood by all team members	✔
Shared responsibility for achieving the goal	✔
Well-defined membership for the whole team or for the core team	
A clear leader, acknowledged by all team members as the leader	
Sufficient hierarchy to enable quick decision making if needed	
Adequate authority for the team to take action to achieve its goal	
Stability of membership	
Team Focus	
Respect for the interests of patients and families, above all other interests	✔
Generation of trust in patients and families	✔
Support for patients as partners in their care or managers of their own care	✔
Team Orientation	
Agreement on common values	✔
Agreement on a common set of work processes	✔
Team identity	✔
Attention to the social climate of the team	✔
Mutual accountability for achieving the team's goal	✔
Spending time on activities that build and maintain the team	✔
Team Collaboration	
Respect by all team members for each other and for the patient	✔
Trust	✔
Active interdependence	✔
Use of scientific evidence in decision making	
Effective communication	✔
Prevention and management of relationship conflicts	✔
Team Management	
Unity of purpose and structure	✔
Favorable social climate	✔
Enjoyment of work	✔
Effective building of the team	✔
Effective team-level operations	✔
Management of unresolved relationship conflicts	✔
Timely and effective training	
Systematic performance improvement	
Effective sponsorship of the team	
Support from the larger organization	

Elements of a Team Building Program

Some teams with serious difficulties or with ambitious development goals will choose to invest in a systematic program to build the team, as opposed to sporadically identifying issues and then addressing them with team building interventions. To begin a team building program, a team should assess its own functioning. A serious and systematic team building cycle includes stages of problem identification, data collection and analysis, action planning, implementation, and evaluation (Dyer et al, 2007).

Data gathering provides a team with the opportunity to develop a foundational understanding of its own problems. Surveys, interviews, and round robin sharing are all examples of how a team can gather data about its problems. Next, to develop an agenda for its team building program, a team should prioritize the information collected and consider how well the team is functioning, what is related to existing problems, and how the team can change. Finally, using findings from the data collection and analysis phase, a team should generate an action plan, implement it, and evaluate its success. Action planning is often as simple as coming to agreement, defining assignments, and following up to ensure that actions have been completed.

As with any infrastructure investment, systematic team building makes more sense, the more permanent the team is. For teams expected to do concentrated work in a delimited time frame, though, team building can accelerate the movement of the team through stages to the performing stage. (See Chapter 8 for a discussion of the stages of team formation.) Such teams may not have the luxury of time to work out those elements of effective teams in the natural course of events. Only in teams of very short duration is systematic team building not an option due to the lack of time. For template teams, where team composition varies over time, team building activities in the pool of potential team members can help develop the template teams. For example, team building could be conducted for a group of 45 physicians, nurses, and technicians who work together in an emergency room in ever-shifting template teams.

Team Building or Team Training?

Relative to team training, there is some indication that team *building* is more effective for teams with relatively lower task interdependence, while team *training* is more effective for teams with higher task interdependence (Shuffler et al, 2011). This may be because specific, isolable problems can be better addressed via particular team building activities, while more complex (highly interdependent) ones benefit from foundational improvement in individual competencies via training. Another occasion for investment in team training, as opposed to team building, is with template teams. Building teamwork competencies in the pool of individuals who can comprise a template team may be a more useful pursuit than running myriad combinations of template team members through team building exercises, when they may not interact with those same people again. For similar reasons, teams with a short lifespan (for example, a 2-month quality improvement project team) may not have time to engage in team building exercises, and prior teamwork training of participants would be valuable for those individuals.

Inside or Outside?

Team building activities can be managed by existing team members, typically the leader, or by external facilitators. Facilitation by the team leader (or another suitable team member) is reasonable under the following conditions (Dyer et al, 2007, p. 80):

1. The leader is comfortable with the activity.
2. The team is experienced in successfully working through difficult issues.
3. The leader is not part of the problem.
4. The activity is easy to understand.

Team leaders may be comfortable with some of the shorter and simpler team building interventions, while more extensive interventions, or delineation of a systematic team building program, may benefit from expert facilitation.

Another possibility is that an outsider could be used to collect data from the team, interviewing each member to identify problems and concerns. The information could then be discussed by the team as a whole, which could then decide if team building events are needed, and whether an outsider should facilitate them. The team members may feel comfortable addressing the problems and concerns without outside help.

TYPES OF TEAM BUILDING INTERVENTIONS

There are several types of team building activities. We categorize team building activities into the following categories: clarifying goals, building interpersonal relationships, establishing team identity, clarifying roles, or improving processes. The categories are listed in Table 15–2, along with examples of each. We also discuss a popular setting for many team building activities, the team retreat. The team retreat can cover many or all of the different types of team building. It is discussed separately due to its popularity.

Clarifying Goals

A basic foundation of team effectiveness is a shared goal or set of goals, understood by all members. New teams need to directly develop this shared understanding, and long-standing teams need to revisit this shared understanding as membership changes or as goals shift. Relevant team building events can be as simple as an agenda item to review the team's goal (or charter, mission, vision, or values) and going around the room to make sure there is understanding and, ideally, buy-in, on the part of all team members. Such an activity seems indicated for Dr. Richter's long-term care patient management team in the opening vignette.

Table 15–2. Types and examples of team building interventions

Type of Activity	Example(s)
Clarifying goals	As a team, addressing a set of specified questions about the team goal
Building interpersonal relationships	Ice breakers; social events; sharing vulnerabilities; behavioral profiles
Establishing team identity	Honoring team history; telling team stories; celebrating team successes; team symbols
Clarifying roles	Describing roles and expectations in round robin, with questions; responsibility matrix
Improving processes	Using a team process observer; discussing disruptive behaviors and consequences; managing problem members (see Chapter 16 for other examples)

To clarify a team's goal more comprehensively and collectively, a designated team member or the team leader (or team sponsor) can lead a more formal exercise, typically occupying a full meeting. First, someone reads and explains the team goals. A set of questions is then discussed regarding the goals, with each question receiving separate attention. The team then could be divided into sub-groups for discussion purposes, with groups assigned different questions and reporting back to the full team. Questions such as the following allow for probing and understanding of team goals (Scholtes et al, 2003, p. C-28):

1. Is it clear what our sponsor expects of us?
2. Where do we fit in the larger scheme of things? Is our team a priority of the sponsor?
3. Are the boundaries of our work clear? What is outside our jurisdiction?
4. What resources do we need?
5. Does our goal make sense to us based on our knowledge of the area?
6. Do we have the right people on the team to accomplish the goal? What other people who are not on the team will be crucial to our efforts?
7. Who will support us in our efforts? Who will be opposed? Who will be neutral? How should we communicate with them?

Unanswered questions should be assigned out for investigation and follow-up discussion.

Building Interpersonal Relationships

Historically, most team building interventions have focused on building relationships among team members. Building interpersonal relationships typically begins with "ice breakers" for team members who do not know each other. Ice breakers are useful for new teams or teams that need to bond quickly or when members come from quite different backgrounds. Sharing simple information about each other begins the process of establishing a relationship. Dr. Richter's long-term care patient management team (in the earlier vignette) likely would benefit from members sharing some personal information about each other.

Ice breakers come in endless variety, from members taking turns sharing one little known fact about themselves to members meeting in pairs and then introducing each other to the group. One ice breaker exercise has each member answer 4 questions in writing (Biech, 2008, pp. 419-423). Answer sheets then are collected and read aloud, after which the members record their (silent) guesses on paper as to who gave the answers. Then the correct identifications are announced. The 4 suggested questions are:

1. The one thing that nobody in this room realizes about me is...
2. My favorite leisure activity is...
3. A perfect day for me would be to...
4. The actor or actress who should portray me in the movie of my life is...

Any number of other questions, customized to team members, would fulfill the same purpose.

Other relationship-building activities go beyond the ice breaker stage, involving members in a shared activity where teamwork is needed. An Internet search reveals hundreds of such team building activities, including competitions around cooking, golf, building catapults, game shows, and transporting marbles along pipes, or shared experiences, such as ropes courses and other obstacle courses. Some of these activities will seem very pointless (or unprofessional or inane) to many scientists and healthcare professionals, so it is important that team members participate in the design of the activities and that team leaders know their members and tailor activities to their preferences. At worst, some team building activities can waste time, embarrass team members, and even cause physical injuries (for example, paintball games can do some damage). They can create resentment due to lost time and resources spent on the activity.

Social events are additional examples of team building activities that can strengthen bonds among team members. Again, social activities need to be tailored to the team members' time constraints and preferences. Team leaders often learn through trial-and-error the preferences of their team members on the timing and type of social activity that adds value. In Chapter 6, a primary care team, Red Family Medicine, is described. This team had a positive social climate. Each summer Red Family Medicine held a picnic which included joke awards that expressed caring and humor. Social events may or not be appropriate for a team, depending on the permanence of the team and the need for strong bonds among members.

More intensive relationship-building activities begin to cross into the arena of team training. Members can complete behavioral profiles and share self-assessments of traits and preferred styles. Ideally, behavioral profiles give members a reliable and objective means to reveal their strengths and weaknesses and supply a common vocabulary for team members to communicate differences and similarities. Usually, profiling questionnaires should be administered, analyzed, and debriefed by a qualified consultant or trainer. Often, sharing of results within the team aids understanding of different interaction and work styles (Amos et al, 2005).

There are many profiling tools, including StrengthsFinder (strength.gallup.com), Insights Discovery (www.insights.com), and DiSC (www.inscapepublishing.com). DiSC places individuals into one of 4 behavior styles–dominance (direct and decisive), influence (optimistic and social), steadiness (cooperative and supportive), and conscientiousness (cautious and concerned). All individuals possess all 4 styles but differ in the strengths of each. Insights Discovery similarly uses 4 major categories of temperament, matched with colors—fiery red is driving and aggressive, cool blue is formal and deliberate, earth green is caring and relaxed, and sunshine yellow is enthusiastic and sociable. StrengthsFinder identifies areas where an individual has the greatest potential for building strengths based on recurring and consistent patterns of thought, feeling, or behavior. Examples of the areas, which are 34 in number, include: learner (having a great desire to learn and wanting to improve continuously), positivity (having an enthusiasm that is contagious), achiever (having a great deal of stamina and working hard; taking great satisfaction from being busy and productive), and competition (measuring progress against the performance of others; striving to win first place or finish first).

The Myers-Briggs Type indicator (MBTI) is a popular choice for behavioral profiling in professional teams (Quenk, 2009). The MBTI has relatively well-established and adequate psychometric properties. The MBTI classifies individuals into one of 16 types based on the 4 dimensions of introversion-extroversion, sensing-intuition, thinking-feeling, and judging-perception. The types are preferences, with no type better or worse than the others. The MBTI or variations of it that focus on team roles can be useful in launching discussions of team members' preferred styles. For example, extroverts are more likely than introverts to speak up in discussions and to enjoy brainstorming. Perceiving types pay less attention to deadlines than judging types. Since interpersonal conflicts often are related to personality type, knowledge of others' preferences can decrease the likelihood of interpersonal conflict on the team. As well, members can be better matched with tasks depending on their personality traits. For example, compared to most other MBTI types, the Introvert-Sensing-Thinking-Judging (ISTJ) type likely would enjoy tasks requiring extreme attention to detail.

As discussed in Chapter 6, trust in teammates is an important attribute of team members that often is lacking, particularly during the forming and storming (early) stages of new teams. (The stages of new teams are examined in Chapter 8.) Interpersonal trust can be influenced by team building activities. Generally, team building activities to develop trust involve experiential exercises or sharing of personal vulnerabilities. Experiential exercises to develop trust include ropes courses, which involve climbing a rope then being lowered to the group by a teammate, and similar recreational challenges that require dependence on teammates, such as ascending a tall ladder with a partner (all with appropriate safety equipment, of course). The "trust fall" exercise involves a team member falling backwards from table height into the arms and hands of the other team members. We do not recommend this one, for health reasons among others.

One expert, Patrick Lencioni, argues that sharing of vulnerabilities is essential to the development of trust (Lencioni, 2005). Lencioni recommends that in an off-site location, teams go around the room with each member explaining where they grew up, how many siblings they had, and the most important challenge of their childhood. He argues that such sharing can be handled by most individuals without embarrassment and that it is an efficient way to develop empathy. Many healthcare professionals may be uncomfortable sharing feelings, and some degree of facilitation expertise is required for this type of team building exercise. For example, some members may discuss particularly painful memories. Other questions, such as best job and worst job, or biggest mistake at work, can provide a basis for sharing vulnerabilities. The key is to have people reveal something personal about themselves that is relevant but not embarrassing or silly. Guidelines on time per person, such as 1-2 minutes, are helpful, although they need not be strictly enforced.

Establishing Team Identity

A strong team identity, and related characteristics that contribute to identity, such as common values, processes, and shared goals, are critical to team effectiveness (see Chapter 6). Team identity ideally is established early in the development of a team, but if it is not, or if turnover creates uncertainty about identity, team building activities can help. Earlier in this chapter we addressed activities to build shared goals. Other activities to build identity include honoring team history, telling team stories, celebrating team accomplishments, and designing team symbols.

Honoring Team History

Busy teams rarely take time to document their history. Simple information like founding date, team composition, major events, and changes in membership and leadership can be recorded in an "About" section of a website, or in paper documents. Even for template teams, a history of the team's accomplishments, which could be publicized to the pool of potential team members, establishes permanence of purpose and respect for members. Recording membership may not be of major import to past members, but it signifies to current members that their contributions and legacy are valued.

Telling Team Stories

Telling stories about the team lends legitimacy to the identity of a team, and it conveys that aspects of the work of the team will be communicated into the future and to new members and perhaps even to outsiders. Team stories might reveal special actions of a leader or sponsor to save the team, for example, or efforts "beyond the call of duty" on the part of a team member to further team goals. Selfless service to the team can be memorialized through team stories.

Celebrating Team Successes

Publicizing team activities and accomplishments (as opposed to individual member activities and accomplishments) promotes pride and team identity. Team sponsors and leaders should take the lead in communicating and praising team accomplishments, but if they are not actively doing so, other team members can assume that function. A specified physical site (like a bulletin board) or website can be used to store team history and accomplishments. Organizations that promote teamwork are careful to recognize team accomplishments in order to build teamwork into organizational culture (see Chapter 18).

Designing Team Symbols

Symbols of the team convey meaning to members that they belong to the same unit. Recalling the Red Family Medicine vignette from Chapter 6, that team went through a stage where several member wore an article of red clothing on "Ruby Tuesdays" to indicate pride of membership on the Red Team. The practice gradually faded away, after having served a team building function. Requiring the practice would have been counterproductive. In addition to the occasional piece of symbolic clothing, of course, Red Family Medicine had its own distinctive name. Red Family Medicine also could have developed a team logo, or a team slogan or motto. Symbols of team identity include names, logos, mottos, or physical objects that have meaning to team members. Symbols generally should be developed or approved by team members rather than imposed. Distributing baseball caps to team members who never wear caps may just invite concern over the wasted investment. Shirts with a team logo or motto are a popular option. Leaders need to involve team members or know their members well enough to select appropriate symbols that will have meaning and will not be viewed as wasteful.

Clarifying Roles

Symptoms of the need to clarify team roles include widespread conflicts around responsibility for particular tasks. Or, members may wonder what other members are contributing to the team and may suspect that the others do not understand their contributions. Occasionally, a crisis will occur when everyone thinks someone else is responsible for handling a task that falls through the cracks. Role clarification issues are more common in new teams, teams with high turnover, and teams that do not meet frequently, causing members to feel isolated (Dyer et al, 2007, pp. 122-123).

Goals of a role clarification exercise are that members emerge with: (1) a clear understanding of their own roles, (2) comfort that other members understand their roles, and (3) an understanding of what others expect of them. A formal means of *role clarification* is the following exercise (Dyer et al, 2007, pp. 126-129):

1. Going around the room, each member takes turn being the focal member, describing her or his role—what is expected, when it is expected, and how it is expected to be done.
2. Clarifying questions from other members follow, after which other members indicate that they understand the focal member's role.
3. Finally, the focal member talks directly to each person in the team, specifying what he or she needs from the other member.

Researchers claim that this is one of the easiest and most effective team building exercises (Dyer et al, 2007, p. 127). A similar exercise, labeled *role negotiation*, has each team member post a list of her or his principal activities (West, 2012, pp. 100-101). Other team members write on the list, indicating whether they think the focal member should do more, do less, or maintain each activity at the present level. Comments are signed. Pairs of team members then discuss the end results.

A less comprehensive exercise, the *responsibility matrix*, helps teams identify and assign responsibility for tasks to appropriate team members (Scholtes et al, 2003, pp. C-11 to C-12). The activity begins with the identification of tasks that are not clearly assigned to a team member or set of team members. Together, the team creates a list of unclear tasks. The list is posted or circulated, and team members record whom they believe is responsible for each task. Finally, the team collectively discusses each of the tasks and the responses from team members. Team members must reach a consensus on each task assignment.

Improving Teamwork Processes

Chapter 16 covers methods of improving team performance by using formal process improvement methodologies. These could be considered team building activities. In addition, less formalized interventions can help build the team's capacity to process information, solve problems, and make decisions.

To identify potentially problematic patterns of interaction within the team, individual team members can be assigned to observe team processes during a meeting, watching for specific behaviors, and taking notes. At a designated point in the meeting agenda, the observers then report findings, and the team discusses the observations together. Observers should have clear guidelines about what they are looking for, and the measured behaviors should be explained to the team in advance. Examples of such checklists are available (Scholtes et al, 2003). Observers can record the types of contributions made by members, for example, or record the pattern of interaction during a team meeting.

Confronting Disruptive Behavior

Team processes may be hampered by members holding side conversations, reading during meetings, talking at length, or other potentially disruptive behaviors. Such issues can be addressed by team building activities. In one disruptive group behavior exercise, the team develops a shared understanding for acceptable team behavior through agreement on how to manage group problems, how much disruptive behavior is allowed, and how much a leader can do to deal with a problem (Scholtes et al, 2003, pp. C-16 to C-18). The activity is best used after the second or third meeting of a new team, when team members are more familiar with one another, or when team member' behaviors begin to disrupt team activities. The exercise should be introduced to team members as a method of creating guidelines for meetings and developing ways to manage disruptive behavior. The exercise begins with brainstorming about behaviors that may disrupt team activities. (See Chapter 10 for a discussion of brainstorming.) Voting reduces the list to a manageable number. The team then discusses possible responses to the behaviors, ranging from prevention, to minimal intervention, to strong intervention. The team reaches consensus on ways to deal with the key disruptions. The activity sensitizes team members to pay attention to the flow of their meetings and other team activities, and encourages them to confront and manage disruptive behaviors.

Managing a Problem Team Member

Sometimes disruption of team processes is due to the continuous actions of one or more problem members. Such team members consistently may miss team activities, take a negative position on team consensus issues, or fail to complete their tasks. A first consideration is to consider the value that challenge can bring to the team, particularly in the form of creativity. A certain degree of task-related disruption through questioning can be healthy for the team. (Chapter 10 on creativity discusses this in more detail.) However, if the disruption is persistent and does not provide value, then some action is often warranted to stop the disruptive behavior. In Chapter 17, various options are discussed. In extreme cases, it may be necessary to remove the member from the team. This often requires support from the team sponsor.

Retreats

For the first time, Russell MacIntyre, MD, a psychiatrist, left a team retreat with a feeling of accomplishment. His adult behavioral health team held annual retreats whether they needed them or not. Under the team's previous leader, a psychiatrist colleague of Dr. MacIntyre's, retreats were occasions for promoting pet ideas and surprises that his colleague had run across in his readings or travels. The leader fancied that the team would enjoy and benefit from her pet ideas. Last year, for example, 6 hours of "authentic engagement" exercises were the main activity at the all-day retreat, which was preceded by a long dinner the evening before. The exercises were embraced by a small minority of team members, mostly newer ones, while Dr. MacIntyre and the majority of his fellow teammates looked for excuses to check their voicemail or take a long walk. He felt that he already knew his teammates well, maybe too well.

Recently, psychologist Miriam Adelman, PhD, had assumed the team leader role. Unlike her predecessor, Dr. Adelman solicited team feedback to guide the content of the retreat, well in advance of the retreat. Most of the retreat was spent debating the merits of a relatively new therapy for depression, vagus nerve stimulation, and whether or not to add a team member who had knowledge of that therapy. Social time consisted of a short luncheon.

A follow-up survey and team discussion (another new activity implemented by Dr. Adelman) would confirm whether Dr. MacIntyre's conclusions were shared by other team members.

Retreats are extended team meetings, typically held away from the work location and lasting anywhere from several hours to several days. At retreats, social activities frequently accompany review of the team's performance, problems, and opportunities. Retreats often are useful in the start-up stage of team development, because accelerated progress can be made on a variety of foundational issues, in a short time period. Some teams use annual retreats to review performance and plans. Other teams use retreats to examine issues that are "stockpiled" or "put in the parking lot"—issues that deserve intensive examination but cannot be addressed during normal operations.

At worst, retreats can be a major source of dissatisfaction in teams, if members conclude they are a waste of valuable time. Dr. MacIntyre and many of his colleagues in the adult behavioral health team in the vignette held that view of retreats for their team. This is very common but largely preventable. Several guidelines increase the probability of successful retreats (Clevenger, 2007). Table 15–3 outlines the guidelines. First, team members in addition to the leader should plan the retreat, with the help of an outside facilitator if needed. Team members should own the retreat. Second, attendance should be required, particularly of all key players. Scheduling to allow for maximum attendance is critical. If members are reluctant to contribute full days, a one-half day retreat still can be useful. Retreats generally should be held away from the normal workplace, to minimize work distractions and provide a degree of symbolism of the importance of the event. The location needs to be accessible, though.

Perhaps most critical for successful retreats is to have multiple planning meetings months before the retreat, including gathering of input on topics, speakers, activities, or team performance issues. Data collected on the opinions and preferences of team members is particularly useful. Topics that require face-to-face interaction are ideal for retreats, while communication of information that could be done in the normal workflow is not. Finally, both for instrumental and symbolic reasons, note-taking is important.

Table 15–3. Guidelines for effective team retreats

Involve team members in planning the retreat.
Require attendance, particularly of all key players.
Go off-site.
Have multiple planning meetings months before the retreat.
Pick topics based on team input. Focus on topics that require face-to-face interaction and participation.
Communicate the goals of the retreat well in advance.
Take and distribute notes.
Follow up any decision.

Source: Data from Clevenger K. Improve staff satisfaction with team building retreats. *Nurs Manage.* 2007;38(4):22,24.

Instrumentally, the notes communicate content to those who cannot attend, provide a historical record, and form the basis for continuing discussions. Symbolically, taking notes means the activity is important, and that people should take it seriously. Finally, any decisions taken at the retreat should be followed up, again to avoid criticism of retreats as temporary "feel-good" occasions that have no lasting impact.

EFFECTIVENESS OF TEAM BUILDING

Although the practice of team building has been popular for the last several decades and is often discussed in conjunction with team performance, until recently there has been little evidence concerning the effectiveness of team building, particularly with regard to improving team performance. Historically, findings have been relatively inconsistent on the effectiveness of team building interventions (Salas et al, 1999). There have been conflicting findings among researchers, as well as variability regarding the effects of team building on objective and subjective measures of performance. In general, subjective reports often suggest improved performance while objective measures often do not indicate a positive effect of team building on performance.

However, more recent findings are more promising, providing evidence that team building can result in improved outcomes, particularly "affective" outcomes, which include feelings of trust among team members (Klein et al, 2009). Researchers have studied the impacts of different types of team building (for example, clarifying goals or building interpersonal relationships) on specific outcomes (for example, cognitive, performance, process, and affective outcomes). Interventions that emphasize role clarification, in particular, notably improve performance. More recent research syntheses have found support as well for goal clarification activities (Klein et al, 2009; Shuffler et al, 2011). Role clarification is particularly important to improve individual performance, while goal clarification enhances the achievement of team outcomes.

Finally, researchers believe that team building is more effective in larger teams (defined as larger than 10 members), possibly because larger teams exhibit more of the problems that team building can vitiate, such as groupthink and confusion over goals and roles (Klein et al, 2009, p. 213).

The effectiveness of team building is linked to the quality of the team building effort. To improve the chances that a team building event will have a positive effect, the activity should be linked to overall team processes or outcomes—it has to be relevant. The team building activity should be followed up with meaningful changes in the team's processes or with demonstrable improvements in outcomes. Team building activities with no follow-up or evaluation are viewed as a waste of time and energy by team members. Successful team building activities generally should be planned by team members in addition to team leaders or sponsors. The planning process should reflect the culture of teamwork.

CONCLUSION

Team building activities are directed at improving the capacity of a team to be effective. Team building is growing in importance concurrently with the importance of team effectiveness, as teams ordinarily do not become effective without deliberate attention to their effectiveness. Team building activities typically involve goal or role clarification, interpersonal relationship building, identity building, or team process improvements. Retreats are a common setting for accomplishing team building. Teams can increase the chances of successful team building activities, including retreats, by involving team members in planning well in advance of events, maximizing attendance, and following up with changes and evaluation of the activities.

REFERENCES

Amos JA, Hu J, Herrick CA. The impact of team building on communication and job satisfaction of nursing staff. *J Nurses Staff Dev.* 2005;21:10-16.

Biech E, ed. *The Pfeiffer Book of Successful Team-Building Tools: Best of the Annuals.* 2nd ed. San Francisco, CA: Pfeiffer; 2008.

Clevenger K. Improve staff satisfaction with team building retreats. *Nurs Manage.* 2007;38(4):22, 24.

Dyer WG, Dyer WG Jr, Dyer JH. *Team Building: Proven Strategies for Improving Team Performance.* 4th ed. San Francisco, CA: Jossey-Bass; 2007.

Klein C, DiazGranados D, Salas E, et al. Does team building work? *Small Group Research.* 2009;40:181-222.

Lencioni P. *Overcoming the Five Dysfunctions of a Team: A Field Guide.* San Francisco, CA: Jossey-Bass; 2005.

Quenk NL. *Essentials of Myers-Briggs Type Indicator Assessment.* Hoboken, NJ: John Wiley & Sons; 2009.

Salas E, Rozell D, Mullen B, et al. The effect of team building on performance: an integration. *Small Group Research.* 1999;30:309-329.

Scholtes PR, Joiner BL, Streibel BJ. *The Team Handbook.* 3rd ed. Madison, WI: Oriel Incorporated; 2003.

Shuffler ML, DiazGranados D, Salas E. There's a science for that: team development interventions in organizations. *Curr Dir Psychol Sci.* 2011;20:365-372.

Venneberg DL. An eclectic approach to building effective teams: eight separate but interrelated components. *Advances in Developing Human Resources.* 2010;12:3-6.

West MA. *Effective Teamwork: Practical Lessons from Organizational Research.* 3rd ed. Chichester, UK: John Wiley & Sons, Ltd.; 2012.

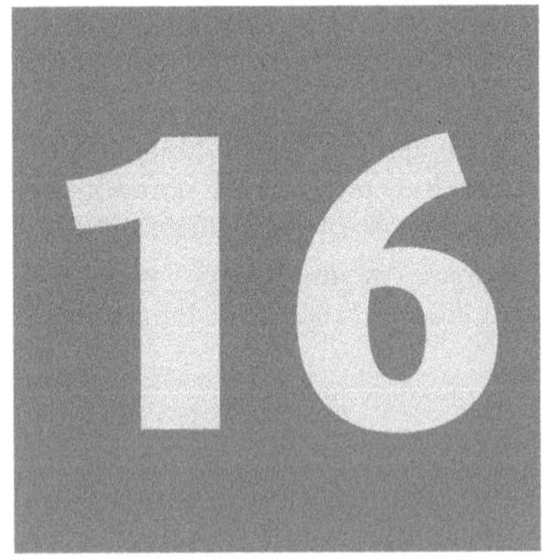

Process Improvement in Healthcare Teams

Chapters 14-17 deal with action for improvement of team performance. Chapter 14 covers training, and Chapter 15 examines team building. This chapter provides an account of process improvement, beginning with how it fits within the larger category of performance improvement. Chapter 17 deals with troubleshooting.

PERFORMANCE IMPROVEMENT

The phrase *performance improvement* refers to a cycle of management activities that consists of measuring performance, identifying areas for improvement, settings goals for improvement, taking a variety of actions aimed at achieving the goals, and measuring performance again—followed by identifying new areas for improvement, setting goals again, and so on in unending repetitions of the cycle.

The first step in the cycle is to measure performance. The measurement of performance in a team should include assessment of the team's success in achieving its goals as well as assessment of the quality of its teamwork. Chapter 13 deals with evaluation of team performance and emphasizes the measurement of teamwork quality, in keeping with the topic of this book. The details of measuring how well teams perform in achieving their goals is outside the scope of this book, but the general nature of this measurement can be stated briefly. For a clinical team, measuring goal attainment consists of measuring how well the team succeeds in achieving the Institute of Medicine's 6 aims discussed in Chapter 6. For example, a clinical team will want to know the quality of its clinical outcomes such as the quality of obstetrical outcomes in the Labor and Delivery Unit described in Chapter 13. For management teams, the goals vary widely from team to team, and measuring goal attainment varies accordingly. To take one example, a hospital finance team will want to know how well the hospital is performing on various financial indicators, including the hospital's debt-to-equity ratio and its cash-on-hand. Considering teams of all kinds, the list of appropriate performance measurement topics includes many widely varying topics: patient satisfaction, waiting times, postsurgical infection rates, costs for common procedures (for example, total hip replacement), rates of revenue growth and operating margin growth, and so on. One of the topics on the list is the quality of teamwork.

After measurement of performance has revealed areas for improvement, the next step in the cycle is to take action for improvement. The list of potential actions consists of a broad and diverse array: coaching, training, team building, process improvement, culture change, and many other management actions. Coaching is explained in Chapters 8 and 12. Training and team building are covered in the previous 2 chapters. Chapter 18 covers creating a team-based organizational culture and using compensation systems to foster organizational alignment. The list of possibilities is long. Some actions can be very simple and straightforward. For example, if a hospital supplier can no longer consistently meet its delivery schedule, a change to a more reliable supplier will improve performance.

In recent years, discussions of performance improvement in health care have often emphasized a particular cluster of activities that collectively are called *process improvement*. The primary field of knowledge underlying process improvement is systems theory.

A system, in this context, is a group of interacting, interdependent parts unified into a whole that has a single purpose or a coherent set of purposes. Systems theory is the study of these groupings of parts, including how they are structured, how they function, the ways in which the parts interact, the determinants of system performance, and other properties of systems. Besides systems theory, process improvement makes extensive use of statistics and scientific method as well as a few other fields of knowledge such as human factors knowledge (Ransom et al, 2008).

PROCESS IMPROVEMENT

The focus of this chapter is process improvement in teams, that is, improving the team's performance by directly improving the processes used by the team to achieve its goal.

The origin of knowledge about how to improve processes is different from the origin of most of the knowledge about teams in this book. Most of the content of this book originated in sociology, organizational behavior, social psychology, and management science. Knowledge of process improvement, in contrast, originated in systems thinking and engineering. Important foundational contributors were W. Edwards Deming (1986), Joseph M. Juran (1988), and Taiichi Ohno (1988) among others. In the United States, the use of systems thinking and process improvement in health care has been championed by Donald M. Berwick (2004) and others. A systems approach to improving the quality of health care is prominent in the work of the Institute of Medicine (2001).

The application of systems thinking specifically to healthcare teams has been pioneered by Paul B. Batalden and colleagues (2003). Their concept of the clinical microsystem is discussed in Chapter 12.

METHODS FOR PROCESS IMPROVEMENT

Over the past 60 years, many systematic approaches have been devised for improving the performance of processes in manufacturing, service industries, financial services, and other sectors of the economy. The methods most commonly espoused in health care have been Continuous Quality Improvement (CQI), Lean Production, and Six Sigma (Ransom et al, 2008, pp. 63-83). CQI calls for: (1) understanding a system as a set of processes, (2) identifying opportunities for process improvement, (3) making process changes in order to improve performance, (4) measuring the effects of the changes made, and (5) stabilizing those changes that have been found to improve performance (McLaughlin and Kaluzny, 2006). Lean Production is similar except that this method is focused on the elimination of waste in a system. The elimination of waste results not only in improved efficiency but also in higher reliability of the system in achieving its goals (Liker, 2004). Six Sigma is also similar to CQI, but it focuses on the reduction of errors to extremely low levels, thereby improving consistency of performance and improving efficiency by eliminating the need for rework (Barry et al, 2002).

All of these process improvement methods are comprehensive approaches to managing the processes that an organization uses to provide for the needs and wants of its customers. All of the methods share 7 several general principles:

- Good performance means meeting the needs of the customer.
- An organization is a system of interacting processes or sequences of events.
- Improvement in performance is achieved by improving processes.
- Performance of the system is assessed by collecting and analyzing data and not by using impressions or subjective judgments.
- Engaging those who participate directly in the processes is central to improving those processes.
- Improvement can be achieved only through the commitment of the senior leaders of the organization.
- Pursuit of improvement never ends; it is both perpetual and relentless.

As suggested by the generality of these statements, each of the different process improvement methods has a management philosophy underlying its approach to improvement. These philosophies differ somewhat, and some are more developed than others. This chapter, however, is not focused on the general underpinnings of process improvement. Instead, its chief aim is to explain the mechanics of process improvement, that is, the actions that teams can take at a detailed level to improve their work processes. Broader organizational considerations are nonetheless important and are discussed briefly later in the chapter.

The Model for Improvement

Heartland Medical Group was a primary care practice of 12 family physicians, 7 internists, 8 adult nurse practitioners (NPs), and 1 obstetrician who cared for women with high-risk pregnancies. Heartland had 1 clinic site in a town of 12,000 people. It served people from this town as well as several smaller towns nearby. The 19 physicians and 8 NPs in Heartland were divided into 3 groups with separate front desk staff and separate medical assistant staff. In other words, there were 3 teams of clinicians and support staff. In addition, a group of registered nurses (RNs) and administrative staff supported all 3 teams. Heartland used an electronic health record (EHR) to which it had access as a result of an affiliation agreement with the hospital where the physicians also practiced.

Public reporting of medical group performance was becoming a reality in the state where Heartland was located. A project had been underway for 3 years to introduce the idea. Medical groups' performance in preventive care and chronic disease care had been measured and reported back to the medical groups but not more widely. All medical groups knew that the quality of care measurements would soon be reported on a public website, starting in 1-2 years.

One component of chronic care being measured was care for patients with asthma. The 2 measures reported were the percentage of patients who had high scores on a self-administered questionnaire about their asthma symptoms (a high score indicating that the patient had few symptoms) and the percentage who reported that they had been hospitalized for asthma during the past year or had visited an emergency department (ED) twice (or more) for asthma. In the most recent report, Heartland had scored poorly relative to other medical groups on both measures. Only 20% of their patients had high scores on the self-administered questionnaire, and 14% of their patients had been hospitalized during the past year or had 2 more ED visits. The physicians and NPs wanted to improve these scores.

With the approval of Heartland's Clinical Services Committee (the day-to-day operations committee), a quality improvement (QI) team was formed to serve all 3 primary care teams. The QI team consisted of a physician from one primary care team, an NP from a second team, another NP from the third team, an operations manager, a medical assistant, an RN, and a staff member from the hospital's EHR support group. The general aim of the QI team was to improve Heartland's scores on the asthma measures so that Heartland could "hold its head up with pride" in the company of the other medical groups in the state.

The team met for the first time to review its charge and get to work.

Like the story about surgical safety training in Chapter 14, this story is recurring throughout the United States as clinics and hospitals become motivated to improve their performance. In many cases, the motivation of the clinics and hospitals stems from their concern for their reputations. The concerns are being generated by public reporting of how well patients fare under their care. Sometimes insurance company payments are also tied to meeting certain thresholds on quality measures although not in the case of Heartland and its asthma care. There was no question that Heartland wanted to achieve better results for its patients with asthma. What they sought was a pathway to better results. What approach did they use?

The traditional method for Heartland was the Model for Improvement, which is shown in Figure 16–1 (Langley et al, 2009, pp. 15-25). The Model for Improvement is one interpretation of the CQI approach to process improvement. It derives from the work of Deming and Shewhart, who originated the cycle of *Plan-Do-Study-Act* or *PDSA* (Langley et al, 2009, p. 465). The Model also includes 3 preliminary questions to be answered before beginning cycles of PDSA. In the United States, the Model for Improvement has become very widely used. It was devised and has been taught by Associates in Process Improvement (API), Austin, TX, and is sometimes referred to as the *API Improvement Model*. The model has been disseminated and promoted by the Institute for Healthcare Improvement, Boston, MA.

The first step in the Model for Improvement is to answer the question "What are we trying to accomplish?" In other words, the first step is to state as clearly as possible the aim of the improvement project or endeavor. General statements of aim are not useful without further specification because they do not lend themselves to careful determination of whether

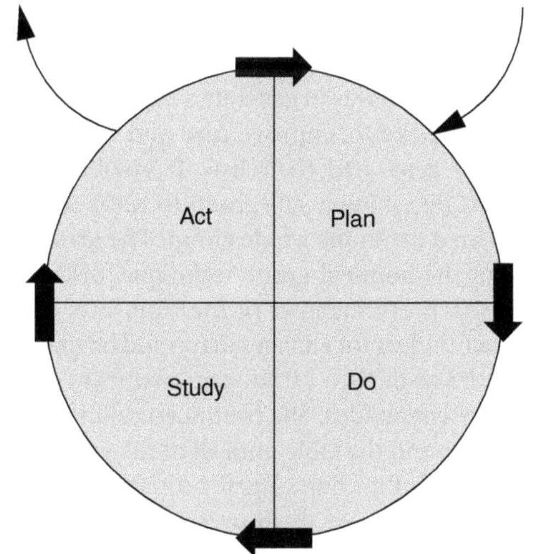

▲ **Figure 16–1.** The Model for Improvement. Langley GJ, Moen RD, Nolan KM et al. *The Improvement Guide: A Practical Approach to Enhancing Organizational Performance*. 2nd ed. San Francisco, CA: Jossey-Bass; 2009:24. Reproduced with permission of John Wiley & Sons, Inc.

progress is being made. For example, in the case of Heartland's asthma care project, the team might have decided that they were trying to accomplish an improvement in their care of patients with asthma. Although this statement is, of course, correct, it would have afforded the team little direction and little basis for knowing whether they were succeeding. To some people at Heartland, accomplishment of this aim might have meant that asthma education should be improved. To others, it might have meant that more patients should be treated with medication having long-term effects, for example inhaled corticosteroids (beclomethasone, fluticasone, and similar drugs delivered with an inhaler). Still others might have been thinking of improving the assessment of the severity of patients' disease. Any of these actions might have been appropriate; but in the end, how would the QI team know with confidence whether they were making progress toward their goal of improving asthma care?

As it happened, the Heartland QI team was not tempted to settle for a general statement of its aim because the organization measuring their performance had in essence assigned them a twofold aim: (1) to reduce the burden of symptoms in their patients with asthma, and (2) to reduce their asthma patients' needs to obtain care for their symptoms in the inpatient portion of a hospital or in an ED. The statement of these 2 aims provided an adequate answer to the question of what the team was trying to accomplish. These 2 aims are not the only defensible aims that the team could have chosen. For example, they might have settled on symptom reduction as one aim but decided that improvement of actual breathing capacity (speed of airflow into and out of the lungs) would be their second aim, to be measured by devices used by the patients at home or in the clinic. But the team was content with the 2 aims stipulated by the reporting organization.

And yet stating the twofold aim was not enough to enable the team to chart its progress. The team needed to answer the Model's second question, "How will we know that a change is an improvement?" In other words, for each aim, they needed to have a well-defined measure that would enable them to quantify their progress and know whether the changes they were making in the clinic were lessening their patients' symptom burdens and decreasing the patients' needs for emergency care. Again, the measurement question was defined for them by the reporting organization, which had adopted detailed specifications for the measurement of symptom burden and use of emergency care. Briefly, the specifications started with a definition of the population of asthma patients in Heartland's practice. This definition was needed for the measurement of progress on both aims. Next, the use of a specific questionnaire was called for, enabling a symptom score to be obtained for each patient indicating the patient's level of symptoms during the week prior to the date when the patient completed the questionnaire. The proportion of symptom-free patients was then defined as the number of patients with a high score (above a specified threshold) on the questionnaire divided by the number of asthma patients. The use of emergency services was to be determined by using hospital and ED records as reflected in billing statements sent to insurance companies. The proportion of patients needing emergency care was defined as the number of patients with a hospitalization or 2 ED visits (or more) for asthma during the past year divided by the number of asthma patients. Additional details were also spelled out in the specifications. Again, various team members might have preferred different measures of attainment of the aims. For example, they might have preferred to use a different questionnaire or to define use of emergency services so that the number of ED visits in the definition was 3 instead of 2. But the team was satisfied enough with the definitions used by the reporting organization.

The next step in the Model for Improvement is to answer the question "What change can we make that will result in improvement?" This question is open to misinterpretation because it provides no indication of how an idea for a change is to be obtained. It might be tempting for a QI team to seize upon the first idea that is voiced by anyone on the team. It would be imprudent to proceed with the first idea offered or with someone's pet idea not subjected to any evaluative thinking. But it also would be wasteful to delay taking action while the possibilities for changes are investigated at great length. Some systematic approach to generating ideas for changes and evaluating them is appropriate at this stage in using the Model.

It is always useful to inquire what other organizations have done to solve the problem at hand. If the problem is a clinical problem, sometimes the inquiry can be done by searching the literature, using MEDLINE or an alternative database. However, it is often faster and more productive to inquire of other medical groups or hospitals that are facing or have faced the same challenge.

The other approach commonly employed to generate ideas is to use one or another of the tools for creativity presented in Chapter 10, for example, some version of team brainstorming. Alternatively, a QI team can ask 2 or 3 of its members to confer and present a few possibilities to the whole team for consideration. This approach assures that possible process changes receive some critical appraisal even before they are presented to the team and that further debate and critique occurs in the whole team—provided that the small group of 2 or 3 is asked to present some well-considered possibilities and not what they have firmly concluded are the best change ideas.

The QI team at Heartland proceeded first by gathering some background information that could be collected quickly. First, they wanted to know how many asthma patients Heartland cared for. They learned from a review of their electronic records that there were 2521 asthma patients in the practice. They suspected that the practice actually had more asthma patients, but 2521 was the number that could be verified by using their data. Because the approach to assessment and treatment is different for children and adults, they also determined how many patients were in each age group.

Their next step was to generate a list of changes that they might make to improve care and achieve their aims. They generated their list of possibilities as a group, not by asking a sub-group to meet separately and present a list to the whole group. The team used a version of the nominal group technique, discussed in Chapter 10. Every member of the team was asked to write down 3 ideas for changes that could be made. The chair of the team then asked team members one at a time to present an idea. She continued calling on team members around the table until all of the group's ideas were listed on a flip chart. The list consisted of 26 possible changes, some of them overlapping. Among the suggested changes were:

- Assure that every clinic visit by an asthma patient includes a formal assessment of the patient's asthma symptoms.
- Contact asthma patients who have not returned to the clinic for 6 months and ask them to return for a visit.
- Assure that inhaled corticosteroids are prescribed for all asthma patients whose symptoms are not well controlled by short-acting inhaled medications (β_2-agonists).
- Track ED use and contact patients seen in an ED for asthma symptoms to assure that they come to the clinic within 1 week of the ED visit.

Some of the change ideas came from reading done by QI team members, and some were solely the results of individual insight and creativity. Other ideas were taken from other medical groups in the state, whose efforts to improve asthma care were known by some of the QI team members.

After a list of possible changes was generated, the next step was a discussion of criteria to use in choosing among the possibilities. The criteria might have been devised before the list of possible changes was generated, but it is usually easier for teams to deal with the criteria after they have a concrete list of possible changes in front of them. Criteria often considered in making choices among possible changes are:

- The change under consideration has a reasonable likelihood of success.
- Compared with other possible changes, the change is likely to have a greater impact in achieving the project's aim(s).
- The healthcare practice or hospital has the resources necessary to make the change.
- There is evidence that the change was effective when it was used in other similar settings.

The QI team's next step was to discuss how the possible changes in the list compared with one another when they are judged against the criteria. Some teams go so far as devising a matrix to make explicit the scores for each possible change with respect to each of the criteria, with the scores usually assessed only roughly as "high," "medium," or "low." Sometimes different possible changes are combined, and some possibilities may be dropped at this point if they are deemed by consensus to be unpromising.

Finally, the QI team chose a change to test. Sometimes more than one change is chosen for testing simultaneously. The final choice is usually made by consensus. Alternatively, there are several voting procedures that can be used, as explained in Chapter 10. One popular voting method is multivoting (Scholtes et al, 2003, pp. 3-20 to 3-21). Team members multivote by voting for 2-5 of their top choices, thus avoiding an artificial forced choice by each member of a "top choice." This procedure recognizes that preferences among possibilities usually are not black-and-white but differ like shades of gray. The votes are tallied as usual, and the top choices for the team are those with the highest numbers of votes. The team may choose to test the change that received the highest number of votes, or it may choose the top 2 or 3 changes to test.

The steps described here, from posing the question "What change can we make that will result in improvement?" to choosing a change to test, may appear time consuming. However, provided that team members have done some homework in advance to inform their discussion, the entire sequence can usually be completed in a single meeting of 90 minutes or so.

The Heartland asthma QI team first chose to test whether performance could be improved by reaching out to patients who had not had a clinic visit for 6 months. The medical assistant on the QI team plus one of the NPs proceeded to identify which of the 2521 patients with asthma had not been seen in the clinic for 6 months. They discovered that only a tiny proportion of the 2521 patients had not been seen, and so this approach was abandoned. However, there was benefit for the team in that they learned that the low performance scores for Heartland were not due to poor follow-up of patients. The clinicians were seeing the patients on a timely basis, but they needed to change what they were doing during the visits.

The next change to be pursued was to assure that inhaled corticosteroids were prescribed for all patients whose symptoms were not well controlled by short-acting inhaled medications. The medical assistant and RN worked with the EHR expert to obtain a list of all asthma patients who had been prescribed medication for their symptoms but not corticosteroids (or more potent medication). They examined a sample of these patients' records and found that at the most recent visit it was usually not possible to determine whether the patient's symptoms were controlled or not. Formal assessments of symptom severity were generally not done or, if done, were not recorded in the record. The team decided to test whether improvement could be achieved by increasing the frequency of both routine formal assessment of symptoms and prescription of inhaled corticosteroids when needed.

At this point, the QI team had reached the beginning of the PDSA cycle in Figure 16–1. The next step was to *Plan*, that is, plan the change. They decided to add a prompt to the EHR that would remind the medical assistant to have all patients with asthma complete the customary symptom questionnaire at every visit, construing the administration of the questionnaire in the same way that they regarded measuring a patient's blood pressure, that is, as a routine element in every visit for patients with asthma. At the same time, they planned to promote the prescription of inhaled corticosteroids for appropriate patients, to be identified by their poor scores on the symptom questionnaire. This promotion would be done by *academic detailing*, that is, by having 2 highly interested physicians initiate conversations with all other clinicians in the medical group to remind them about the appropriate prescription of inhaled corticosteroids (Soumerai and Avorn, 1990). In addition, the QI team decided to distribute short e-mail updates on the improvement project to all clinicians and medical assistants at Heartland.

The next step in the Model for Improvement is *Do*, that is, make the change in a limited or test environment. The QI team decided to try this 2-pronged change (using symptom questionnaires and academic detailing) in just one of the 3 teams in the clinic. The EHR prompt was added and the academic detailing was carried out within the test setting within a few days. (Meanwhile, the e-mail updates on the project were distributed every 2 weeks to those on all 3 clinical teams.)

The next step in the Model is to *Study*, that is, find out what has happened as a consequence of instituting the test change. Some years ago, this step in the PDSA cycle was called "Check," and the cycle is still sometimes called the *PDCA cycle*. The first part of this step is to check to see whether the planned change was implemented as intended. The second part is to inquire whether the change had its intended effect. At the end of 2 weeks, the QI team assessed its test of the change by simply inquiring of those working in the test setting, first, whether the EHR prompts were appearing on the computer screens as intended. Second, they asked whether the medical assistants were administering the symptom questionnaires and whether the clinicians were using the questionnaires to decide whether to prescribe inhaled corticosteroids. Everyone on the QI team presumed that the reports about the function of the EHR would be reliable but that the medical assistants and clinicians were likely to exaggerate how well they were following through with the planned change—not because they deliberately misreported their actions but because of optimism or selective memory. But, at this stage, a subjective check on progress was sufficient. A more thorough investigation came at 6 weeks when 3 members of the QI team reviewed a sample of records for visits by asthma patients occurring after the start of the test of change. There had been 105 visits by patients with a diagnosis of asthma. One hundred visits were reviewed. For 94 visits, a symptom questionnaire score was recorded in the record. For 14 of these 94 visits, the patient's symptom score was poor and the patient had not been prescribed inhaled corticosteroids previously. In 13 of these 14 cases, the clinician prescribed an inhaled corticosteroid at the time of the visit. (In the one case that was a failure, the physician said with a wink that she had "lost my head"—made a mistake.) The test of the change was judged a success.

The final step in the PDSA cycle is *Act*. In the Model, to act means to take broader and more long-lasting action. In the case of the Heartland project, acting meant extending to the other 2 clinical teams the EHR prompts, routine use of the symptom questionnaire, and routine prescription of inhaled corticosteroids to patients whose symptoms were poorly controlled with short-acting inhaled medication.

After 4 more months, the QI team did a full audit of its performance on the 2 measures that would soon be reported publicly. The audit showed that both the symptom burden and the use of emergency services by asthma patients had improved—but not enough for those at Heartland to be satisfied. This result, in turn, raised the question of returning to the PDSA cycle to consider more possibilities for process changes, to choose 1 or 2 more changes to test, to plan them, and to continue on through the cycle again. As in this case, the quest for quality usually continues indefinitely.

This story of Heartland Medical Group's pursuit of improved performance in caring for its patients with asthma illustrates the Model for Improvement. In other medical groups, the story would have been different. The range of process changes considered might have been different. The changes first chosen for testing might have been different, resulting in different details during the Study phase of the first turn of the cycle. But the steps traversed would have been the same.

There is a good deal more to using the Model for Improvement than the events described in Heartland's story. For example, no mention was made of the use of statistics, which would help determine whether the apparent improvement in quality scores was real and not simply a result of random fluctuation. The basic statistical tools for analyzing process improvement scores are run charts and control charts. A run chart is a simple plot of measurements over time with no statistical calculation results included in the chart except for the average of the measurements (Brassard and Ritter, 2008, pp. 124-127). A control chart includes results of statistical calculations that permit large, real changes to be distinguished from random fluctuations (Montgomery, 2009, pp. 179-343). A third type of chart for tracking process changes, commonly used in manufacturing and service industries but seldom used in health care, is the cumulative sum chart or cusum chart. A cusum chart includes more complex calculation results that permit small but persistent, real changes to be distinguished from random fluctuations (Hawkins and Olwell, 1998; Montgomery, 2009, pp. 400-419).

In the Heartland story, there is also no mention of the many diagrammatic tools that are used in process improvement, for example, process maps, cause and effect diagrams, and project management charts (Nelson et al, 2007, pp. 296-307, 313-320, 362-368). Finally, there is no discussion in the story of the organizational supports that are needed for a team to be able to succeed consistently in improving its processes. These supports include an organizational culture that nurtures perpetual improvement and construes clinical work as encompassing not only the care of patients but also work to improve the processes of patient care. These topics are covered in works by Deming (1986), Ohno (1988), Harry and Schroeder (2000), and Nelson and colleagues (2011).

Some of the organizational supports needed for effective process improvement are the same as those needed for teams to succeed in general. Chapter 18 deals with the roles and responsibilities of senior leaders in supporting teams. Some of the necessary supporting actions aid process improvement.

OTHER APPROACHES TO PROCESS IMPROVEMENT

As mentioned earlier, the Heartland QI team could have used a different step-by-step process improvement method to improve the care it provided for Heartland's patients with asthma. Two other choices are described here briefly. These methods are the only other methods that currently receive frequent attention in the healthcare literature. They are less commonly used in the United States than the Model for Improvement.

Lean Production

The Lean Production approach to process improvement focuses on eliminating waste or "fat" in processes, hence the name. This approach is often called the *Toyota Production System (TPS)* because it was developed in the Toyota Motor Company beginning in about 1950. The system is a fully developed method for the leadership and management of any enterprise, and it includes all aspects of performance improvement. Embedded within the system is a methodical approach to process improvement in particular (Liker, 2004).

Forms of Waste

In the Lean approach to improvement, processes are improved by ridding them of 7 different types of waste (Ohno, 1998, pp. 19-20). The types of waste, listed in Table 16–1, are:

Waste of Overproduction: Overproduction is the production of goods or services that are not needed. An example in health care is a tray of paper forms that go unused because a new one is printed from the computer whenever it is needed. Pharmacies sometimes continue to order medications that have gone out of use. Hospital admissions offices sometimes collect information from patients that is never used, for example, their mothers' maiden names.

Waste of Time on Hand (Waiting): Health care is replete with obvious, wasteful waiting. Patients wait to see clinicians in their offices. Physicians wait for laboratory results. Social workers wait for telephone calls to be returned by agencies that they contact for services. Administrators wait for other administrators

Table 16–1. Types of waste in the Lean approach to process improvement

Type of Waste	Example
Overproduction	Collect patient information that is never used
Time on hand (waiting)	Wait for team members to arrive late to meetings
Transportation	Moving a patient a long distance from the ED to Radiology
Processing	Taking a patient's medical history multiple times during a hospital stay
Stock on hand (inventory)	Holding prostheses in inventory months ahead of need
Movement	Having families of patients in an ED go to the admissions office on another floor and return to the ED
Defective products	Repeating x-ray imaging because it was improperly performed

and clinicians who are late to meetings or who cannot be found for a planned telephone call. All of this waiting is waste. Some of it cannot be eliminated, but processes are improved whenever waiting can be eliminated or decreased.

Waste in Transportation: The process of moving a patient in a wheelchair down 3 hallways to go from the ED to the radiology department is wasteful. If the ED were located next to the radiology department, far less transportation of patients would be needed. Moving paper documents by mail or courier is also wasteful if the documents could be moved electronically. Transporting clinicians from one hospital to another is wasteful if their work could be all done at one hospital.

Waste of Processing Itself: This is the waste of doing more than necessary. Taking the medical history of a patient 4 times during the first 2 hours of a hospital stay is wasteful. Needing to write down the same telephone number 3 times in a paper form is wasteful. Overprocessing also occurs when what is done or produced is of higher quality than what is needed; for example, wiping down the counter at a nurses' station once an hour is overprocessing. Repeating clinic visits or laboratory tests frequently often contributes nothing to the care of the patient and thus counts as overprocessing. These excesses are in fact not examples of high quality; they are examples of defects.

Waste of Stock on Hand (Inventory): In health care, it is tempting to build up inventories of equipment, supplies, and person-hours just in case, that is, to cover the possibility that something will be needed without warning. While covering contingencies makes sense, covering them too well is a fault. Surgical supply rooms stocked with sterile kits to last for 2 years are wasteful. It is wasteful to stock several different prostheses for hip replacement procedures, each one waiting to be used by a particular orthopedist. Negotiating agreement to use 1 or 2 prostheses would reduce the waste. So would ordering prostheses to arrive immediately before surgery. In this way, inventory of prostheses for elective hip replacement can be eliminated altogether.

Waste of Movement: People working in health care often move around far more than is necessary to accomplish their tasks. Frequently this happens because the physical design of their workspace does not facilitate the flow of work processes. Laboratory technicians walk back and forth across laboratories to take specimens from one machine to another when the machines are used in sequence many times a day but have been placed on opposite sides of the room. The families of patients sometimes arrive with the patient at an ED, are directed to an admissions office located on a different floor in the hospital, and then return to the ED. If there were a satellite admissions office in the ED, this movement would not be needed.

Waste of Making Defective Products: This form of waste is the most obvious of all. Chest x-rays that need to be repeated because part of the chest was not included in the field of view are waste. Surgical infections that could have been prevented are waste. Meetings for decision making that run overtime and reach no conclusion are waste.

Using Lean Production in Health Care

TPS has been adopted by many healthcare systems across the country. Particularly prominent among these adopters has been Virginia Mason Medical Center in Seattle (Kaplan and Patterson, 2008). Nelson-Peterson and Leppa (2007) have described the application of Lean Production methods to the care of patients in an inpatient unit of the Virginia Mason Hospital. To improve the nursing care for patients, nursing leaders and a team of 6 frontline nursing staff focused on eliminating waste from the processes of care. As part of their project, they used a highly organized event called a *Rapid Process Improvement Workshop (RPIW)*. RPIWs are a routine part of TPS. Preparation for an RPIW begins weeks before the event. It includes identification of the process or cluster of processes to be improved, planning of the RPIW event, and assignment of responsibilities for the event and for follow-up. The RPIW usually lasts 3-5 days. During this time the improvement team of 6-8 people creates a clear depiction of the processes to be improved using flowcharts and other diagrammatic tools. They identify as many sources of waste as they can. In the case of the nursing care RPIW at Virginia Mason, the team identified unneeded inventory, wasted movement of nurses moving around the inpatient unit, and many other examples of the 7 forms of waste. Some processes were redesigned during the workshop, and others were flagged for redesign later. At the conclusion of the workshop, the leaders met to set target dates for completing the work planned in the workshop, to be followed by spreading the successful changes throughout the hospital. Improvements achieved included a reduction in unnecessary walking by nurses during each shift, increased levels of patient satisfaction with nurse responsiveness, and increased time spent directly with patients. The improvements in patient satisfaction and nurse-patient time nicely demonstrate how TPS improves quality even though the focus is on reducing waste.

Imagining Lean Production at Heartland Medical Group

The Heartland QI team used the Model for Improvement and not TPS. If it had used TPS, the approach would have been more elaborate and would not have begun with setting the 2 aims derived from the agency reporting measurement of Heartland's care for people with asthma. Instead, team members would have studied their processes for providing asthma care and identified all instances of the 7 types of waste they could find. Two of those instances of waste would have been ED visits and undesirably high levels of symptoms in their patients. In order to minimize or eliminate these 2 instances of waste, the redesign of processes then might have proceeded in much the same way as it did with the Model for Improvement. However, the redesign would almost certainly have been more thorough, and the team would have identified many other areas of waste to be eliminated.

Use of the Model for Improvement enables QI teams to proceed directly to the aim they have in mind when initiating a project. It is simpler to explain and to use, and it requires fewer resources. In particular, less time is required from staff and clinicians. TPS, on the other hand, is more thorough from the onset.

Six Sigma

Six Sigma originated with Motorola in about 1980. While TPS focuses on waste, Six Sigma focuses instead on eliminating defects in producing goods or services. Six Sigma includes a management philosophy, but it is less elaborate than that of TPS. The core of Six Sigma thinking is the relentless and uncompromising eradication of defects. The goal of a Six Sigma organization is to reduce its defect rates in all processes to less than 3.4 errors per million opportunities. (The target was chosen by reference to a statistical concept. The area under a normal or Gaussian curve outside of 6 sigma, that is, 6 standard deviations, on either side of the mean is 0.00034% or 3.4 per million. The intent of this choice is to set the target extremely low, but the exact choice is arbitrary. See Montgomery, 2009, pp. 28-29, for a more complete explanation.)

Table 16–2. Five steps in the Six Sigma approach to process improvement (DMAIC)

Steps	Description
Define	Identify the opportunity to improve and document the processes
Measure	Define measures and collect data
Analyze	Analyze data to identify deviations from intentions and root causes
Improve	Devise and test potential solutions; select which ones to use
Control	Error-proof and monitor the new processes

Each Six Sigma project proceeds through a series of 5 steps, depicted in Table 16–2:

1. *Define*: Identify the opportunity to improve performance for the patient or customer; define what is important to the patient; document the processes used.
2. *Measure*: Decide what to measure; collect data; establish the baseline error rates.
3. *Analyze*: Analyze the data to determine why processes deviate from what is intended and to identify the root causes of those deviations.
4. *Improve*: Devise potential solutions for the problems; test and evaluate different options; select which solutions to implement.
5. *Control*: Develop plans for managing the improved processes long-term; error-proof the processes; monitor the processes and plan what to do in the event that they malfunction.

The mnemonic for this sequence is DMAIC, pronounced "duh-MAY-ic" (Montgomery, 2009, pp. 45-60).

The distinctive feature of Six Sigma's method is its extensive use of statistical methods at steps 2, 3, and 4 of DMAIC. Six Sigma uses not only control charts but any relevant statistical method that might be used in a research investigation. For example, if it is suspected that patients admitted to the hospital during changes of nursing shifts are more vulnerable to medication errors during their stays, then a Six Sigma approach would call for assembling records of admission time and medication errors for, say, all patients in the past 6 months, followed by analysis of the data using a chi-square test (or alternative) to determine whether admission time is associated with the occurrence of a medication error during the patient's stay. This investigation could lead eventually to the institution of special precautions for patients admitted during shift change. Analysis of variance, logistic regression, and other statistical methods are also used. The methods are used both for determining root causes of errors and for estimating the capacities of processes to handle flow volumes, for example, for the capacity of an admissions office to admit patients without generating a waiting time of a specified number of minutes.

Using Six Sigma in Health Care

Six Sigma has been adopted by some healthcare organizations but not by as many as have adopted TPS. The literature contains some reports of success using this approach. For example, Yale New Haven Hospital adopted the Six Sigma method in 2001.

Frankel and colleagues reported on the use of Six Sigma methods in reducing the rate of catheter-related bloodstream infections in the Yale New Haven's surgical intensive care unit (Frankel et al, 2005). These infections occur in patients who have an intravenous catheter in place for the administration of fluid and medications. In most cases, the tip of the intravenous catheter is located in the large vein just outside the heart. The infections are assumed to be caused in some way by the presence of the catheter. The project used the DMAIC procedure. A measure of outcome was selected—the number of catheters placed between catheter-related bloodstream infections. In other words, following each infection, Frankel and colleagues counted the number of catheters placed before the next infection. An increasing number indicated improvement in performance. Factors contributing to development of infections were displayed on a cause-and-effect diagram. Control charts were used to assess the effects of process changes that were instituted serially over a 2-year period. As the project progressed, statistical analyses were performed to determine causes of new infections. The rate of infections was reduced from the baseline rate of 11 infections per 1000 catheter days to a rate of 1.7 per 1000 catheter days.

Kelly and colleagues reported on the use of Six Sigma to decrease treatment time for patients with myocardial infarction (heart attack) at Wake Forest University Baptist Medical Center (Kelly et al, 2010). The treatment used was percutaneous coronary intervention (opening of one or more arteries supplying blood to the heart). In this procedure, an artery is opened by inflating a small balloon at the end of a catheter that is inserted through the skin, slid through a large artery, and positioned inside the artery that is blocked. Inflating and then collapsing the balloon decreases or eliminates the obstruction to blood flow. The "door-to-needle time" is the time elapsed between the patient's arrival at the ED entrance and the insertion of the needle through which the catheter is inserted. Better results in minimizing the consequences of a heart attack are achieved with shorter door-to-needle times. The project used process-mapping (flowcharting) and set time goals for each segment of the sequence of events from door to needle. Factors contributing to delay in each time segment were meticulously identified and eliminated. Control charts were used to track progress as various interventions were used to improve performance. The overall door-to-needle time and the durations of the time segments were monitored. No statistical testing was done to identify causes of defects. The door-to-needle time was reduced from 128 minutes to 56 minutes over 6 years. The variation in door-to-needle time from patient to patient was also reduced.

Imagining Six Sigma at Heartland Medical Group

In theory the Heartland QI team could have used the Six Sigma method in doing its work on asthma care. They would have started by laying out the key characteristics of good care for asthma as seen by both patients and clinicians. They would have mapped the events in the care of the patients, identifying opportunities for defects to occur. At that point, however, they would have encountered difficulties. Six Sigma requires the availability of substantial amounts of data and the ability to analyze the data using statistical methods that are not used in most hospitals, medical groups, and other delivery settings (for example, analysis of variance and logistic regression). Heartland would have needed, for example, to be able to identify patients who had used an ED and then to determine whether these patients, compared with other asthma patients, had higher rates of various possible causal factors in their histories. Possible causes would have been absence of a prescription for an inhaled corticosteroid, lack of a clinic visit for 6 months, absence of an asthma action plan for use by the parents of a child with asthma, and so on. While these data could be obtained in principle, the resource requirements would have been great, and in any case Heartland very likely did not have access to a statistician to perform the necessary calculations. A thorough Six Sigma approach was not feasible for this QI team although some of the tools used in Six Sigma, for example, flowcharts and cause-and-effect diagrams, would have been very useful and not expensive or time consuming. In any case, most of diagrammatic tools used in Six Sigma are also used in the Model for Improvement, the method used by the Heartland team (Langley et al, 2009, pp. 409-451).

Six Sigma is a powerful method for process improvement. However, at the present time it is beyond the reach of most healthcare organizations because of the extensive data requirements and the need for statistical expertise. Some of its tools, however, can be added easily and usefully to simpler approaches to process improvement.

Lean Six Sigma

Not surprisingly, many process improvement experts now advocate taking the best from the Model for Improvement, Lean Production, and Six Sigma and using whatever methods fit with the problem at hand and the resources available. The British National Health Service has taken this position explicitly and is promoting use of both Lean and Six Sigma, calling the method *Lean Six Sigma* (Bevan et al, 2005). And, in fact, at the core of all of the process improvement methods is a cycle of performance measurement, problem identification and clarification, goal setting, process change, and monitoring of the effects of the changes. Elements of the Model for Improvement, Lean Production, and Six Sigma can be used together whenever mixing the methods is useful.

ESTABLISHING A PROGRAM OF PROCESS IMPROVEMENT

This chapter focuses on the methods that the individual teams can use to improve selected processes. While teams can and do pursue process improvement projects in isolation from any broader endeavor, a more systematic and more desirable approach is to pursue projects in the context of an organizational program of process improvement, one that is part of a general program of performance improvement. Teams operating in large healthcare systems are usually not permitted to pursue process improvement projects at will because the staff supporting these projects is limited in number and the use of staff time needs to be carefully allocated for maximum benefit in improving care. In Heartland's case, moving forward with project selection would be much simpler than it would in a large organization. Regardless of the size of the organization, it is desirable for potential projects to be identified and for choices among the possible projects to be made based on explicit, agreed-upon criteria, for example, availability of resources for the project, the gains in healthcare outcomes that can be reasonably anticipated, the gains in patient satisfaction that can be anticipated, and the organizational needs that would be met (for example, improvement of Heartland's reputation caused by improvement in their publicly reported scores on asthma care). In large organizations, projects are often chosen by the senior executive group in the organization. In smaller organizations like Heartland, projects can be chosen by the executive or management committee of the medical group.

CONCLUSION

Healthcare teams can improve their performance by using systematic performance improvement. Several different options are available for taking action for improvement, including training, team building, and culture change. One important option is process improvement, which uses well-defined methods to understand processes, set goals, and improve the processes by making changes in the processes and measuring the effects of these changes. There are currently 3 models for process improvement in use in US healthcare: the Model for Improvement, Lean Production (also called the Toyota Production System), and Six Sigma. The most widely used of these 3 is the Model for Improvement. The core of the Model for Improvement is Deming's cycle of Plan-Do-Study-Act. Lean Production focuses on waste reduction and is a more elaborate approach using more staff and clinician time. Six Sigma is more complex and resource-intensive than both the Model for Improvement and Lean Production; it employs a variety of statistical tools.

At this time the more complex methods of process improvement (Lean and Six Sigma) are outside of the capabilities of many healthcare organizations.

However, it is not difficult to imagine that some decades from now these methods will be as commonly used in health care as they now are in manufacturing, retailing, communications, and other sectors of the economy. It would seem that both the welfare of patients and the ever growing cost of health care require the use of these methods to secure improvement. Yet, broad use of the more powerful methods will need to await changes in how health care is organized in the United States and in the mindset of clinicians and managers. In the meantime, healthcare practices and hospitals will continue to use the methods they find feasible.

REFERENCES

Barry R, Murcko AC, Brubaker CE. *The Six Sigma Book for Healthcare.* Chicago, IL: Health Administration Press; 2002.

Batalden PB, Nelson EC, Edwards WH, et al. Microsystems in health care: part 9. developing small clinical units to attain peak performance. *Jt Comm J Qual Saf.* 2003; 29:575-585.

Berwick DM. *Escape Fire: Designs for the Future of Health Care.* San Francisco, CA: John Wiley & Sons, Inc.; 2004.

Bevan H, Westwood N, O'Connor M, et al. Lean 6 Sigma: Using Common Sense and Common Science to Achieve Uncommon Results. Presentation at: 17th Annual National Forum on Quality Improvement in Health Care; December 11, 2005; Orlando, FL. http://www.institute.nhs.uk/images//documents/FinalVersionLeanSigmaDec11Orlandopresentation.pdf. Accessed September 7, 2012.

Brassard M, Ritter D. *The Memory Jogger II: Healthcare Edition.* Salem, NH: GOAL/QPC; 2008.

Deming WE. *Out of the Crisis.* Cambridge, MA: Massachusetts Institute of Technology Center for Advanced Engineering Study; 1986.

Frankel HL, Crede WB, Topal JE, et al. Use of corporate Six Sigma performance improvement strategies to reduce incidence of catheter-related bloodstream infections in a surgical ICU. *J Am Coll Surg.* 2005;201:349-358.

Harry M, Schroeder R. *Six Sigma: The Breakthrough Management Strategy Revolutionizing the World's Top Corporations.* New York, NY: Doubleday; 2000.

Hawkins DM, Olwell DH. *Cumulative Sum Charts and Charting for Quality Improvement.* New York, NY: Springer-Verlag New York, Inc.; 1998.

Institute of Medicine. *Crossing the Quality Chasm: A New Health System for the 21st Century.* Washington, DC: National Academy Press; 2001.

Juran JM, Gryna FM. *Juran's Quality Control Handbook.* 4th ed. New York, NY: McGraw-Hill; 1988.

Kaplan GS, Patterson SH. Seeking perfection in healthcare: a case study in adopting Toyota Production System methods. *Healthc Exec.* 2008;23(3):16-18.

Kelly EW, Kelly JD, Hiestand B, et al. Six Sigma process utilization in reducing door-to-balloon time at a single academic tertiary care center. *Prog Cardiovas Dis.* 2010;53:219-226.

Langley GJ, Moen RD, Nolan KM, et al. *The Improvement Guide: A Practical Approach to Enhancing Organizational Performance.* 2nd ed. San Francisco, CA: Jossey-Bass; 2009.

Liker JK. *The Toyota Way: 14 Management Principles from the World's Greatest Manufacturer.* New York, NY: McGraw-Hill; 2004.

McLaughlin CP, Kaluzny AD, eds. *Continuous Quality Improvement in Health Care: Theory, Implementations, and Applications.* 3rd ed. Boston, MA: Jones and Bartlett Publishers; 2006.

Montgomery DC. *Introduction to Statistical Quality Control.* 6th ed. Hoboken, NJ: John Wiley & Sons, Inc.; 2009.

Nelson EC, Batalden PB, Godfrey MM, eds. *Quality by Design: A Clinical Microsystems Approach.* San Francisco, CA: Jossey-Bass; 2007.

Nelson EC, Batalden PB, Godfrey MM, et al, eds. *Value by Design: Developing Clinical Microsystems to Achieve Organizational Excellence.* San Francisco, CA: Jossey-Bass; 2011.

Nelson-Peterson DL, Leppa CJ. Creating an environment for caring using lean principles of the Virginia Mason Production System. *J Nurs Adm.* 2007;37:287-294.

Ohno T. *Toyota Production System: Beyond Large-Scale Production.* New York, NY: Productivity Press; 1988.

Ransom ER, Joshi MS, Nash DB, et al, eds. *The Healthcare Quality Book.* 2nd ed. Chicago, IL: Health Administration Press; 2008.

Scholtes PR, Joiner BL, Streibel BJ. *The Team Handbook.* 3rd ed. Madison, WI: Oriel Incorporated; 2003.

Soumerai SB, Avorn J. Principles of educational outreach ('academic detailing') to improve clinical decision making. *JAMA.* 1990;263:549-556.

Troubleshooting Healthcare Teams

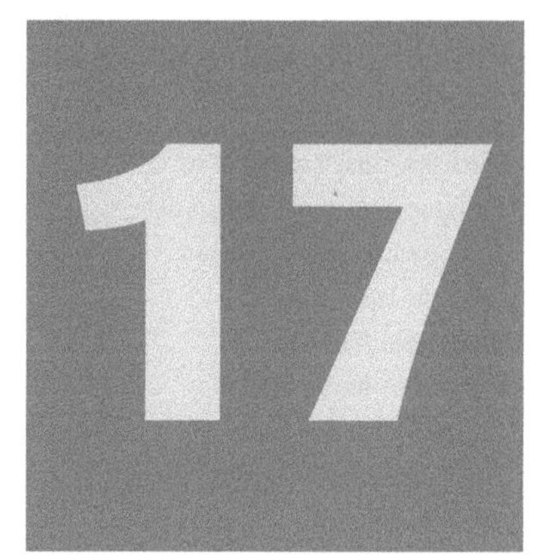

Chapters 14-16 explain 3 different means for improving the effectiveness of healthcare teams. These means—training, team building, and process improvement—all require a methodical approach and are often time consuming. Sometimes the necessary time is not available, and sometimes the problem at hand will not yield to these methods. This chapter provides a fourth approach to problem solving, namely, troubleshooting, which is more direct and usually faster. It also commonly carries more risk.

Troubleshooting involves responding to specific problems and solving them. There are many different avenues available to individuals who do troubleshooting, ranging from making gentle suggestions to disbanding teams. This chapter deals with 9 different actions that can be used to address problems; the actions are listed in Table 17–1. Other actions could be added to the list. The actions chosen for presentation are ones that hold promise in circumstances commonly encountered in teams.

Troubleshooting is an activity to be performed by team leaders and team sponsors and only very occasionally by team members other than the leader. Sometimes more senior leaders in an organization need to troubleshoot problems in a team within the organization, but troubleshooting from afar tends to be ill-informed interference or tampering, and so senior leaders are usually more effective when they prompt action by a team leader or a team sponsor instead of taking action themselves.

COACH INDIVIDUAL TEAM MEMBERS

Team leaders often have occasions to correct problems in the team by coaching individual team members. Individual team members can provide coaching too.

Granite Hills Health Center, a rural hospital, was considering expanding its cardiovascular service line to provide more emergency heartcare services, possibly including a medical intensive care unit (ICU). An ICU would enable Granite Hills to care for patients with myocardial infarction (heart attack), eliminating the need to transfer these patients by air ambulance to a larger hospital. The advent of ICU telemedicine had made this expansion of Granite Hills' service worthy of consideration. With telemedicine, cardiologists can provide ICU care at a distance by using electronically communicated x-ray images, electrocardiograms, and other information. The senior leadership of the hospital had charged a task force with considering the medical ICU as well as other possible additions to the cardiovascular service line.

The task force was led by Gita Juntasa, RN, MSN, the hospital's Director of Nursing. The other members were mainly nurses and physicians, including Peter Olsen, MD, a general internist. The discussion quickly focused on providing ICU care for patients with myocardial infarction. Beth Rappaport, MD, a family physician, spoke enthusiastically in favor

Table 17-1. Troubleshooting actions for healthcare teams

Coach individual team members
Intervene with difficult team members
Resolve relationship conflicts
Coach the team leader
Use focused team building
Reframe the team's task
Change the team leader
Change the composition of the team
Disband the team

of investigating the possibility. She emphasized the value of keeping the patients at Granite Hills, where they would have the support of their families. Current practice was to transfer these patients to a hospital that was 125 miles away.

Dr. Olsen spoke next. He was opposed to creating an ICU, and he had done his homework. He reported a series of facts and figures to the task force. He addressed most of his remarks to Dr. Rappaport, speaking in her direction and looking directly at her. He reported that the number of myocardial infarction patients during the previous year had been 27. This number, he said, was too low for nurses to able to maintain their skills in caring for these patients. No other rural hospital in the state was using telemedicine for ICU care, he reported. Based on a telephone call he had made to a hospital in another state, he related that the cost for the necessary equipment and training would be in excess of $2 million, a sum that Granite Hills could not afford. He continued on for 10 minutes, speaking in his usual confident, declarative manner, expressing no doubts. Although Dr. Olsen did not say so, his manner suggested that anyone who had reached a conclusion different from his conclusion was either poorly informed or foolish.

When Dr. Olsen had finished, initially there was silence in the room for nearly a minute. Then various doubts were expressed about the conclusions Dr. Olsen had drawn. For example, the number of myocardial infarction patients might be increased if Granite Hills received similar patients from hospitals in surrounding towns, avoiding the need for these patients to be transported 100 miles or more.

Dr. Rappaport said nothing. She felt overwhelmed and embarrassed. She thought that other people in the room probably saw her as naive, even mawkish, for suggesting that myocardial infarction patients should be treated closer to their families. She looked dejected, as Ms. Juntasa noticed. Dr. Olsen did not notice that she looked dejected. However, he did notice that she was silent, and he inferred that he had won the argument.

To some people in the room, Dr. Olsen appeared to be bullying Dr. Rappaport. Dr. Olsen would have been dismayed if anyone had later told him that he acted like a bully. He intended only to present reasons not to establish an ICU, supported by the many facts he had assembled. He did not intend to humiliate Dr. Rappaport and had given no thought to how his remarks might affect her. He did not consider her feelings (or his feelings) to be relevant to the discussion. The purpose of the task force, in his mind, was to reach the conclusion that best served Granite Hills' patients.

Ms. Juntasa noted that Dr. Olsen could have achieved his short-term goal—reporting a host of relevant information—without causing the damage he caused. She had observed Dr. Olsen behave in similar ways in the past. The next day, she sought him out and asked to speak with him alone. Ms. Juntasa and Dr. Olsen held each other in high esteem. Recently, they had worked together to see the hospital through a difficult time, dealing with community relations and with funding. Ms. Juntasa told Dr. Olsen that Dr. Rappaport was quite upset the previous day. Initially Dr. Olsen was skeptical that his remarks had had any ill effect, but then he said that he was sorry for unintentionally upsetting Dr. Rappaport. He added that, in his opinion, she should set aside her feelings and deal with the work of evaluating the possibility of establishing an ICU. Ms. Juntasa told Dr. Olsen that Dr. Rappaport was very unlikely simply to set aside her feelings and probably could not. The incident during the meeting was likely to have ill effects on Dr. Rappaport's participation in the task force and ill effects on her working relationship with Dr. Olsen well into the future. Dr. Olsen had alienated Dr. Rappaport and thereby diminished his own capacity to work effectively in the hospital.

Dr. Olsen was astounded, but Ms. Juntasa had been persuasive. Her comments were a revelation for

Dr. Olsen. Four years ago, he had finished his residency in internal medicine at an academic medical center. The milieu in the training program rewarded clinical observation, medical knowledge, and logic. The feelings of patients were important, but the feelings of colleagues during discussions of diagnosis and treatment were not important. All professional staff were expected to act with dignity, calm, and logic. Humor was encouraged, but feelings were not to be displayed because they were irrelevant and threatened to interfere with clear thinking.

Dr. Olsen had never considered that his assertive, direct manner might be intimidating and might create barriers to the achievement of his own goals. He regarded Ms. Juntasa as having done him a great service by coaching him on his behavior in dealing with colleagues. In the weeks that followed, Dr. Olsen asked her several more questions about how he might make his behavior more effective.

In one of their follow-up conversations, Ms. Juntasa introduced Dr. Olsen to the notion of an *emotional bank account* (Covey, 1989, pp. 188-203). An emotional bank account is a reservoir of trust that someone can develop in a colleague by keeping commitments, respecting what is important to the other person, and other positive interactions. Each of these trust-generating actions makes a deposit in the bank account. These feelings of trust facilitate joint action. If one team member has a high balance in his emotional bank account with another team member, collaboration or at least serious consideration can be expected from the other team member. If the balance is negative, opposition or indifference is far more likely.

In this case, the team leader (Ms. Juntasa) was the coach, but Ms. Juntasa could have coached Dr. Olsen even if she had been a team member without being the leader.

Sometimes dysfunctional actions that appear to be fully considered and deliberate are in fact performed without any attention to their effects. The possibility that dysfunctional behavior lacks full awareness should always be kept in mind by those who are in a position to coach. Sometimes, with the permission of the person being coached, additional team members can be enlisted to point out the undesirable behavior tactfully as it is happening or shortly afterward.

On the other hand, some dysfunctional behavior is fully conscious and intentional; and in these situations, more skill is required in the coach, as discussed next.

INTERVENE WITH DIFFICULT TEAM MEMBERS

Imagine now that Dr. Olsen's behavior had been much worse—that he was fully aware of the effects of his forceful manner and that, although he did not deliberately seek to intimidate and to humiliate, he was quite willing to accept these secondary effects if they happened to be the price of reaching what he saw as the correct answer to whatever question was being considered. Imagine further that Dr. Olsen sometimes deliberately used intimidation to win arguments and that he engaged in this and similar behavior often. In other words, imagine that Dr. Olsen was a "difficult person" or that he was frankly abusive.

The handling of difficult team members is discussed briefly in Chapter 9 in connection with a vignette about physicians and nurse practitioners considering whether to stop distributing pharmaceutical samples provided to the clinic by pharmaceutical representatives. Several options are offered in that discussion for how a team leader can deal with someone whose behavior as a team member is objectionable.

West offers several more considerations about difficult team members (West, 2012, pp. 195-197). First, he observes that some people are labeled "difficult" when they are simply consistent dissenters. If the person in question often disagrees with other team members but does not dominate, demean, or otherwise inflict psychological or physical harm, then his or her dissenting remarks actually should be regarded as a help to the team in its attempts to examine choices carefully. Second, a team leader should not try to deal with a difficult person by immediately excluding the person from team meetings or other team activities. This approach will not eliminate the offending behavior and may cause resentment that makes the behavior worse. Third, at the outset of dealing with the problem, the team leader (or a delegate) should assume that the problem behavior is not fully conscious and that it may yield to coaching as did Dr. Olsen's behavior in the earlier vignette. One attempt at coaching is not sufficient. It may be desirable for more than one person to try coaching because different people in the team and elsewhere in the organization will have different kinds of personal connections with the difficult person, opening the door to coaching in unpredictable ways. Fourth, persistent difficult behavior or abuse of others in the workplace should not be tolerated. In some cases, the departure of the person from the team or the organization is warranted. Leaving the person and the behavior in place continues the harm to the team and encourages more behavior in the same vein since there is no adverse consequence for the wrongdoer. Avoiding dealing with the problem may even encourage dysfunctional team behavior in other people.

Dyer and colleagues (2007, pp. 136-139) present an escalating series of options for dealing with the problem when the difficult person is not receptive to coaching:

1. Direct confrontation by the leader with the individual member in private, describing the offending behavior and specifying consequences if the behavior does not change
2. Direct confrontation by the team as a whole, describing the behavior and its effects
3. Cooptation of the member by assigning him or her to special roles, such as summarizing discussions, or even serving as acting team leader
4. Restricting participation, such as allowing attendance at team meetings but no participation in discussion during the meetings
5. External assignment, that is, after full explanation of the situation and the ill effects of the individual's behavior, assigning the difficult person to perform tasks separately from the rest of the team and to participate in the team only through individual effort carried out independently of the team's collaborative activities

If none of these approaches results in a satisfactory resolution of the problem, then removal of the person from the team should be considered. Removing a stubbornly disruptive team member is always awkward and sometimes painful. The team sponsor's support is often required, and the sponsor may be able to provide useful advice about how to achieve the removal. Removing the team member not only from the team but also from the organization often raises legal issues, and an attorney may need to be consulted. In larger organizations, the Human Resources Department will be able to help. And in some situations in health care, removing the difficult person may not be possible. For example, if one among several owners of a medical practice is persistently abusive to the point that everyone in the practice wants him or her to leave (but he or she is not behaving illegally), it may be impossible to force a departure without the practice making an intolerably large severance payment or running a substantial financial risk due to a law suit. In such a case, the coaching should then be directed to those who are being harmed by the disruptive person, teaching them means for coping with the disruptive person's behavior.

RESOLVE RELATIONSHIP CONFLICTS

Carol Reyerson, RN, PhD, FAAN, was recruited to take the position of Vice President for Patient Care Services at Crispin University Medical Center. In this position, she would oversee all nursing services, pharmacy services, the operating rooms, respiratory therapy, occupational therapy, and several other services provided directly to patients. Before accepting the job offer, she requested that social services also be included within the scope of her job. Social services previously had been included among the services overseen by the Vice President for Support Services, Michael Balcerzak, MHA. David Laferte, MBA, the Chief Operating Officer (COO) of the medical center, agreed to Dr. Reyerson's request, and Dr. Reyerson soon joined the senior leadership team. Mr. Balcerzak was informed of the organizational change and the rationale for it, but he was not given an opportunity to object to the change or to offer reasons for maintaining social services as part of Support Services.

As soon as Dr. Reyerson began work at the medical center, Mr. Balcerzak's antagonism to her was apparent to everyone in the senior leadership team. He often made sarcastic comments in response to her statements in team meetings. When she distributed written proposals for comment, he usually responded at length with trenchant criticisms. Soon Dr. Reyerson responded in kind, forming alliances with other team members to oppose Mr. Balcerzak's proposals. Within 9 months, the conflict between the 2 of them was disrupting not only discussions at meetings but also the smooth function of the team in addressing issues that were important for the medical center.

Managing conflict is discussed in Chapter 11, where relationship conflict is distinguished from task conflict and process conflict. Both task conflict and process conflict are ordinarily useful for team effectiveness. Resolving task conflict helps to clarify the team's goals. Resolving process conflict helps to clarify roles and the methods used by the team to accomplish its goals. In contrast, relationship conflict concerns personal or social issues that are not parts of the team's work.

Relationship conflicts, unless they can be shelved for the sake of smooth team function, are almost always damaging to the effectiveness of the team. Since they are not concerned with issues that constitute the work of the team, it is not necessary for the whole team to deal with these conflicts. In fact, it is normally best to deal with them privately, as discussed in Chapter 11. Either party to a relationship conflict can, in principle, initiate discussions to resolve the conflict, and the ability to resolve conflicts to which one is a party is a competency to be sought by all team members (see Chapter 7).

The team leader has reason to intervene if the parties do not seek to resolve the conflict or if they try and fail. Task conflicts and process conflicts are properly matters for the whole team to address, but unresolved relationship conflicts ordinarily call for troubleshooting by one person, usually the team leader but sometimes the team sponsor if the leader is a party to the conflict. The methods for addressing relationship conflicts are discussed in Chapter 11.

In the case of Dr. Reyerson and Mr. Balcerzak, Dr. Reyerson was in the best position to initiate discussion of the conflict since she had gained by the organizational change while Mr. Balcerzak was a passive victim of the change. In any case, if Mr. Laferte, the COO, were to encourage the quarreling parties to settle their conflict and no resolution was reached, then Mr. Laferte would need to troubleshoot. Incidentally, any unpleasantness for Mr. Laferte would be, in a sense, well deserved since he handled the organizational change poorly and in effect caused the conflict.

COACH THE TEAM LEADER

Martin Santiago, PharmD, was the Director of Inpatient Pharmacy Services at a large, urban health system with 4 hospitals and an interprofessional healthcare group of 550 physicians and nurse practitioners (NPs). Dr. Santiago led a management team of 6, including the Manager of Pharmacy Services at each of the 4 hospitals and 2 additional pharmacists at the largest hospital, one a specialist in nutrition support pharmacy and the other a specialist in pharmacotherapy. Dr. Santiago was accountable to Nicholas Borovsky, PharmD, the Vice President of Pharmacy Services, for the whole health system.

Dr. Santiago had become the head of inpatient pharmacy services 18 months ago. His previous position was Manager of Pharmacy Services at the smallest of the system's 4 hospitals.

Dr. Borovsky frequently spoke with the managers of the 4 inpatient and 4 ambulatory pharmacy services throughout the system. He had several reasons for speaking with them, for example, he needed to be sure that these 8 operational units were well coordinated with the centralized contracting, purchasing, and business sections of the system's Department of Pharmacy Services. During the first year that Dr. Santiago was head of all inpatient pharmacy services, from time to time Dr. Borovsky received positive comments from the 4 inpatient pharmacy managers about Dr. Santiago. Dr. Santiago was seen as energetic, thorough, and fair.

However, Dr. Borovsky lately had begun to receive gentle but negative reports, usually embedded in accounts from pharmacy managers about recent events at their hospitals. The managers described Dr. Santiago as overly energetic, disposed to instructing individual managers about how to do their work, and prone to presenting system-wide changes for pharmacy procedures to his team without requesting or even permitting their input. The managers were sure that Dr. Santiago had the best of intentions, but he was perceived as "micromanaging." Two of the managers also perceived Dr. Santiago as neglecting to develop the management team as a source of collective knowledge and professional support for each of the team members.

Dr. Santiago had fallen victim to one of the hazards for team leaders discussed in Chapter 8. He was managing the individuals on his management team and not the team as a whole. This mistake is common, especially in team leaders who formerly worked in settings where they could supervise and direct all aspects of the work within their scopes (Hill, 2007). Dr. Santiago formerly managed the inpatient pharmacy services in a small hospital. In that position, he could and did oversee everything that happened in the pharmacy. (His team members in this pharmacy also thought he micromanaged, but they accepted his style.) In his new position, Dr. Santiago could not succeed by directing the activities of the inpatient pharmacy services of all 4 hospitals because his scope of work had become too large for him to supervise all aspects directly. He needed the team to function well as a team.

Having learned of the problem, Dr. Borovsky needed to initiate discussions with Dr. Santiago about the difference between leading a team and supervising the individual members of the team. In other words, Dr. Borovsky needed to coach Dr. Santiago about this specific issue. As Dr. Santiago's superior in the pharmacy hierarchy, Dr. Borovsky was the sponsor of the team. The sponsor is normally best positioned to provide coaching for the leader, especially when there is a clear and functional reporting relationship between the sponsor and the leader.

Dr. Borovsky ideally would devise a way to raise the issue without generating ill will between Dr. Santiago and any members of his team by implying that one of pharmacy managers was complaining about him. One way would be to ask about progress in making a recent change in system-wide inpatient pharmacy procedure. Dr. Santiago's answer likely would reveal that he had formulated the change alone, without the participation of his team members, and that he simply had instructed the pharmacy managers to make the change. Dr. Borovsky then would have occasion for talking about leading a team instead of instructing team members as individuals. This discussion would likely lead to a more general discussion about developing the team. Dr. Borovsky might then also suggest some reading for Dr. Santiago or even suggest a training course, as discussed in Chapter 14.

Coaching a team leader falls under the heading of guiding the team, one of the 3 elements of the sponsor's role, discussed in Chapter 12. When coaching is provided in order to deal with a specific problem, it is a form of troubleshooting.

USE FOCUSED TEAM BUILDING

Although most team building activities are time consuming—requiring interviews of team members and other preparation for the team building event—team building can be used to focus on a particular issue, using only a few hours.

It was Wednesday morning. As usual, the Patient Care Team on 6 West was having a care conference to discuss their patients. 6 West is a portion of Livorno Regional Medical Center. It is the unit where patients with strokes and brain injuries receive care after they are managed acutely in one or another intensive care unit. When ready for discharge from 6 West, patients with strokes and brain injuries depart for a variety of care settings and need care plans that differ widely. Some patients return home and follow up with a neurologist in 2 weeks as outpatients. Some need occupational and physical therapy for several months. Some need care indefinitely in a long-term care facility. Many need mental health care, usually because of depression. For many of the patients, a central consideration is whether there are family members who are available and willing to be caregivers.

The 6 West Patient Care Team consists of the 10 registered nurses working on 6 West, 2 social workers, a physical therapist, an occupational therapist, 2 hospitalists, a physiatrist (physician specializing in rehabilitation), and a neurologist. The 2 hospitalists are general internists who serve as the primary physicians for patients while they are hospitalized on 6 West. The physiatrist and neurologist function as consultants to the hospitalists. Sometimes a neurosurgeon, speech therapist, pharmacist, or mental health therapist is asked to participate in the care conference, depending on the needs of the patients considered at a particular meeting. The chair of the meetings is Renee Snyder, RN, MSN, CNS, the head nurse of the unit. She is a co-leader of 6 West; the other co-leader is Rob Thurber, MD, the senior hospitalist.

On this Wednesday morning, the meeting attendees were Ms. Snyder, Dr. Thurber, 2 of the staff nurses, 1 social worker, and the physical therapist. The 2 staff nurses reported on the patients they cared for directly. For other patients, one or the other of the staff nurses reported information provided to her by other staff nurses who were direct care givers for those patients. Similarly, Dr. Thurber relayed reports from the other hospitalist and from the neurologist and physiatrist who provided consultations on 6 West. The physical therapist relayed information from the occupational therapist. For one of the patients, a staff nurse relayed information from a mental health therapist about the needs of that patient. Each patient was discussed in turn, and for those to be discharged within the next few days, a tentative care plan was formulated. Decisions were made by Ms. Snyder and Dr. Thurber jointly although this method of decision making had never been discussed and agreed upon explicitly. Both Ms. Snyder and Dr. Thurber were entirely open to input from the others attending the meeting. The care plans decided upon were tentative because the next step in the process was for each patient's primary hospitalist and primary nurse to meet with the patient and family, solicit their wishes and other input, and propose a care plan. Plans were then finalized after working through the issues with the patients and their family members.

The attendance at the team meeting this Wednesday was typical, but those attending did change from week to week. Sometimes different staff nurses attended. Sometimes the occupational therapist attended but not the physical therapist. The neurologist and physiatrist almost never attended. The second hospitalist attended about half of the meetings.

Ms. Snyder and Dr. Thurber debriefed as usual after the meeting. As their one-on-one meeting ended, Ms. Snyder voiced her concern that the Patient Care Team was not functioning as a true interprofessional team. Dr. Thurber agreed. The other members of the team were serving as advisers to Ms. Snyder and Dr. Thurber. Some team members routinely provided their advice indirectly without attending the meetings, so there was only limited interprofessional interaction and creative planning, and occasionally the team would learn after a care plan had been devised that the input of the neurologist, physiatrist, speech therapist, or other absent professional had been misunderstood.

Ms. Snyder and Dr. Thurber discussed their observations and concerns privately in 2 more meetings. They then proposed to the whole team that a 1-day off-site meeting be held to review the purpose of the team and how it could best operate to achieve its purpose. They made their concerns clear to the other team members. The team building exercise was carried out 2 months later.

Sometimes the correction of a problem in the function of a team cannot be achieved by the team leader or any other single person intervening to troubleshoot. Sometimes the intervention needs to involve the whole team or a substantial part of it. In these cases, one might say that the troubleshooting consists of intervening to initiate action taken by the whole team.

In this case, Ms. Snyder and Dr. Thurber considered several options for intervention. They might have approached the second hospitalist, the staff nurses, and others to learn why they were not attending the meetings and urge them to begin attending. They might have initiated a team discussion of the process for decision making. After conferring, however, they decided to use a team building approach in order to engage the whole team and to address the issues in a setting in which the team members' attention was relatively unlikely to be distracted by other patient-care concerns. They realized that some team members might not want to take the time required, that some members actually were not needed (for example, the night-shift staff nurses, who did not participate in forming care plans), and that changes in the composition of the group meeting each Wednesday might result from consideration of how best to make decisions in the team.

Team building is discussed in Chapter 15, where several different purposes for team building are considered. The purpose for the team building exercise contemplated by Ms. Snyder and Dr. Thurber was goal clarification, to be followed by exploration of how team processes should be redesigned to enable achievement of the goal. In other situations, more extensive team building might aim instead to build interpersonal relationships, to strengthen team identity, or to clarify the roles of team members, as discussed in Chapter 15.

REFRAME THE TEAM'S TASK

Cindy Meller, NP, MSN, and James Beinborn, DO, practiced together in a practice of 6 rheumatologists and 4 NPs. For several months, they had noted in conversation with each other that the patient education materials in the practice were inadequate. They were interested in particular in the pamphlets and videos for people with rheumatoid arthritis. They regarded these materials as too limited in scope and not sufficiently engaging for patients. Their underlying concern was that many patients seen in the practice did not exercise adequately and often did not use the foot orthotics (supports) and wrist splints that were prescribed for them.

Ms. Meller and Dr. Beinborn raised the topic of educational materials at a monthly meeting of all NPs, physicians, and several staff members. There was general support for updating the materials. Ms. Meller and Dr. Beinborn, joined by a second NP, volunteered to investigate the availability of materials, their costs, and other related topics. Within a few months, the practice had a much improved supply of pamphlets and videos, which were well received by the patients.

However, after another year, the trio who had taken on the project shared with each other that they saw no difference in the behavior of patients who received the new materials. They were somewhat frustrated. They decided to consult with Nancy Schriver, CHES, the head of patient education at the large nearby hospital where the physicians were on staff. They thought that Ms. Schriver would probably know of additional materials.

Ms. Meller and Dr. Beinborn met with Ms. Schriver. She did know of additional materials and showed them pamphlets and videos that were new to them. However, her principal advice was to shift the aim of their project and to focus on establishing a support group for patients with rheumatoid arthritis, that is, a group in which patients would share with each other how and why they exercised and the details of using orthotics and wrist splints in ways that minimized inconvenience. The ultimate objective of Ms. Meller's and Dr. Beinborn's initiative, Ms. Shriver noted, was to change the behavior of patients. Ms. Schriver said that a support group carried more promise of achieving this objective than the use of updated education materials—although both could be used together. She also said that a self-management education program would hold even more promise than a support group but that she realized that Ms. Meller's and Dr. Beinborn's practice did not have the resources to offer a self-management education program to its patients.

Ms. Meller and Dr. Beinborn had heard presentations about support groups at national meetings, but all of the examples they knew were support groups conducted in hospital settings or in very large medical groups with health education departments. Ms. Meller and Dr. Beinborn had never considered that a small practice like theirs could host support groups. Later that week, they began exploring the feasibility of creating a support group in their practice.

In the context of organizational behavior, the term *reframing* means using a new conceptual lens to characterize and orient the planning, activity, or evaluation being pursued (Bolman and Deal, 2008, pp. 12-14). Reframing usually does not imply discarding the theory or model formerly used. Instead reframing adds a new way of viewing the issues, suggesting fresh insights and different ways to proceed. Ms. Meller and Dr. Beinborn had been using a conventional clinician-as-teacher approach. They supplemented this approach with a patient-self-help or patient-as-teacher model—a model in keeping with the patient-centered approaches discussed in Chapter 4. As soon as Ms. Meller and Dr. Beinborn saw their project through the new lens, they were able to move ahead with a course of action that was more likely to succeed than the simpler approach they had been using.

In this case, the troubleshooting was accomplished almost by chance by someone who was outside of the team and who was simply reacting to the story provided by the team members. One can imagine that one of the NPs or physicians in the practice but not involved in the project could have observed the frustration of the 3 team members and reframed the project in the same way. There was no sponsor for this project team because the practice was small and there was no internal hierarchy. In other circumstances, the team sponsor often is well positioned to troubleshoot by reframing. In situations in which a team is a temporary sub-group of a larger team (for example, a planning group within a Department of Family Medicine), the leader of the larger team often has enough distance from the team's task to be able to use reframing to move the team past a sticking point.

CHANGE THE TEAM LEADER

The Obstetrics and Gynecology Department of Redstone Clinic consisted of 5 obstetricians, 3 midwives, and 5 NPs. The department provided a full range of women's health services except for obstetrical care for women with high-risk pregnancies. Women with high-risk pregnancies were referred to a sub-specialty group across town.

The department had existed for 15 years, ever since Redstone had been founded. Initially there was only 1 obstetrician. The department grew steadily. During the whole 15 years, the chair was Tison Newbury, MD, an excellent leader who was well loved by all.

When Dr. Newbury retired, the heir apparent was Amanda Takata, MD. Dr. Takata was regarded by everyone in the department as the most proficient obstetrician in the group, a truly gifted clinician whom others consulted with when they needed help with diagnosis or obstetrical management. Michael Greene, MD, was the medical director of Redstone. After consulting with department members, Dr. Greene appointed Dr. Takata as the new department chair.

Within 6 months, the department was in shambles. An additional NP and obstetrician were needed to handle the workload. Dr. Takata had interviewed 2 candidates for the NP position and 1 for the obstetrician position, but she had taken no other action. The monthly department meeting had been cancelled 3 times in the last 4 months. Questions had arisen about the scope of practice of the NPs, but no approach to dealing with these questions had been chosen and the NPs were frustrated and angry.

Dr. Greene faced a difficult situation. In retrospect, he realized that his basis for appointing Dr. Takata as chair was unsound. A fine clinician is not necessarily a fine leader. He considered his options: coach Dr. Takata, arrange a mentor for her, arrange some training for her, or replace Dr. Takata with someone else. He asked Dr. Takata to meet with him, and he was not looking forward to the meeting.

Sometimes the team leader is simply not suited to the job. This appears to be the case with Dr. Takata. The appropriate person to change the team leader is normally the team sponsor. In organizations with poorly developed sponsor roles (for example, many medical groups), the task commonly falls to someone senior in the organization. It often is not clear which senior person or committee should have the duty, and this lack of clarity can cause unfortunate delay.

Before concluding that the leader needs to be changed, the sponsor or other responsible party needs to consider what might be done to make the leader's performance at least acceptable. Dr. Greene considered the main options, that is, to coach Dr. Takata or provide her with a coach, to arrange for Dr. Takata to have a mentor, or to ask Dr. Takata to obtain some training, which could include reading that she would do on her own. For any of these options to be good choices, the sponsor needs to have confidence that there is at least some chance of success. Simply delaying a change of leader does both the leader and the team a disservice.

Dealing with a poorly performing leader is usually easier than dealing with a difficult team member in that personal behavior faults are usually not at issue. Most of the time, the problem is lack of fit between the poorly performing leader and the job. Lack of fit is not a personal failing; and so, if the situation can be presented as a case of poor fit, the discussion can proceed more easily.

Let us assume that Dr. Greene has concluded that Dr. Takata is not suited to her position as leader of the department. He will then need to meet privately with Dr. Takata to explore the situation and take some action. It usually works well for the sponsor to begin by asking for the leader's perceptions about how she or he is faring in the position of leader. At some point, the job expectations need to be reviewed—hopefully not for the first time. The sponsor can then ask the leader how she or he views her or his performance with respect to the principal job expectations. If the leader acknowledges that she or he is not performing well, the conversation can move along smoothly with the sponsor then asking whether the leader and the job are well matched. It might even happen at this point that Dr. Takata would say that the match is poor and that she wishes to be relieved of her responsibilities as leader. She might say that she did not understand the job properly before taking the position. Sometimes a poorly performing leader is simply waiting for the question to be called. If, on the other hand, the leader claims excellent performance and the sponsor believes otherwise, the conversation can become awkward because the sponsor will then need to put forward information from other sources who do not agree with the leader's own assessment of his or her performance. The sponsor needs to be prepared in advance with information about poor performance that can be shared with the leader. The best evidence is evidence based on direct observations by the sponsor or on written records, but sometimes the sponsor has no choice but to report what others have told her or him. If the leader accepts that his or her performance is inadequate, the conversation can then turn to the question of whether it might be improved by coaching, mentoring, or training. However, the sponsor needs to avoid the pitfall of considering help for improvement if the sponsor believes that the leader's performance will remain inadequate even if help is provided. If the leader does not accept that his or her performance is inadequate, the conversation can reach an impasse. The sponsor may then chose to propose to the leader that he or she continue as leader on condition that one or more means (for example, coaching) is used to improve performance—subject to review at some suitable interval, say, 2-3 months. Again, the sponsor needs to avoid this approach if she or he believes that there is no realistic hope that the problem can be solved. If the sponsor does not believe that performance will improve even with help, then the sponsor must remain firm and tell the leader that he or she may not continue in the position. Plans can then be made for an orderly change of leader, including withdrawal of the poorly performing leader in a manner that avoids humiliating the leader or subjecting him or her to hurtful public criticism.

CHANGE THE COMPOSITION OF THE TEAM

In Chapter 2, a hospital project team is described. The team is led by Eric Shelstad, MHA, an administrator. It is charged with planning the expansion of space in an emergency department (ED). The members of the team are Mr. Shelstad, the nurse manager of the ED, 2 staff nurses, 3 physician assistants (PAs), 1 pharmacist, 1 ED scribe, 1 radiology technician, 1 laboratory technician, 1 ED health unit coordinator, the materials manager for the hospital, 1 housekeeping supervisor, a financial analyst from the Chief Financial Officer's (CFO's) office, and an architect from the firm engaged for the project. There are no nurse practitioners on the team because the ED does not employ nurse practitioners. There are no ED physicians on the team because of the time required, although the physicians are consulted often by the team.

In the hospital's hierarchy, Mr. Shelstad reports to Nancy Cunningham, RN, MSN, the Vice President for Patient Care at the hospital. Mr. Shelstad reports progress to Ms. Cunningham each month.

After the team had been meeting biweekly for 5 months, Mr. Shelstad presented his progress report in a meeting with Ms. Cunningham. At their meeting, Ms. Cunningham reviewed the working floor plan proposed by Mr. Shelstad's team. She was surprised and alarmed by an apparent major oversight by the team, resulting in her telling Mr. Shelstad that the physician work space would need to be redesigned because it was too small and located too far from the patient examination rooms. She gave this directive reluctantly because she realized that she was interfering with the autonomy of the team. However, she was quite certain that the floor plan's provision for physician work space was inadequate. Over the next 2 days, she thought about how the physician work space could have been so poorly designed by the team. Tentatively, she arrived at 2 possible causes and asked to meet again with Mr. Shelstad to discuss her hunches.

This planning team had a major problem. Although the problem was recognized in time by the team sponsor, the team sponsor's intervention did threaten the team's effectiveness. Moreover, the occurrence of one problem raised the question of whether other problems might occur if the underlying causes were not addressed.

Ms. Cunningham speculated that the team was having difficulty for 2 reasons. First, there were no physicians on the team. Second, the team was too large. In other words, she thought that the team's composition would need to be changed in order for it to become fully effective.

The reasons for not including a physician were plausible enough. Physician time was expensive, and the ED was understaffed with physicians. However, it appeared that the mechanism for obtaining physician input by consultation was not effective. In addition, the team of 16 people was too large. Ms. Cunningham suspected that sometimes the protracted discussions led the group to make a decision simply to be able to move on to the next issue.

Ms. Cunningham and Mr. Shelstad discussed Ms. Cunningham's hunches. Mr. Shelstad agreed that a physician was needed on the team; he had always thought so but had no power to change the original decision to proceed without a physician. He also agreed that he had been too permissive in accepting team members from departments that wanted representation on the team. Together Ms. Cunningham and Mr. Shelstad decided to add a physician and to reduce the team size to 12, including the physician. Ms. Cunningham undertook to talk with the ED medical director to clear the way for a physician team member to be recruited. Ms. Cunningham and Mr. Shelstad decided that one of the PAs, the radiology technician, the laboratory technician, the materials manager, and the housekeeping supervisor were not needed on the team. They realized that removing these team members would be a delicate matter, and they made plans for how to handle the change.

In this case, the composition of the team needed to be changed because one of the essential constituencies was not represented and because the team was simply too large. A team may need to have its membership changed for other reasons as well. For example, essential expertise may be missing even though the right constituencies are represented. In Mr. Shelstad's planning team, a financial analyst was needed; but if the CFO's office had sent a financial analyst who was expert in handling accounts receivable but not in cost estimation, a change likely would have been needed at some point. Inadequate ethnic diversity may need to be corrected if the team's work requires knowledge of several ethnic groups and the ability to interact with people from those ethnic groups. For example, a primary care team whose members all have Hispanic or Northern European backgrounds will probably have difficulty serving a Somali refugee population. Adding a Somali nurse, health education specialist, or other healthcare professional is likely to help.

DISBAND THE TEAM

Lilli Schiffer, MD, was the chair of a task force aimed at reducing the frequency of breast cancer patients seeking health care for the first time with late-stage disease, that is, with cancers at stage III or IV. Specifically, she and 7 others at Hillman Health System were working to decrease the proportion of new breast cancer patients with stage III-IV tumors seen at their hospital and clinics. Hillman consisted of a 425-bed hospital and 6 clinics, including a specialty center, where Dr. Schiffer practiced oncology.

The project had been chartered by the senior leadership of the health system, including Barbara Bergeron, MD, the system's Chief Medical Officer (CMO). The duration of the project was expected to be about 5 years.

The task force used several methods for pursuing their goal. Three initiatives were instituted in quick succession during the first 2 years. First, a campaign was started to promote screening breast examinations and mammography. The hospital served primarily people living in the northeastern quadrant of a metropolitan area in the eastern United States. The campaign for screening focused on this population. Breast cancer screening clinics were established, staffed by nurse practitioners. Waiting time for screening mammograms was eliminated by increasing the hours of operation and changing scheduling procedures.

Second, a training program was established for NPs and physicians doing breast examinations. Examination skills were assessed and taught with simulation methods, using breast models with different types of simulated breast tissue (for example, fatty tissue or fibrous tissue) and different sizes of breast lumps. Clinicians were invited to test their skills, and training was offered.

Third, a systematic follow-up program was instituted for women with borderline abnormal mammogram results who had been advised to have another mammogram performed after an interval of some weeks or months. Patients were reminded in advance of their due dates for the follow-up mammograms. Patients who did not return were contacted, and, if they still did not return, they were contacted 2 more times.

During the first 2 years of the project, the proportion of new patients with stage III-IV cancers fell. However, the actual numbers of these patients remained about the same as before, and the numbers of patients with stage I-II tumors rose. Dr. Schiffer and her colleagues concluded that the proportion of patients with more advance cancers probably had fallen because more early cancers were being detected and not because the later cancers were decreasing. They hoped that in time the detection of early cancers would result in a decrease in stage III-IV cancers.

The proportion of stage III-IV cancers actually increased in the fourth year compared with the third year. The number of new patients with later cancers remained about the same, and number of patients with early cancers decreased compared with the number detected in the third year. In years 5-8, the proportion of later cancers remained unchanged compared with year 4. The task force was able to do a survey of women aged 50-75 in Hillman's customary catchment area. They learned that 84% of women in this area were up-to-date with respect to breast cancer screening. This figure was higher than the figure for the whole state but about the same as it was about 7 years earlier, when an academic research group had done a similar survey.

Dr. Schiffer and her colleagues were frustrated. Eight years of work appeared to have produced no benefit. The team's goal was not achieved, and yet they had no other feasible ideas for what might be done to achieve the goal. Drs. Schiffer and Bergeron discussed the situation with the whole task force and many others. They decided to end the task force.

The media relations group at Hillman was concerned about how the end of the task force might be received by the press and television stations. The beginning of the project had been announced with great fanfare. Everyone agreed that avoidance of adverse publicity was not a sound reason to continue the project, but they also agreed that the project's end should not be announced. The media relations staff prepared answers to questions that the press might raise if they learned that the project had ended. The answers emphasized the numbers of mammograms performed, the numbers of clinicians whose skills were upgraded, and other results that could be cited to put the project in the best possible light.

Sometimes a team is no longer needed, and continuing the team is wasteful or has other ill effects.

It was somewhat puzzling that the project described in the vignette apparently failed, but perhaps the dominant consideration was the screening rate, which was high by national standards at the outset and was affected only temporarily by the campaign to promote screening. In any case, Drs. Schiffer and Bergeron decided that continuing the task force was a waste of the task force members' time and thus of the organization's resources. Moreover, continuing the project in the face of several years without progress would run the risk of generating cynicism because it might be perceived within Hillman that the project was being continued solely to avoid adverse publicity, that is, solely to avoid action that might suggest admission of failure.

Disbanding the team in this case was fairly straightforward. In other cases, disbanding a team because of failure can be highly controversial since determining that success is no longer possible can be difficult and can generate sharp differences of opinion.

There are many other reasons to disband a team in addition to failure to achieve the goal despite best efforts. Sometimes the expense of a project turns out to be higher than anyone expected and higher than the organization can afford. Sometimes a team is performing so poorly that its continuation threatens the health of patients served by the team and threatens the reputation of the larger organization. For example, some cardiac surgery programs have been ended because of high death rates following surgery (Siddique, 2010). Sometimes the leader of a project team or consultative team resigns and there is no one available to lead the effort successfully. Sometimes a merger that looked promising is revealed to be a poor idea from both parties' points of view, and so the group exploring the merger is disbanded. In all of these cases, the sponsor and the leader of the team—as well as others in the organization—need to exercise judgment about whether the team's task might be achieved by making some change in the definition of the task, the leadership of the team, the composition of the team, or some other aspect of the team and its work. But sometimes the best next step is to disband the team.

CONCLUSION

Troubleshooting is direct action taken by the team leader or sponsor—and occasionally by others—to correct a problem in team performance. Troubleshooting is suitable when other corrective means, for example, training, conventional team building, and process improvement, are either unlikely to succeed or are not advisable because faster action is needed. Many different action options are available to troubleshooters. This chapter explains 9 of these options, which are listed in Table 17–1. The choices range from simple coaching to reframing or revising the team's task to disbanding the team.

REFERENCES

Bolman LG, Deal TE. *Reframing Organizations*. 4th ed. San Francisco, CA: Jossey-Bass; 2008.

Covey S. *The Seven Habits of Highly Effective People*. New York, NY: Simon & Schuster; 1989.

Dyer WG, Dyer WG Jr, Dyer JH. *Team Building: Proven Strategies for Improving Team Performance*. 4th ed. San Francisco, CA: Jossey-Bass; 2007.

Hill LA. Becoming the boss. *Harv Bus Rev*. 2007;85(1):49-56.

Siddique H. Heart surgery 'must stop' at John Radcliffe after baby deaths. *The Guardian*. July 28, 2010:5.

West MA. *Effective Teamwork: Practical Lessons from Organizational Research*. 3rd ed. Chichester, UK: John Wiley & Sons, Ltd.; 2012.

Senior Leaders and Teamwork in Their Organizations

Section III (Chapters 13-17) presents ideas for improving teams and teamwork. It assumes that teams are present and regarded as standard practice in organizations. In many organizations, however, this is not the case—in fact, organizational policies and practices often work against rather than promote the success of teamwork. Senior leaders of these organizations are responsible for creating the cultures and structures in which teams thrive and also for providing needed resources for teams to succeed. In this section of the book, we first (in Chapter 18) provide guidelines for senior leaders committed to improving team presence and performance in their organizations. Then in Chapter 19 we discuss the potential for a future in which teamwork is expected and rewarded throughout the healthcare sector.

THE SENIOR LEADER'S ROLE

Senior leaders of healthcare organizations are not those with the highest age or tenure, but those in the highest positions of authority in the organization. They are the leaders with the power to allocate scarce resources, set and enforce organizational values and norms, and represent the organization to external constituents. Typically, the term *senior leader* includes those at the level of vice president and above in large organizations, or department director and above in smaller organizations. In some organizations, like medical group practices, the senior leaders may include all of the partners if the group is small, or a small elected group from among the partners if the group is large.

Senior leaders of healthcare organizations face a difficult challenge when they commit to improving their organizations through expanded use of teamwork. Improvement comes with risk, because it requires change from the status quo, and change often meets resistance. Some healthcare leaders are content to sustain the status quo and not "rock the boat," particularly if change involves upsetting existing patterns in clinical care delivery developed by powerful and largely autonomous professionals. However, to the extent that improvements in team-based care and teamwork effectiveness depend on changes in the organization, senior leaders must be willing to step up to the challenge.

Senior leaders are responsible for creating a context that builds, supports, and nurtures interprofessional teams. With respect to supporting teams, senior leaders have 3 major tasks: (1) creating and sustaining a team-based organizational *culture*, (2) creating and sustaining a team-based organizational *structure*, and (3) providing key resources. The 3 tasks are listed in Table 18–1. The first of these tasks is paramount, because cultures set the philosophy and operating assumptions that guide behavior in the organization, independent of how work is structured. Organizational *culture* refers to the prevailing beliefs and values in an organization. These beliefs and values drive "the way we do things around here," which is a common interpretation of the meaning of culture in organizations (Deal and Kennedy, 1982, p. 4). Organizational cultures can encourage, discourage, or ignore teamwork. For example, the MIT Media Lab, a futuristic research laboratory for engineers, artists, designers, and scientists, states that it is a "highly collaborative and antidisciplinary environment," reflecting the organization's efforts to break down barriers among disciplines in order to produce innovative technologies (MIT Media Lab, 2012).

Table 18–1. Tasks for senior leaders

1. Create and sustain a team-based organizational culture
2. Create and sustain a team-based organizational structure
3. Provide key teamwork resources

Organizational *structure* is comprised of the policies and practices that define roles (descriptions of activities expected of incumbents in job positions), reporting relationships and work flow in the organization. In most organizations, structure is formally documented in organizational charts, job descriptions, and compilations of policies and procedures. Roles typically are grouped into departments or divisions, which are hierarchically arranged. Grouping roles into separate departments based on the professional education of the incumbents, such as departments of medicine, nursing, and pharmacy, makes interprofessional teamwork harder, as discussed in Chapter 5 on healthcare administration. Organizational structures can be modified to promote effective teamwork.

A third task of senior leaders is to provide key organizational resources for team-based activity. These organizational resources can make it easier for teamwork to thrive. Teams need resources for information and communication flow and for training and education, among other activities.

The 3 tasks that define the senior leader's role in relation to teamwork serve well to categorize the competencies needed by senior leaders. Senior leaders need to be able to perform the 3 tasks, each of which requires certain competencies.

COMPETENCIES FOR SENIOR LEADERS

Regina Simpson, MSN, MBA, was still feeling her way into her new job as CEO of Rockaway Heights Hospital, a position she had attained 3 months ago. The organization was missing something, but she couldn't put her finger on it. Everybody she talked to seemed to want to do the right thing—they generally were very caring, hardworking professionals. Surveys by the Human Resources Department showed that employees, with the possible exception of nurses, generally were happy to be at Rockaway Heights. But hospital performance was poor, and she had been hired to fix that. "Culture of safety" scores for the hospital were in the lower quartile compared to national norms.

The governing board was concerned that the hospital was losing market share to competitors in the large metropolitan market area of Rockaway Heights, particularly in cardiac services, orthopedics, and obstetrics. "Minute clinics," staffed with nurse practitioners, and urgent care centers were popping up all over the town. Rockaway Heights usually was last on the scene for new programs, like the minute clinics, urgent care centers, and the new palliative care program announced yesterday by a competitor hospital.

The Rockaway Heights Hospital employed over 200 physicians, but Ms. Simpson understood that they didn't always work well with other physicians in the community. Nurses were angry over a failed effort to gain Magnet recognition for the hospital, an effort that many physicians and administrators opposed, or at least did not openly advocate. And some of the senior leaders of the organization seemed content to keep their heads down and worry about their own departments rather than the organization as a whole.

Create and Sustain a Team-Based Organizational Culture

Poor organizational performance often has its genesis in poor organizational culture. Ms. Simpson is right to wonder about the root causes of poor performance at Rockaway Heights Hospital. She can begin by assessing the culture of the organization, the first of 5 competencies to create and sustain a team-based culture (Table 18–2).

Assess the Organizational Culture

If senior leaders are interested in improving the culture of their organizations, they must first understand the existing culture of the organization. Likely, if leaders

Table 18–2. Competencies for senior leaders: creating and sustaining a team-based organizational culture

1. Assess the organizational culture
2. Emphasize teamwork values: collaboration, respect, patient focus, and innovation
3. Hire and promote for teamwork values
4. Make teamwork highly visible
5. Relate effectively to clinicians

have been in the organization for a year or more and have been listening, they have a good handle on "the way we do things around here" and the values and beliefs that underlie those typical ways or patterns. However, if leaders are new to an organization, like Ms. Simpson in the vignette, they can accelerate their learning by targeted examination of the cultures of their organizations.

Organizational culture, or underlying beliefs and assumptions, can be diagnosed by examining the artifacts of culture, including stories and myths, rituals and ceremonies, formal organizational vision and value statements, heroes and heroines, logos, physical facilities, and commonly used metaphors for the organization. All of these indicators of culture are directly observable. For example, members of the organization may refer to it as a "well-oiled machine" or a "three-ring circus," perhaps reflecting an emphasis on order in the well-oiled machine and a tolerance of autonomy in the three-ring circus. Another sample indicator of culture is stories about the organization. The founder of the organization, and the founder's values, may be presented as a heroic figure in stories, as Dr. William Worrall Mayo and his 2 sons are represented in the history of Mayo Clinic.

Social psychologist Edgar Schein suggests investigating organizational culture more deeply by identifying *tacit* or unspoken assumptions, which may vary from beliefs formally espoused by the organization in documents and announcements to employees and the public (Schein, 2009). An organization may claim to promote teamwork in its formal value statement, for example, but leaders may not work actively to support it. Employees may be quite cynical about the degree to which teamwork is supported and may behave inconsistently with that value. To uncover tacit assumptions, Schein recommends that senior leaders conduct individual and group interviews, rather than relying on large surveys. The interviews allow leaders to probe more deeply into differences between behavior and espoused values. Hopefully Ms. Simpson, in the preceding vignette, will spend much of her time talking to individuals and small groups rather than relying on hospital-wide surveys for insights into the culture of Rockaway Heights Hospital.

Another fairly obvious fact to those in healthcare settings is that strong sub-cultures, such as cultures of the different health professions, are present in healthcare delivery organizations. The sub-cultures have different underlying beliefs and assumptions. Ms. Simpson will need to be alert to identifying and working with those sub-cultures at Rockaway Heights. In her institution, acknowledging differences among the nursing, physician, and administrator sub-cultures would be an obvious initial step.

Once leaders understand the organization's existing culture, they have a better grasp on the challenge they face, as well as levers for change. Changing a culture is difficult and painstakingly slow. Values and assumptions take years to develop and to change. They cannot be imposed by senior leaders (Kouzes and Posner, 2012, p. 66). To accelerate the change process, senior leaders need to draw on the strengths of the existing culture rather than starting over with a blank slate (Katzenbach et al, 2012; Schein, 2009). In most healthcare organizations, there are underlying assumptions, beliefs, and past accomplishments to celebrate, honor, and reinforce. Most healthcare professionals are committed to serving the best interests of patients, for example. And most health professionals value respect and collaboration among the members of their own profession. In both cases, there is an organization-wide strong foundation for promotion of the core values.

Emphasize Teamwork Values

What key underlying assumptions and beliefs generate teamwork in organizations? We note 4 values that help improve the interprofessional teamwork culture—collaboration, respect, patient focus, and innovation.

First, senior leaders should aim to establish *collaboration* as "the way we do things around here." Maximizing collaboration means considering everyone in the organization to be a valued contributor to the organizational mission, including those lowest in the formal hierarchy (for example, clerks and custodians). The preference for collaboration as a way to get things done can be explicitly promoted by top management in ways that will be discussed later, but first collaboration needs to be established as a priority and explicit value of the organization.

Another organizational value that is foundational to teamwork, as covered in several other chapters, is *respect*, in particular, respect for members of other professions. Hammick and colleagues (2009, p. 23) argue that interprofessional teamwork requires that individuals hold 5 values, all of which relate to respecting others:

1. Respect for everyone in the collaborative team
2. Confidence in what you know, what you do not know, and what others know

3. A willingness to engage with others rather than taking a detached view of proceedings
4. A caring disposition toward your colleagues
5. An approachable attitude and showing a willingness to share what you know as a means to the best possible outcome for the user of your service

Mutual respect allows for the knowledge bases of the different professions to be optimally used for the benefit of patients. The importance of respect as a primary value in health services delivery also has been noted recently in relation to establishing a culture of safety (Leape et al, 2012a; 2012b). Disrespect is signaled in healthcare organizations by such actions as disruptive behavior, humiliation of nurses, students, residents, and others, and dismissive treatment of patients, such as not providing information needed to make informed decisions. To demonstrate that respect is expected, organizations can adopt a zero-tolerance policy for abusive behavior by team members, letting everyone in the organization know that shouting at colleagues, relentless personal criticism, harsh treatment of subordinates, and other forms of abuse will not be ignored or accepted—and then taking action when instances of abuse occur even if they are rare.

A third critical organizational value is *patient focus.* Senior leaders should repeatedly and effectively convey that the patients' interests (as defined by the patients) are the primary interests of the organization. This is not just a priority (which can change over time) but a permanent core value of the organization. If team members perceive that profit or market share or personal power or other interests are more important than patient service and quality of services, they will become cynical and disengaged.

A fourth component of an interprofessional teamwork culture in most organizations is that *innovation* is supported. Effective teams discover new and unexpected ideas and solutions. If those ideas and solutions are not valued by the larger organization, team members become dispirited and disengaged from the change process. If organizations do things the way they have always been done, teams will have more difficulty being successful (Whelan, 2013, p. 8).

All 4 of these values are present to some extent in healthcare organizations. Often it is the responsibility of leadership to highlight and accentuate these values rather than others—to "shine light on them." In the vignette earlier, Ms. Simpson could engage individuals and small groups in discussions about the degree to which collaboration, respect for other professionals, patient focus, and innovation are exhibited in behaviors of hospital employees and affiliated clinicians.

Hire and Promote for Teamwork Values

Business consultant Jim Collins popularized the importance of "getting the right people on the bus" before embarking on an organizational change journey (Collins, 2001, pp. 41-64). Because many personal values are deeply held, some individuals will find it hard to change them. If individuals are unable to embrace teamwork values, and they serve in roles where teamwork is expected, they may need to depart or to work in areas where teamwork is not important. In the long run, hiring and promoting people who embrace and demonstrate teamwork values eliminates the need to remove some individuals from the organization.

Collins also notes that discharging employees can be more difficult in the social sector than the business sector, as many social sector organizations are not-for-profit or public entities, and some have significant proportions of unionized employees (Collins, 2005). Decisions to terminate employees can be anguishing and costly, but necessary, in order to alter culture. If removing employees is difficult, rigorous application of early assessment—the typical probationary period for employees—is even more critical. As it is impossible to know a new hire fully at the outset, testing and assessing for teamwork values are essential in the early months of employment.

Make Teamwork Highly Visible

Cultivating a culture of teamwork requires visible demonstration of the use of teams by top leadership. Putting the middle and lower reaches of an organization in teams is not enough to create successful team-based organizations (Harris and Beyerlein, 2005, p. 152). Teams must "cascade" throughout the organization. Having teams at all levels of the organization models and reinforces the team concept. Thus, the top management group must become a team. They need to "walk the talk" of teamwork by using teams, particularly interprofessional teams and teams including patients and family members, to do their own work in the organization. They need to demonstrate teamwork in the culture change effort itself by being widely inclusive, particularly of the clinician and patient populations.

Top leaders are watched and noticed by clinical professionals, as well as by junior leaders, so role modeling by top leaders is critical.

Under-communication of basic messages is a primary reason that change efforts lose steam or fail (Kotter, 1996, pp. 85-100). Kotter's advice to senior leaders for communicating a change vision is relevant to creating a teamwork culture: (1) keep the message simple, avoiding jargon, (2) use metaphors, analogies, and examples that people can visualize, (3) promote the message in multiple forums, both formal and informal, (4) repeat the message over and over, (5) lead by example, (6) address any inconsistencies (for example, that teamwork may cost more), and (7) listen to feedback, including questions and suggestions. Senior leaders can repeatedly communicate the desirability of using teams for many (but not all) tasks in delivering care and managing the organization. They can communicate the clear expectation that teamwork and collaboration will be used. They can communicate continually about the goal of creating a teamwork culture, the activities to achieve it, and the progress made.

To make teamwork visible, senior leaders need to be proactive in demonstrating successes from the use of teamwork. Senior leaders can demonstrate pride in teams by tying team identity to the organization's identity. This means celebrating team successes publicly and widely disseminating their accomplishments. Senior leaders can tell stories about individuals who lead or contribute to successful teams. They can create organizational awards for team performance, for example, for improvements in safety measures in clinical units of the organization, making sure that, as with any award, the selection criteria are transparent and the selection process is fair. Small and symbolic awards still can be quite meaningful, and celebrations need not be costly. Team members appreciate knowing that the organization recognizes their collaborative efforts.

Relate Effectively to Clinicians

Senior leaders cannot promote interprofessional teamwork without connecting to the professionals who comprise teams. Some senior leaders, whether they have a clinical background or not, shy away from associating with clinical professionals and understanding clinical processes. This makes it less likely that they can serve as role models or connect with clinicians. Of all the professions involved in interprofessional teams, administrators particularly need to strive to engage the clinical culture. Overcoming the traditional divide between administrative processes and clinical processes in many healthcare organizations, discussed in Chapter 5 on healthcare administration, requires that administrators learn enough about clinicians and clinical processes to engage clinicians and patients as equal partners on interprofessional teams. By the same token, clinical professionals need to connect proactively with administrators and understand administrative functions to be constructive partners on management teams.

Create and Sustain a Team-Based Organizational Structure

After 6 months of exploration, Ms. Simpson, CEO of Rockaway Heights Hospital, concluded that the Rockaway Heights organizational culture needed serious revamping and that she would focus on "innovation through collaboration" as a theme of her leadership tenure. She appointed 3 leadership task forces, with a variety of representatives, including clinical professionals and patients, to study the feasibility of opening new ventures or redesigning services in the areas of cardiac services, orthopedics, and obstetrics. Ms. Simpson talked about innovation through collaboration at every chance that she got, and she hired a new Director of Marketing to spread the concept throughout the organization and community.

A year later, the marketing campaign was in full gear. The governing board had given its formal endorsement of the marketing effort. The tagline, "innovation through collaboration" was attached to most of the hospital's internal communications and several advertisements, and the 3 task forces received some positive publicity in the community. Three of the more traditional senior leaders in the organization had left to pursue other opportunities, at the urging of Ms. Simpson.

However, Ms. Simpson was having trouble delivering on her vision of innovation through collaboration. The 3 task forces had finished their work and had been disbanded, though Ms. Simpson continued to meet with key physician leaders in the orthopedics, cardiac services, and obstetrics areas. The task force reports were awaiting review at the board level, and the reports included some interesting ideas. The orthopedics task force, for example, had recommended designing an orthopedics center with the whole range of related services, including physical therapy and some radiology and other diagnostic services, in a single physical facility, jointly run by the hospital and a large group of orthopedists in the community. But employees in the organization were expecting more and expecting it faster. They were starting to grumble about the "all talk, no action" administration. Senior leaders who were not part of the cardiac services, orthopedics, or obstetrics areas were feeling excluded from the action and were worried that their jobs were in jeopardy. Ms. Simpson knew that she needed to push further, and quickly.

An organizational culture without corresponding organizational structures and resources that reflect and reinforce the culture invites frustration and discord. Senior leaders need to execute on the promise of a new vision and values by redesigning organizational structures and providing key resources. Altering structures to support teamwork begins with conceptualizing the organization as a cluster of interacting teams. This competency and the 5 others needed for creating a team-based structure are listed in Table 18-3.

Design the Organization as a Cluster of Interacting Teams

A first step in transforming organizational structure to support teamwork requires a change in perspective by many managers and leaders. In the traditional organization, the individual employee is the unit of production. That individual reports to a supervisor, who reports to another supervisor, and so on up the chain of command. A primary task of supervisors in the traditional organization is to motivate and provide performance feedback to individuals. In most of health services delivery, however, a team is the unit of production, whether it is a caregiving team, a clinical support team, a management team, or some combination. In many large healthcare delivery organizations today, patient care is organized around service lines—operating units designed around patient-focused care for related disease groups and similar medical specialties—such as cardiac services or orthopedic services or bone marrow transplants. Within those service lines, teams are the central organizing principle, rather than the individual (White and Griffith, 2010, pp. 3-4, 82). Supervisors are concerned not only with motivating and managing individuals, but also with doing the same for teams of individuals.

Not everyone has to be in a team, of course. As discussed in Chapter 1, some tasks may be more appropriately assigned to individuals. In clinical teams, for example, often individuals in highly specialized roles are utilized occasionally rather than serving as permanent team members.

Following through with team-based organizational design requires several further steps, beginning with assuring accountability for teams.

Table 18-3. Competencies for senior leaders: creating and sustaining a team-based organizational structure

1. Design the organization as a cluster of interacting teams
2. Assure accountability up the hierarchy of teams
3. Manage cross-connections among teams
4. Manage connections to external entities
5. Align the reward system with teamwork
6. Support team sponsors and hold them accountable

Assure Accountability Up the Hierarchy of Teams

In team-based organizations, teams not only are the basic unit of production, they are the basic unit of accountability. Teams are connected and arranged in a hierarchy for accountability purposes. Teams need to know where to go for decisions, what approvals are needed, and so on, in the same way that individuals do. Senior leaders are responsible for establishing and maintaining the accountability hierarchy—a reporting path that allows members and teams to communicate with each other and with the broader organization. Among the organization's responsibilities for assuring accountability are: (1) developing appropriate measures of team performance, aligned with the organization's goals, (2) clarifying purpose for the team, and (3) clearly defining boundaries that identify the team's scope, responsibilities, authority, and resources (Harris and Beyerlein, 2005, p. 151). Team sponsors can help assure that the organization meets these or similar requirements.

Manage Cross-Connections Among Teams

In team-based organizations, communication and interaction among teams need to be facilitated. Teams dealing with one part of a larger work process need to connect to teams engaged in other parts of the process.

Much of clinical health care requires that patients work with multiple teams, meaning that someone must oversee coordination among different teams. Breakdowns occur with "hand-offs" from one team to another. For example, following care by a surgical team in a hospital, a patient may be cared for by a nursing unit team, followed by a rehabilitation unit team, followed by a home care team. Communication channels need to be assured among the teams so that problems can be managed well, should they arise (for example, readmission of the patient). As well, organizations need policies and training for conflict management among teams in the same way that conflict management within teams is supported. It is as important that interprofessional teams not become isolated silos in organizations as it is that traditional departments comprised of members of the same profession not become silos. When the core organizational unit is the team, attention must be focused on promoting communication and good working relationships among teams.

Manage Connections to External Entities

Links to community organizations and other healthcare organizations are another arena in which senior leaders proactively can support teams internal to their own organizations. Senior leaders of organizations represent the organization to external constituencies. They typically have experience dealing with, for example, the media and philanthropic organizations. Such linkages can benefit teams and patients. For example, senior leaders may suggest sources of publicity or funding for teams developing innovative models of care. Connections with local, state, and federal government agencies, accrediting organizations, and professional associations may be useful to specific teams in the organization. Linkages to peer healthcare delivery organizations can be a source of insight and counsel for some teams. If peer healthcare delivery organizations in the community are not accessible because they are competitors, other organizations outside of the market area can be sources of best practices or advice. For many clinical delivery teams, reimbursement issues are a major concern. Senior leaders or their staff can represent the interests of the organization's teams to healthcare payers.

Align the Reward System with Teamwork

Most compensation systems in organizations primarily evaluate and reward individual goal achievement, not team goal achievement. Senior leaders can ensure that teamwork competency and team performance are used as determinants of individual compensation and bonuses. Team members can be compensated for meeting individual goals, exhibiting teamwork competencies, and working on teams that meet their team goals. This may be difficult if individuals work on multiple teams, or only occasionally work on teams. At the other extreme, in organizations where stable teams are the unit of work production, linking individual rewards to team outcomes can be straightforward. For members who work full time on one team, team achievements can be the basis of a large portion of salary. Or, team goal achievement can be part of bonus compensation for individuals.

Compensation models for clinicians can be altered so that payment provides an incentive for teamwork instead of discouraging it. Using salary for payment removes an obstacle to collaboration that is present in many settings. Paying nurse practitioners (NPs), physician assistants (PAs), and physicians on the basis of their fee-for-service billings encourages each clinician to maximize her or his own billings regardless of whether the work might serve patients better if the work were shared with other professionals. Paying clinicians salaries eliminates this incentive. Of course, using a salary system is accomplished more easily if the payments to the organization come as capitation payment or some other form of "per-beneficiary per month payment." As noted in Chapter 19, changes are needed in insurance companies and government agencies to reform payment to delivery organizations. Nonetheless, some healthcare organizations already use salary for paying their clinicians even though the organizations receive nearly all of their revenues as fee-for-service payments (for example, Virginia Mason Medical Center in Seattle and Mayo Clinic).

If bonus payments are used in compensating clinicians, the payments can be made to teams rather than to individuals. Making bonus payments to individuals signals that teamwork is unimportant in the eyes of those leading the healthcare practice or institution. Individual bonuses encourage each clinician to focus on the measures used to assess his or her own performance, regardless of the team's performance. If bonus payments to individuals are drawn from a fixed sum available for bonus payments, the system creates an even stronger disincentive for teamwork.

Compensation is only one component of the incentive and reward system of organizations. Senior leaders are responsible for ensuring that human resources policies regarding promotion, performance review, and employee selection are aligned with teamwork culture. Formal criteria for hiring, promotion, and performance review should include teamwork competencies.

Support Team Sponsors and Hold Them Accountable

Team members, leaders, and sponsors all are important to teamwork success. Team members and leaders in effective teams hold their fellow members accountable, and team sponsors hold team leaders accountable. Who holds team sponsors accountable? Senior leaders of the organization are responsible for ensuring that team sponsors are capable of executing the sponsor competencies described in Chapter 12, relating to designing, evaluating, and coaching the team. Senior leaders should foster excellence in team sponsorship. To do so, senior leaders should: (1) support team sponsors in their role, that is, coach them and provide resources, and (2) hold team sponsors accountable. Senior leaders need to set clear expectations about team output, quality, and timing.

Provide Key Teamwork Resources

A multitude of diverse organizational resources and support systems is important to successful teamwork (Lawrence, 2002, pp. 137-141). For example, in growing organizations, meeting space may be difficult to find. Allocation of space for team meetings is not a priority in the design of most healthcare physical plants. In such settings, designation of space for team meetings, renovation of physical facilities, and a coordinated reservation system are responsibilities of leaders in the area of support resources. Senior leaders need to assure that the space needs of teams are met.

More broadly, researchers have found 3 types of organizational support systems to have particularly high leverage for promoting teamwork: the reward system, the information system, and the educational system (Hackman, 2002, p. 134). We have dealt with the reward system earlier under the category of *Create and Sustain a Team-Based Organizational Structure*. Next, we discuss the need for senior leaders to assess and improve the information system and educational systems that support teamwork. In addition, if they are serious about promoting excellence, senior leaders will ensure that organizational support for teamwork is evaluated and improved regularly. These 3 competencies are important in following through on a commitment to improving teamwork (Table 18–4).

Table 18-4. Competencies for senior leaders: providing key teamwork resources

1. Assess and improve resources for information and communications
2. Assess and improve resources for education and evaluation
3. Assess and improve organizational support for teamwork

Assess and Improve Resources for Information and Communications

Senior leaders can assure that resources for information exchange and communication among members meet teamwork needs by assessing and improving organizational capacity in this arena. Clinical and management teams require effective communication among team members and between patients and team members, which means providing whatever communication technologies are utilized by patients. These technologies can include face-to-face meetings, telephones and faxes, as well as computer access for e-mail, clinical databases, online support groups for patients, and customized health education for patients (Institute of Medicine, 2001, p. 164). Improved technology can help clinical teams achieve the 6 Institute of Medicine goals (see Chapter 6). For example, patients and clinicians can improve the *timeliness* of team care through e-visits and telemedicine and immediate access to results of diagnostic tests and treatment results.

In clinical health care, a critical information tool is a common body of information on patients that can be shared securely by clinicians. The electronic health record (EHR) increasingly is a preferred source for basic clinical information. The shared EHR is needed to move information about patients among team members, including patients, and from one team to another. Some clinical teams, including patients in the teams, have centralized web-based communication and access to full medical records (Mitchell et al, 2012). Many healthcare teams still rely on paper copies of basic records, which are long overdue for digitizing. Sizable capital investments usually are required to transition to a common EHR or shared information systems across different entities of the same healthcare organization.

Privacy and confidentiality issues are paramount in the sharing of patient information, and all team members should be trained in ethical and legal responsibilities for patient data privacy. Senior leaders need to enforce such training organization-wide, so that all team members share the same concerns and norms about patient information privacy and confidentiality.

We have noted the importance of having evaluative information on individual and team effectiveness in order to improve teams in organizations. Often, support from centralized information systems and data analysis staff is critical to producing such information efficiently and conveniently. Electronic surveys can collect information quickly from multiple sources, and standard software packages can generate statistics and presentations of the statistics. Staff support may be needed to capture clinical data that monitor the health of a team's patient base and promote safety and quality. Teams also often need information systems support to establish a web presence for external audiences or for internal communication (for example, posting of shared articles or updates to a project or minutes of meetings). Access to information systems staff for teams enables that need to be fulfilled with minimum delay and aggravation to the team. Members of clinical teams also benefit from shared access to the same basic and current sources of evidence on clinical care, including digital repositories of journals and reference material, so that they can refer to materials that all members can access. Members of management teams need similar access to evidence on management practices.

Assess and Improve Resources for Education and Evaluation

Chapters 13-16 detail the need for teams to evaluate individual and team performance, educate and train members, and conduct team building and process improvement activities. Large organizations can provide these services, or support for these services to teams, through their Human Resources Department and their Internal Consulting Department, if they have one. Smaller organizations can provide financial support, contracting, and access to screened lists of external consulting services. Such resources need to be marketed proactively and communicated to teams, or they may go unnoticed and unused. In addition, the services used for team education and evaluation need to be routinely assessed and improved. This is true of educational resources in particular. Poor quality in the delivery of training and education for team members not only inhibits learning and improvement, but it also demoralizes team members as to the value of organization-sponsored education in general and leads them to question the true commitment of the organization to teamwork.

Assess and Improve Organizational Support for Teamwork

As with all organizational functions, it is important to measure and evaluate organizational support for teamwork. Senior leaders are responsible for making sure this happens. Regular surveys of employees or teams should ascertain support for teamwork and proactively solicit suggestions for improvement. Reviews of organizational support energize team members by identifying specific problem areas and assuring them that the organization is a facilitator, not a barrier, to their success. Examples of such review instruments are available (Whelan, 2013, pp. 121-128).

Returning to the Rockaway Heights Hospital vignette, the activities described earlier in regard to improving the team-based organizational structure and providing key resources would help to cement the values of innovation and collaboration into the behavior and attitudes of employees at Rockaway Heights. Working with a team with clinical and patient representatives, Ms. Simpson, the CEO, could focus attention on a large number of service lines that include most of the organization's employees. She could ensure that Human Resources policies, including compensation, contain incentives and rewards for collaboration and innovation. She could accelerate standardization of digital health records and communications technology throughout the hospital, and implement training programs to promote teamwork and innovation. Such steps would help Ms. Simpson and Rockaway Heights successfully execute on the vision of "innovation through collaboration."

HAZARDS FOR SENIOR LEADERS WITH RESPECT TO TEAMS

There are 3 concerns that leaders should anticipate as they work to improve the teamwork environment in their organizations. First, senior leaders may be prone to accept uncritically that patient interest is the prime value in the organization's culture. Second, enthusiastic support for teamwork by senior leaders needs to be balanced with the need for teams to function within the framework of organizational goals. Finally, too much organizational support can diminish the incentives for teams to develop self-sufficiency.

Senior leaders mistakenly may assume that everyone knows that patients' interests are the most important interests in the organization. It is common for healthcare professionals to "mouth the words" that patient interests come first. However, the primacy of patient interests is challenged daily in healthcare delivery organizations, at all levels. For example, as explained in Chapter 3, different professions interpret patient interests in different ways. Administrators may emphasize their commitment to the interests of a population of potential patients in the long term, necessitating painful budget cuts to maintain some services and delete others. Such long-term patient population interests may be counter to the short-term interests of specific patients, whose interests may be championed by their direct care providers. Dialogue and constructive conflict around interpretations of patient interest are healthy for interprofessional teams. If such discussions are absent, different professions may assume that only they are the protectors of patients' interests.

Worse still is the possibility that protection of patient interests is a guise for the pursuit of personal or organizational power or profit. Formal commitment to patient interest as an organizational value, cultural and structural reinforcement of the primacy of patient interest, and transparency of assessment of patient focus all are important in buttressing team-based care.

Second, teams can be given too much autonomy, whether by neglect or by design in a misguided effort to show support for them. Too much autonomy can result in the team becoming disconnected from the organization, such that their accomplishments then collide with other organizational goals. For example, teams with the freedom to market their services may deliver marketing messages contrary to the organization's marketing efforts. Teams need sufficient autonomy to do their work, but they also need guidance from sponsors and senior leaders to align with organizational goals.

Third, it is possible for teams to receive too much support in some areas. Well-resourced and well-supported teams may get help from their leaders, sponsors, and senior leaders, as well as trainers and consultants. Too much help increases dependency on outsiders and reduces the likelihood that individual team members will learn to resolve team issues themselves (Whelan, 2013, pp. 120-121). If the solution to every team problem is to "bring in an expert," the teams will not develop the capacity to solve problems and learn on their own.

CONCLUSION

Senior leaders who strive to promote interprofessional teamwork for clinical health delivery and for management decision making face 3 major tasks in their organizations: (1) creating and sustaining a team-based organizational culture, (2) creating and sustaining a team-based organizational structure, and (3) providing key resources. Leaders can begin by assessing existing organizational culture in their organization, searching for values that support teamwork: collaboration, respect, patient focus, and innovation. They can promote those values by hiring and promoting people who adhere to the values, making teamwork highly visible throughout the organization, and relating effectively to the clinical professions. To cement teamwork in the attitudes and behaviors of employees, senior leaders need to design the organization structure as a cluster of interacting teams, accountable in a hierarchy. They can help teams connect with each other and with external constituencies. Importantly, senior leaders can align the reward system with teamwork competencies and team performance, and support team sponsors and hold them accountable. Finally, senior leaders are responsible for seeing that teams are appropriately provided with communications and information technologies, education and training, and for evaluating and improving the level of organizational support provided to teams. The enthusiastic and material support of team-based activity by senior organizational leaders is critical if team-based activity is to flourish in healthcare organizations.

REFERENCES

Collins J. *Good to Great: Why Some Companies Make the Leap. . . and Others Don't.* New York, NY: HarperCollins; 2001.

Collins J. *Good to Great and the Social Sectors: A Monograph to Accompany Good to Great.* New York, NY: HarperCollins, 2005.

Deal TE, Kennedy AA. *Corporate Culture: The Rites and Rituals of Corporate Life.* New York, NY: Perseus Books Publishing; 1982. Reissued, 2000.

Hackman JR. *Leading Teams: Setting the Stage for Great Performances*. Boston, MA: Harvard Business School Press; 2002.

Hammick M, Freeth D, Copperman J, et al. *Being Interprofessional*. Cambridge, UK: Polity Press; 2009.

Harris CL, Beyerlein MM. Team-based organization: creating an environment for team success. In: West MA, Tjosvold D, Smith KG, eds. *The Essentials of Teamworking: International Perspectives*. Chichester, UK: John Wiley & Sons, Ltd.; 2005:149-171.

Institute of Medicine. *Crossing the Quality Chasm: A New Health System for the 21st Century*. Washington, DC: National Academy Press; 2001.

Katzenbach JR, Steffen I, Kronley C. Culture change that sticks: start with what's already working. *Harv Bus Rev*. 2012;90(7/8):110-117.

Kotter JP. *Leading Change*. Boston, MA: Harvard Business School Press; 1996.

Kouzes JM, Posner BZ. *The Leadership Challenge*. 5th ed. San Francisco, CA: John Wiley & Sons; 2012.

Lawrence D. *From Chaos to Care: The Promise of Team-Based Care*. Cambridge, MA: Da Capo Press; 2002.

Leape LL, Shore MF, Dienstag JL, et al. Perspective: a culture of respect, part 1: the nature and causes of disrespectful behavior by physicians. *Acad Med*. 2012a;87:845-852.

Leape LL, Shore MF, Dienstag JL, et al. Perspective: a culture of respect, part 2: creating a culture of respect. *Acad Med*. 2012b;87:853-858.

MIT Media Lab. The MIT media lab at a glance. MIT Media Lab Web Site. April, 2012. http://www.media.mit.edu/files/overview.pdf. Accessed October 21, 2012.

Mitchell P, Wynia M, Golden R, et al. Core principles and values of effective team-based health care. Discussion Paper. Washington, DC: Institute of Medicine; 2012. http://www.iom.edu/tbc. Accessed March 3, 2013.

Schein EH. *The Corporate Culture Survival Guide*. Revised ed. San Francisco, CA: Jossey-Bass; 2009.

Whelan S. *Creating Effective Teams: A Guide for Members and Leaders*. 4th ed. Thousand Oaks, CA: Sage; 2013.

White KR, Griffith JR. *The Well-Managed Healthcare Organization*. 7th ed. Chicago, IL: Health Administration Press; 2010.

19 The Future of Teamwork in Health Care

Chapter 18 describes actions that senior leaders of organizations can take to invigorate teamwork in their organizations, focusing on the culture of healthcare delivery organizations. In terms of promoting teamwork in health care, direct delivery organizations are only one piece of a larger puzzle. The conviction that better teamwork can improve health care also needs to be embedded in the context that supports and surrounds healthcare delivery organizations in the United States and globally. Health insurance companies, professional associations, educators, researchers, government, the public, and media all can play important parts in accelerating the improvement of healthcare delivery through enhanced teamwork. In this chapter, we review ways that those constituencies can encourage teamwork more proactively.

TEAM-BASED HEALTH CARE IS HERE TO STAY

As stated in Chapter 1, most patients today receive their health care from several individuals practicing different professions. This is particularly true for the growing chronic care component of healthcare delivery. These clinical professionals are supported by an array of other specialists who provide administrative or logistical support or consultation, often regularly and frequently. At the center of the clinical activity is the patient and the patient's family. It is unlikely that any one professional, without support, can provide quality healthcare services except for the simplest and most routine items of clinical care. Even those professionals who provide primary services in nursing, medicine, social work, and pharmacy rely on teams that include support workers from their own profession or other occupations and professions. As knowledge and specialization continue to increase, the pressures for team-based care only will expand. Clinical healthcare delivery is and will continue to be a team activity.

Management work in healthcare delivery, too, is increasingly team-based. Most management decisions impact clinical care delivery, from the choice of strategic plans for organizations to the redesign of organizational processes, for example, the processes that determine patient flow through the organization. Consensus management decision making requires representation from patients and from multiple clinical professions, because management work cannot be separated from clinical care. Managers need to collaborate with clinical professionals and patients to produce safe, effective, patient-centered, efficient, timely, and equitable care—the 6 quality aims of the Institute of Medicine (IOM), discussed in Chapter 6. For managers to make decisions independently of their clinical professionals and patients invites alienation of their core workers—clinical professionals—and their customers—patients—as well as poor quality and poor cost outcomes for the organization. Management of healthcare delivery is and will continue to be a team activity.

The growth of team-based care and the desire for more of it are evident in recent healthcare reform efforts in the United States. Examples include federal support for patient-centered medical homes, accountable care organizations (ACOs), and healthcare information technology development. The Patient Protection and Affordable Care Act (PPACA) of 2010 encourages development and testing of patient-centered medical homes and interprofessional community health teams to support them. As discussed in Chapter 4, medical homes (or health homes) provide patients with a central primary care practice or healthcare provider who coordinates the patients' care across settings and providers. PPACA also supports the development of ACOs (or coordinated care organizations), which are collaborations among primary care clinicians, specialists and other health professionals, hospitals and other providers, who jointly accept responsibility for the quality and cost of care provided to a defined population of Medicare patients. Finally, federal support for information technology development in healthcare delivery is demonstrated in the Health Information Technology for Economic and Clinical Health (HITECH) Act of 2009, which created a national healthcare information technology infrastructure and a strategy for adoption of the electronic health record (EHR). The strategy is predicated on the assumption that coordination of care across time and multiple providers and multiple sites is enhanced by a shared, digital record. The Act contains specific incentives designed to accelerate the adoption of EHR systems among providers. Qualifying information systems have to meet standards for patient engagement, such as identifying and providing patient-specific education resources and sending reminders to patients for preventive and follow-up care.

Around the globe, similar needs for higher quality and cost-effective health care drive efforts to improve teamwork in healthcare delivery. Pressures for improvements in quality, safety, and patient-centered care are global phenomena, as is the shift of the burden of disease toward conditions requiring chronic care (Reeves et al, 2010, pp. 24-38). A global commission of 20 experts, the Lancet Commission on the Education of Health Professionals for the 21st Century, observes broadly that "Patient management requires coordinated care across time and space, demanding unprecedented teamwork," but that "Professionals are falling short on appropriate competencies for effective teamwork" (Frenk et al, 2010, p. 1926). The breadth of these trends across geographic boundaries reflects their foundational nature and relative permanence. It also suggests that change efforts in the United States should be informed by (and contribute to) similar efforts in other countries.

BOLD LEADERSHIP IS NEEDED NOW

As stated in the Lancet Commission report in reference to global health, "A renaissance to a new professionalism—patient-centred and team-based—has been much discussed, but it has lacked the leadership, incentive, and power to deliver on its promise" (Frenk et al, 2010, p. 1926). Throughout the whole of health care, the need for improved teamwork needs to be acknowledged, voiced, and promoted, especially by people in authority—including heads and other senior leaders of healthcare delivery organizations, clinical department chairs, medical group leaders, nursing practice leaders, heads of professional associations, deans of professional schools and colleges, heads of health insurance organizations, and officials in government healthcare programs. Action needs to be taken in every one of the 7 arenas listed in Table 19–1.

Table 19–1 Arenas where change is needed to promote teamwork

Healthcare delivery organizations
Health professional education
Health professional societies
Health insurance companies
Government
• as regulator
• as payer
Health services research
The public

Healthcare Delivery Organizations

The leaders of hospitals, medical groups, health systems, and other direct delivery organizations can take several steps that would remove obstacles to teamwork and promote it. Chapter 18 presents many of the steps. To summarize, the actions divide into the categories of cultural change, structural change, and targeting of support resources to teams. Cultural changes include emphasizing teamwork values, making teamwork highly visible, and relating effectively to clinicians. Structural changes include designing the organization around teams, assuring team accountability, building connections among teams and between teams and external entities, and altering compensation models for clinicians so that payment provides incentives for teamwork instead of discouraging it. Key resources for teams are information and communication support, support for performance evaluation and education, and qualified and accountable team sponsors.

Health Professional Education

At present, almost all medical schools, nursing schools, and other healthcare educational institutions are working actively against teamwork by educating their students separately from students in other professional schools. By the time students have been in training for 2 years or more, they have developed a sense of identity with their own profession, have embraced the values characteristic of that profession, and have acquired a subtle tribal mindset, which includes wariness and sometimes antagonism to individuals with different professional identities and values. Chapter 3 reviews this process and its consequences in more detail.

The walls between healthcare professional schools need to come down. From the outset of professional education, the value of interprofessional teamwork needs to be stressed. Students need to learn in teams that resemble the teams in which nurses, physicians, pharmacists, social workers, administrators, and other healthcare professionals practice their professions in the day-to-day world of healthcare delivery. It is apparent that teaching students in this way is difficult because it has been achieved so seldom. Professional rivalries, long-held traditions about how to teach certain subjects (for example, interviewing of patients), and mundane considerations such as scheduling of classes all interfere with developing interprofessional education. Still, the obstacles can be overcome as is proven by the programs that have been developed at several universities in the United States and around the world (Meads and Ashcroft, 2005, pp. 135-149; Roethel, 2012).

Professional schools also need to teach principles of teamwork directly. This can be done by interspersing didactic sessions and reading with interprofessional team experiences that are parts of clinical curricula. Discussion of case studies can aid in making the principles fully understood, memorable, and useable by students. Substantial investment in new research is needed to develop the evidence base for cost-effective ways to provide such education (Reeves et al, 2008).

Accrediting organizations for health professional educational programs are potential drivers of transformation. Accrediting organizations can work to infuse interprofessional education competencies within profession-specific accreditation requirements (Royeen et al, 2009, p. 445).

Infrastructure investment funding often is necessary for such efforts. The US Health Resources and Services Administration in 2012 provided 5-year funding for a National Center for Interprofessional Practice and Education, housed at the University of Minnesota (University of Minnesota, 2012). The Macy Foundation, Robert Wood Johnson Foundation, Gordon and Betty Moore Foundation, and John A. Hartford Foundation joined the federal government in supporting the new center. Continuing leadership by private foundations and government agencies for infrastructure development is critical to accelerating progress.

The IOM (2003) recommended refashioning healthcare education so that students are prepared to work in interprofessional teams that are focused collectively on the values, preferences, and needs of patients. Moreover, the report called for educational planning to be done in an interprofessional context so that the walls between professional schools are more likely to be removed. This call is some 10 years old. Although some progress has been made, as indicated earlier, much more is needed.

Health Professional Societies

In recent years, many professional societies and associations, including the American Academy of Family Physicians, the American Association of Nurse Practitioners, the American Medical Association, the American Nurses Association, and the American Pharmacists Association, have engaged in energetic promotion of the interests of their members in a manner that inhibits the development of interprofessional teamwork. While it is not surprising that the societies would advocate for their members, the tone of the rhetoric issued by some of the societies is inflammatory (American Academy of Family Physicians, 2012a; American Association of Nurse Practitioners, 2012). Although all of these associations endorse interprofessional practice in general terms—sometimes using different terms such as *multidisciplinary practice*, *transdisciplinary practice*, and *interdisciplinary practice*—the rhetoric of some of their public statements strongly suggests serious misgivings.

If interprofessional practice is to be broadly understood, trusted, and promoted, the societies will need to soften the tone of their more strident pronouncements and begin trying to seek common understandings. This road will not be easy. Obviously, there are economic concerns underlying some of the disagreements. But there are also legitimate professional points of view at stake. Patients' interests will be served by these societies seeking to understand each other's interests and points of view—all of them—and negotiating collaborative agreements that enable all healthcare professionals to contribute to the care of patients using all of their knowledge and skill in interdependent practice. For example, it would be helpful for a group of societies representing practicing nurses, physicians, pharmacists, social workers, and administrators to negotiate a model of collaborative practice and issue a joint statement describing the model. Some will say that such a venture would be naive. It is worth trying.

Health Insurance Companies

Fee-for-service payment of individual clinicians interferes with teamwork. Health insurance companies primarily pay practitioners and healthcare institutions on a fee-for-service basis. It is understandable that institutions use these payments as the basis for paying individual clinicians, paying individuals a percentage of the revenue received for each individual's services. Some healthcare delivery organizations have severed this linkage, using salaries to pay their clinicians instead of paying them a percentage of the fee-for-service billings they generate. But these organizations are few, and severing the linkage has occurred mainly in very large organizations with multiple sources of revenue.

One approach to dealing with the ill effects of paying for clinical activity on a fee-for-service basis is to enlarge the list of services reimbursed so that, for example, visits to nurse practitioners (NPs), visits to physician assistants, e-visits, medication therapy management, and other services are reimbursed. In recent years, insurance companies have expanded the services they compensate, but this approach is not sufficient. First, each new service receives payment only after a lengthy process, sometimes a protracted battle. Second, any revised fee-for-service payment system tends to lock in care arrangements with the components that are reimbursed and thus to inhibit development of new forms of teamwork going forward.

For teamwork to flourish, insurance companies will need to move ahead much further in devising payments methods other than fee-for-service. At one time capitation payment appeared to be the method that would become universal in the United States, but then there was a backlash against managed care, which was associated with capitation in the minds of the public and legislators. This method of payment is again growing in popularity (Frakt and Mayes, 2012), although the word *capitation* is studiously avoided in policy statements. Now that quality of care can be measured with some degree of validity, it may be possible to move back toward payment per person per unit of time with fewer concerns about the serious shortfalls in quality that could arise in health plans using capitation payment. However, other methods need to be explored as well. Payment for an episode of care appears to have promise, especially if the episode is well defined with a clear beginning date, clear end date, and a reliably standard package of elements of care. For example, total joint replacement and normal obstetrical care lend themselves to this form of payment, sometimes called *global payment*. The advantage of this form of payment in fostering teamwork is that the single payment permits use of the funds in any way that a team deems useful for patient care. Other methods receiving attention now are various forms of "shared savings." If the payments for achieving savings are large enough, this method too could encourage teamwork. PPACA explicitly includes provisions to promote shared savings payments for care provided to Medicare beneficiaries. This precedent likely will encourage insurance companies to experiment with similar methods.

Government

Government as Regulator

At present, licensing laws in several states prevent NPs and pharmacists from practicing to the full extent of their education and training. For example, as advocated by the IOM, the laws in some states pertaining to nursing practice need to be updated (Institute of Medicine, 2011, pp. 4-6). Some states limit collaborative drug therapy management by physicians and pharmacists (American Academy of Family Physicians, 2012b; Giberson et al, 2011). Pharmacists are not recognized as healthcare providers for reimbursement purposes by the Social Security Act, which governs Medicare. This policy is contrary to recommendations of the US Public Health Service and others who advocate changing the law to stimulate integration of pharmacists into collaborative medication management activities (Giberson et al, 2011). Examples like these reflect the potential for the federal government to help in regulatory change efforts by making changes that set precedents at the federal level. The federal government could also help by describing best practices at the state level and disseminating this information to the states.

Government as Payer

For about half of the cost of health care in the United States, the federal and state governments are the payers, primarily through Medicare and Medicaid. The same need for changes in payment methods are needed from the Centers for Medicare and Medicaid Services (CMS) and state governments as are needed from private insurance companies. Some limited movement is visible. Examples of CMS's recent initiatives are the per-beneficiary per month payment method contained in the Pioneer Accountable Care Organization (ACO) Model, which has been established as part of the implementation of PPACA (Center for Medicare and Medicaid Innovation, 2011). This CMS initiative may be a powerful precedent influencing companies insuring people under age 65. There are also many experiments being pursued at the state level, for example, a global budget with shared risk layered on top of existing payment mechanisms is being piloted in northern California (Markovich, 2012). An initiative to use community-level global budgeting for Medicaid has recently been announced in Oregon (Reichard, 2012). Several of these changes promise to provide incentives for teamwork. Much more work by payers, including governments, to replace or modify traditional fee-for-service payment still is needed.

Health Services Research

Health services research on teams is in its early stages, much of it motivated in recent years by research funding for improvements in patient safety. In addition to patient safety, though, improved teamwork can contribute to improvements in outcomes, cost-effectiveness, and other aspects of health care. There is a rich foundation of research on small groups and teams in the social sciences and more recently in management research. Health services researchers can draw on this foundation.

Charitable foundations and government funding agencies can heed the call to place increased emphasis on the study of teams and the building of a stronger evidence base for appropriate use of teams and for drivers of team effectiveness. Academic professional associations such as Academy Health and the Academy of Management, through actions of their members and committees, can increase focus on building the evidence base. Training programs in health services research, and those who lead them, are another constituency that can have important effects on the next generation of health services research. Editors and editorial boards of academic journals are also gatekeepers who can stimulate more attention to team performance in clinical care and the management of health care.

The Public

Patients and the public in general need to reframe their expectations for healthcare service in line with new realities. In reference to physicians, surgeons, and writer Atul Gawande asserts that doctors have been celebrated as "cowboys, but what we need is more pit crews" (Gawande, 2010, p. 60). Heroic and caring professionals typically are depicted in books, movies, and television as individuals, presumably because we identify more easily with the stories of individuals than with the stories of teams. While this approach is fine for entertainment, such depictions create skewed expectations for patients and aspiring professionals. Educating the public on the importance and need for team-based care would be a helpful step on the path to healthcare delivery improvement.

When largely served in the past by one healthcare professional, patients knew what to expect. Referring to the shift to team-based care, Batalden and colleagues discern that "As systems change, patients can feel left behind" (Batalden et al, 2006, p. 549). With team-based care, expectations are fuzzy—relationships with providers can be impersonal and multiple and dynamic, with patients being treated by many different professionals. As a result, patients need to exert more control and have more involvement in their own care. Organizations such as the Institute for Patient- and Family-Centered Care provide resources for administrators, clinicians, families, researchers, educators, and others to integrate patients and families in healthcare services (Institute for Patient- and Family-Centered Care, 2013). Educational resources like those provided by the National Diabetes Education Program can introduce patients clearly to the notion that working together with a team of providers is their best chance for improved health outcomes (National Diabetes Education Program, 2011). Such educational efforts will give patients and future professionals a more accurate view of the realities of healthcare delivery.

CAVEATS

We end with 3 cautionary notes for those seeking to lead change toward team-based health care.

First, the advance of teamwork should not be achieved at the cost of damaging the various healthcare professions as institutions. An *institution* is a "significant practice, relationship, or organization in a society or culture" (Merriam-Webster, 2013). Professions, including healthcare professions, are institutions deeply embedded in US society and culture, and for good reason. In the past few decades, healthcare professions have produced astounding progress in their respective areas of professional expertise. Continuing efforts to develop the expertise and knowledge base of the professions of nursing, health administration, pharmacy, medicine, and other clinical professions provide invaluable service to healthcare delivery. The depth of knowledge created by specialization of the division of healthcare labor cannot be discounted. Any progress toward teamwork among these professionals should build on, not subtract from, the accomplishments of specialized expertise. Team-based care should be fashioned on a strong foundation of evidence-based expertise held by each of the component members of the team.

Second, change of institutions that are deeply rooted in culture and society takes years or decades to attain. As stated in Chapter 1, team-based care has been a vision for health care at least since 1955 in the United States. Persistence and patience are necessary attributes for change leaders in this arena.

Third, rhetoric supporting team-based care easily can exceed reality. We reiterate that every healthcare delivery problem does not need a team solution. The healthcare delivery sector and healthcare organizations are prone to fads and fashions in strategies and tactics (Kaissi and Begun, 2008). If team-based care is a fad, it will suffer in the long run. Team-based care needs a much broader and deeper evidence base. Teams need to be subjected to the transparent evaluation provided by science, and teamwork needs to be adopted based on evidence, not rhetoric.

CONCLUSION

The expansion of team-based clinical health care, as well as the use of interprofessional teams to do healthcare management work, is a trend that will not be reversed. The trend is created by the growing complexity of healthcare delivery and the specialization of healthcare labor. This development creates a responsibility for healthcare leaders and practicing healthcare professionals to refashion healthcare delivery so that organizations more effectively coordinate the talents and commitment of the individual healthcare professionals who comprise the system of healthcare delivery. In the coming years, the call for teamwork urgently needs to be answered by all of those who work in the healthcare professions, all who are dedicated to preserving health and caring for the sick.

REFERENCES

American Academy of Family Physicians. *AAFP Cautions Against Stop-Gap Efforts to Solve Primary Care Shortage.* Leawood, KS: American Academy of Family Physicians; 2012a. http://www.aafp.org/online/en/home/media/releases/2012/primary-care-21st-century.html. Accessed October 20, 2012.

American Academy of Family Physicians. *Pharmacists (Position Paper).* Leawood, KS: American Academy of Family Physicians; 2012b. http://www.aafp.org/online/en/home/policy/policies/p/pharmacistspositionpaper.html. Accessed October 30, 2012.

American Association of Nurse Practitioners. *AANP Responds to the American Academy of Family Physicians Report.* Austin, TX: American Academy of Nurse Practitioners; 2012. http://www.aanp.org/press-room/press-releases/28-press-room/2012-press-releases/1082-aanp-responds-to-aafp-report. Accessed October 20, 2012.

Batalden P, Ogrinc G, Batalden M. From one to many. *J Interprof Care.* 2006;20:549-551.

Center for Medicare and Medicaid Innovation. *Pioneer Accountable Care Organization (ACO) Model Request for Applications.* Washington, DC: Centers for Medicare and Medicaid Services; 2011. http://innovations.cms.gov/Files/x/Pioneer-ACO-Model-Request-For-Applications-document.pdf. Accessed October 20, 2012.

Frakt AB, Mayes R. Beyond capitation: how new payment experiments seek to find the "sweet spot" in amount of risk providers and payers bear. *Health Aff (Millwood).* 2012;31:1951-1958.

Frenk J, Chen L, Bhutta ZA, et al. Health professionals for a new century: transforming education to strengthen health systems in an interdependent world. *Lancet.* 2010;376:1923-1958.

Gawande A. Health care needs a new kind of hero. *Harv Bus Rev.* 2010;88(4):60-61.

Giberson S, Yoder S, Lee MP. *Improving Patient and Health System Outcomes through Advanced Pharmacy Practice. A Report to the U.S. Surgeon General.* Washington, DC: US Public Health Service; 2011.

Institute for Patient- and Family-Centered Care. Web site. http://www.ipfcc.org. Accessed March 15, 2013.

Institute of Medicine. *Health Professions Education: A Bridge to Quality*. Washington, DC: National Academies Press; 2003.

Institute of Medicine. *The Future of Nursing: Leading Change, Advancing Health.* Washington, DC: National Academies Press; 2011.

Kaissi A, Begun JW. Fads, fashions, and bandwagons in health care strategy. *Health Care Manage Rev*. 2008;33:94-102.

Markovich P. A global budget pilot project among provider partners and Blue Shield of California led to savings in first two years. *Health Aff (Millwood).* 2012;31:1969-1976.

Meads G, Ashcroft J. *The Case for Interprofessional Collaboration in Health and Social Care.* Oxford, UK: Blackwell Publishing, Ltd.; 2005.

Merriam-Webster. Free Merriam-Webster Dictionary Web site: institution. http://www.merriam-webster.com/dictionary/institution. Accessed March 20, 2013.

National Diabetes Education Program. *Redesigning the Health Care Team: Diabetes Prevention and Lifetime Management.* NIH Publication 11-7739. Washington, DC: NIH; 2011. http://www.ndep.nih.gov/media/teamcare.pdf. Accessed March 3, 2013.

Reeves S, Lewin S, Espin S, et al. *Interprofessional Teamwork for Health and Social Care.* Chichester, UK: John Wiley & Sons Ltd.; 2010.

Reeves S, Zwarenstien M, Goldman J, et al. Interprofessional education: effects on professional practice and health care outcomes. *Cochrane Database Syst Rev* 2008, Issue 1. Art. No.: CD002213. DOI: 10.1002/14651858.CD002213.pub2.

Reichard J. Oregon gets nod for Medicaid "global budget" plan saving $11 billion. The Commonwealth Fund Web site; 2012. http://www.commonwealthfund.org/Newsletters/Washington-Health-Policy-in-Review/2012/May/May-7-2012/Oregon-Gets-Nod-for-Medicaid-Global-Budget.aspx. Accessed November 3, 2012.

Roethel K. A grounding in medical teamwork. *US News & World Report Best Graduate Schools.* 2013 ed. Washington, DC: US News & World Report LP; 2012:47.

Royeen CB, Jensen GM, Harvan RA. Interprofessional education: themes and next steps. In: Royeen CB, Jensen GM, Harvan RA. *Leadership in Interprofessional Health Education and Practice.* Sudbury, MA: Jones and Bartlett Learning, 2009:439-448.

University of Minnesota, Academic Health Center, Office of Education. National Center for Interprofessional Practice and Education Web site. http://www.ahc.umn.edu/OofE/nexus-ipe/. Published December 10, 2012. Accessed March 25, 2013.

Index

Page numbers followed by f refer to figures; page numbers followed by t refer to tables.

W

Y

Z

Lightning Source UK Ltd.
Milton Keynes UK
UKHW05f0822121018
330318UK00003B/66/P

9 780071 791953